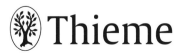

Orthopedic Biomechanics

2nd Edition

Paul Brinckmann
Institute of Experimental Biomechanics
University of Münster
Münster, Germany
Federal School of Prosthetics and Orthotics
Dortmund, Germany

Wolfgang Frobin
Institute of Experimental Biomechanics
University of Münster
Münster, Germany

Gunnar Leivseth
Institute of Clinical Medicine
UiT The Arctic University of Norway
Tromsø, Norway

Burkhard Drerup
Institute of Experimental Biomechanics
Department of Orthopedic Technology and Rehabilitation
University of Münster
Münster, Germany
Federal School of Prosthetics and Orthotics
Dortmund, Germany

367 illustrations

Thieme
Stuttgart • New York • Delhi • Rio de Janeiro

Library of Congress Cataloging-in-Publication Data
Brinckmann, Paul, author.
  [Orthopädische Biomechanik. English]
  Orthopedic biomechanics / Paul Brinckmann, Wolfgang
Frobin, Gunnar Leivseth, Burkhard Drerup. — 2nd edition.
    p. ; cm.
  Preceded by: Musculoskeletal biomechanics / Paul
Brinckmann, Wolfgang Frobin, Gunnar Leivseth. c2002.
  Includes bibliographical references and index.
  ISBN 978-3-13-176822-3 (alk. paper) —
ISBN 978-3-13-176832-2 (e-book)
  I. Frobin, W., author. II. Leivseth, Gunnar, author.
III. Drerup, B., author. IV. Brinckmann, Paul.
Orthopädische Biomechanik. English. 2002. Preceded by
(expression): V. Title.
  [DNLM: 1. Biomechanical Phenomena. 2. Movement—
physiology. 3. Orthopedics—methods.
WE 103]
  QP303
  612.7'6—dc23
                        2015013841

Contents

Foreword vi

Preface vii

Part I   **Mechanics: Some Basics** 1

    1   Basic Concepts from Physics and Mechanics 3

    2   Mechanical Properties of Solid Materials 36

    3   Deformation and Strength of Structures 51

Part II   **Mathematics: Some Basics** 67

    4   Vector Algebra 69

    5   Matrix Notation 86

    6   Translation and Rotation in a Plane 88

    7   Mathematical Description of Translation and Rotation
       in Three-Dimensional Space 103

Part III   **Mechanical Aspects of the Human Locomotor System** 139

    8   Mechanical Properties of Bone and Cartilage 141

    9   Structure and Function of Skeletal Muscle 179

   10   Mechanical Aspects of Skin 224

   11   Dimensions, Mass, Location of the Center of Mass, and Moment
       of Inertia of the Segments of the Human Body 236

   12   Determination of Joint Load in a Model Calculation 250

   13   Mechanical Aspects of the Hip Joint 272

   14   Mechanical Aspects of the Knee Joint 297

   15   Mechanical Aspects of the Lumbar Spine 326

   16   Mechanical Aspects of the Shoulder 362

   17   Biomechanics of the Foot 380

   18   Gait 414

Part IV   **Solved Problems** 439

   19   Solved Problems 441

       Notation 481

       Index 483

Foreword

Biomechanics plays an important role in understanding the musculoskeletal system. After all, human function depends on the intricate coordination of muscles and joints to create the forces and moments necessary to accomplish even the simplest activity. Further, bones, tendons, and ligaments must withstand the occasional high-intensity activity and accident forces as well as the repetitive forces caused by walking, running, lifting, throwing, grasping, and so on.

As a clinician I need biomechanical information to prevent and treat injuries to and pain arising from the musculoskeletal system and to effectively guide rehabilitation. As a surgeon I need to understand the material and wear properties of implants. Biomechanics is equally important for physical and occupational therapists, ergonomists, industrial engineering specialists, and rehabilitation and non-surgical practitioners in the field of musculoskeletal health such as rheumatologists, physiatrists, osteopaths, and chiropractors.

Paul Brinckmann, a physicist well known for his work in the field of biomechanics, has partnered with three outstanding collaborators to write the second edition of a book that is valuable for both clinicians and basic scientists. The result is a comprehensive yet appropriately detailed text on this broad subject.

Beginning with chapters on basic biomechanics, biomaterial science, and mathematical theory, the book moves on to the fundamental biomechanics of musculoskeletal tissues. Locomotion is covered extensively followed by a beautifully written chapter on muscle and muscle function. The modeling of joint loads is discussed separately as are the biomechanics of the hip, knee, spine, shoulder, and foot. Gait and gait analysis is the subject of a separate chapter. Finally, the book includes a chapter on problem solving, which covers a number of clinically relevant situations and examples.

The book expands on the previous edition and is more detailed at almost 500 pages. It is well referenced and beautifully illustrated. It can be used for study or for reference. I found it easy to read and highly relevant.

I congratulate the authors.

I also congratulate the readers. Enjoy!

Gunnar B J Andersson MD, PhD

Preface

This book is intended for readers working in orthopedics, physiotherapy, orthopedic technology, and rehabilitation. It gives an accurate account of the thought processes and procedures employed in orthopedic biomechanics, and of the current state of knowledge about loads and demands on the human locomotor system and the ways in which tissue reacts to mechanical influences, while keeping the mathematics and physics content to a minimum. The intention is to allow insights from mechanics into the structure and function of the human locomotor system to help clinicians identify potentially damaging factors and influences and develop concepts for prevention, treatment, and rehabilitation.

The authors will be content if the book helps readers to understand past and present research in orthopedic biomechanics, form an opinion of its significance, and make use of it in solving practical problems in physiotherapy and orthopedics. Perhaps they may even find stimulation for their own contributions to the field of orthopedic biomechanics.

The book is divided into four parts:

I   Mechanics: Some Basics
II   Mathematics: Some Basics
III   Mechanical Aspects of the Human Locomotor System
IV   Solved Problems

I Mechanics: Some Basics

Chapters 1 to 3 go over fundamental elements of physics and mechanics with which readers need to be acquainted if they are to understand the biomechanical relationships and follow the scientific arguments. Readers not in need of a brush-up on these topics may skip them and turn directly to Parts II and III.

II Mathematics: Some Basics

There is almost no subdomain of biomechanics where the vectors force, torque, velocity, and acceleration do not come into play. Understanding the vector algebra that forms the content of Chapter 4 is therefore indispensable. However, readers for whom description of the three-dimensional motion of the human body and its segments—as, for example, in gait analysis—is not the primary field of interest may skip Chapters 5, 6, and 7 (on matrix calculation and translations and rotations in two- and three-dimensional space) without finding themselves at a disadvantage in the subsequent chapters on mechanical aspects of the locomotor system.

III Mechanical Aspects of the Human Locomotor System

Chapters 8–10 elaborate on the mechanical properties of the tissues of bone, cartilage, muscle, and skin. Chapter 11 presents data on the masses, location of the centers of mass, and inertial properties of the segments of the body. These data are fundamental for estimating static and dynamic joint loads and designing orthopedic aids and appliances. Chapter 12 outlines how to determine joint load by using model calculations, a classical problem in orthopedic biomechanics. The techniques used for this purpose range from grossly simplified static model calculations to complex static and dynamic calculations based on detailed anatomical models and employing various objective functions. Simplified model calculations are dealt with in detail in Chapter 12 as well as in the following chapters on individual joints. This should enable even readers with no previous knowledge of mathematics and mechanics to grasp the principles of these methods. Chapters 13 to 18 are devoted to the mechanical aspects of hip, knee, lumbar spine, shoulder, foot, and gait.

IV Solved Problems

The collection of problems illustrates how to solve biomechanical questions with the help of mathematical and mechanical reasoning. Readers without training in mathematics and mechanics are not expected to solve these problems on their own, but if they follow the detailed solutions step by step, they will deepen their understanding. Readers with the appropriate previous knowledge, on the other hand, can cover up the solutions and compare their own solutions with those provided by the authors.

A list of references at the end of each chapter lists the scientific papers cited in the text or the figures. These studies were selected because the present authors regarded them as particularly interesting or instructive. Naturally, the selection is bound to be subjective. Nowadays, complete and up-to-date literature surveys on particular topics can be researched quite easily with the help of databases such as PubMed.

The authors would like to thank the editorial team, Martina Habeck and Kersti Wagstaff, for their expert help with editing the manuscript, Geraldine O'Sullivan for translation assistance, and Charles Wolstenholme for assistance with the illustrations. The authors are grateful to Thieme Publishers and thank the Executive Editor, Angelika-Marie Findgott, for making our collaboration such a pleasant experience during the preparation of this book.

Paul Brinckmann
Wolfgang Frobin
Gunnar Leivseth
Burkhard Drerup

Part I

Mechanics: Some Basics

1 Basic Concepts from Physics and Mechanics

Basic concepts like *force*, *torque* (also termed *moment of force*, or, for short, just *moment*), *mechanical stress*, *energy*, or *work* are unambiguously defined in physics and mechanics. These concepts have the same meaning in the field of biomechanics. A detailed treatise of the laws of mechanics and material properties can be found in any textbook on physics or mechanics (see for example Alonso et al[1] and Nelson et al[2]). This chapter, therefore, reiterates only those items that are important for an understanding of later chapters in this book, illustrated by examples from the human body.

When discussing biomechanical problems in orthopedics or physiotherapy, the term *mechanical load* (or, briefly, *load*) is frequently used. In its strict sense (as used in this book), the term *load* designates a force or a moment. For example, it may designate the force transmitted by a joint or the bending moment exerted on a bone. When used in this way, loading by a force is measured in *newtons* [N], and loading by a moment in *newton meters* [Nm] (see Eq. 1.1 below). The term *mechanical load* is, however, occasionally used in the literature to designate just some mechanical effect on the biological tissues; it is then up to the reader to find out what is actually meant. When used in this fashion, *mechanical loading* of cartilage or skin might, for example, designate pressure, friction, or deformation. Obviously these are quite different effects which require their own specific description and evaluation. To avoid confusion, it is preferable to adhere strictly to the well-defined mechanical terms when discussing biomechanical problems; only in rare instances are new technical terms required.

1.1 Force

Forces can be neither measured nor observed directly; forces are merely a theoretical concept of physics. However, the effects of forces are measurable and observable. For example, as an effect of a force, the acceleration or deformation of a body can be observed. In this context, the term *body* designates some object composed of inert material or the human body (or a part of it). The term *rigid* designates a body that does not deform, or deforms only negligibly, under the action of a force.

Newton's second law

(1.1)
$$F = m \cdot a$$

describes the relation between a mass m, its acceleration a, and the force F which effected the acceleration (**Fig. 1.1**). Mass is measured in units of kilograms [kg]. Acceleration is the change over time in velocity. Velocity is measured in units of meters per second [m/s], and the change in velocity over time in meters per second squared [m/s^2]. Since the units (or *dimensions*) on the two sides of an equation must be identical, force is thus measured in units of kilograms times meters per second squared [kg · m/s^2]. This unit has been given its own name and is called the *newton* [N].

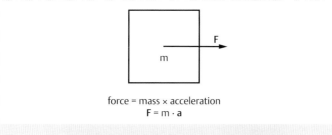

force = mass × acceleration

$$F = m \cdot a$$

Fig. 1.1 Effect of a force: acceleration of a mass. Newton's second law relates the force **F**, the mass m, and the acceleration **a**.

One example: A body of 5 kg mass may have zero velocity at the beginning of the observation period and one second later it may have a velocity of 20 m/s. Thus, during the observation period the object has been accelerated by 20 m/s per second = 20 m/s^2. On the assumption that the velocity increased linearly in the observation period, the force that effected the acceleration is calculated as F = 5 · 20 kg · m/s^2 = 100 N.

In anticipation of the chapter on vector algebra (Chapter 4), it should be pointed out that Newton's second law is really an equation between the vector of the force **F** and the vector of the acceleration **a**.

(1.2) $$\mathbf{F} = m \cdot \mathbf{a}$$

In this form, the law states that the magnitude of the acceleration is proportional to the magnitude of the force. The mass m is the proportionality factor. As an equation between two vectors, Newton's law states that the acceleration is effected in the direction of the force.

The deformation of a body by a force is illustrated in **Fig. 1.2** by the example of a coil spring. When loaded by a force, the spring shortens. For an elastic spring, the relation between the deformation and the magnitude of the force is given by Hooke's law:

(1.3) $$F = c \cdot dL/L$$

In this equation L designates the initial length of the spring and dL its change in length. L and dL are stated in units of meters [m]. The value of the constant c depends on the material properties and the form of the spring. c designates how much the spring deforms under a given force; that is, whether the spring is "hard" or "soft." Any force acting on a body effects a deformation. Depending on the material properties of the body, the deformation can be elastic (reversible), viscoelastic (time-dependent), or plastic (irreversible). In the case of viscoelastic or plastic materials, the relation between force and deformation is no longer described by Hooke's law, but by formulae adapted to the specific materials (see Chapter 2).

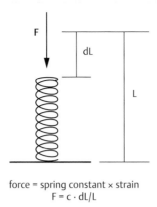

force = spring constant × strain
F = c · dL/L

Fig. 1.2 Effect of a force: deformation of a body. Hooke's law relates the magnitude of force **F**, the initial length L, and the change in length dL of the spring.

Experience shows that when a body 1 exerts a force $\mathbf{F}_{12}$ on a body 2, the body 2 exerts a force $\mathbf{F}_{21}$ of equal magnitude but opposite direction on body 1 (Newton's third law):

(1.4)
$$\mathbf{F}_{12} = -\mathbf{F}_{21}$$

In the static case (that is, when no accelerated movements occur), the force and counteracting force add up to zero. In the example shown in **Fig. 1.3**, the downward-directed gravitational force of the mass is of equal magnitude and opposite in direction to the upward-directed force of the spring.

Both effects of a force, acceleration and deformation, can be observed in the course of the gait cycle when the heel strikes the floor (**Fig. 1.4**). After a heel strike, the velocity of the body decreases; in addition, the heel deforms. Deceleration (negative acceleration) of the body and deformation of the heel are caused by a force exerted by the floor on the foot. There is an equal, opposite force exerted by the foot on the floor. This force deforms the floor. The deformation of a concrete floor is small, but still measurable. The deformation of an elastic floor in a gymnasium can be seen with the naked eye.

Forces exerted in specified directions with respect to a given surface receive additional designations (**Fig. 1.5**). A force directed perpendicularly onto a surface is called a compressive force. A force directed perpendicularly away from the surface is called a tensile force. A force acting in or parallel to the plane of the surface is called a shear force. Occasionally, forces are named according to their origin. Gravitational force (weight) originates from the gravitational attraction between a body and the earth. Muscular force originates from biochemical processes in the muscle tissue. Frictional force originates from surface irregularities and electrochemical properties of the materials in contact.

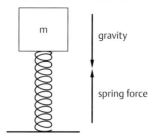

Fig. 1.3 Illustration of Newton's third law. In equilibrium the force of gravity and the elastic force of the spring are opposite in direction and equal in magnitude.

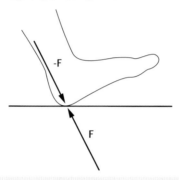

Fig. 1.4 When the foot hits the floor, a force **F** decelerates the body and deforms the foot. An equal but opposite force acts from the foot onto the floor. This force deforms the floor.

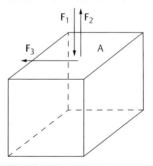

Fig. 1.5 A force directed perpendicular to a surface A is described as a compressive (F_1) or tensile (F_2) force, depending on its direction. A force acting parallel to the surface (F_3) is called a shear force.

In the dynamic case (that is, when accelerated movements are encountered), inertial forces come into play. If the acceleration of a mass m equals **a**, the inertial force **F** amounts to

(1.5)
$$F = m \cdot (-a)$$

The inertial force has the magnitude m · a and its direction is opposite to the direction of the acceleration. **Fig. 1.6** illustrates the effect of the inertial force (or *inertia*) when a mass is lifted from the floor. During lifting, the acceleration is directed upwards. The inertial force is directed downwards and is of magnitude m · a. The object thus appears to be "heavier" in the initial phase of lifting than it does when it is simply being held.

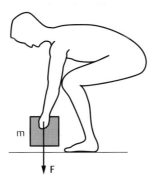

Fig. 1.6 Illustration of the effect of inertial force. When the mass is held, the gravitational force of magnitude F = m · g acts. When the mass is lifted with an upward-directed acceleration **a**, the inertial force m · (−**a**) acts in addition. At this moment, the hand feels a downward-directed force of magnitude F = m · (g + a).

Inertial forces become apparent when the human body is decelerated (that is, negatively accelerated), for example when hitting the floor after jumping from a wall or from gymnastic apparatus. The magnitude of the force between the body and the floor depends on the acceleration **a**. The magnitude of the acceleration can be calculated approximately by dividing the change in velocity Δv by the time interval Δt required to decelerate the body

(1.6)
$$a \approx \Delta v / \Delta t$$

This approximation rests on the assumption that the magnitude of the acceleration is constant during the time interval Δt. For a given change in velocity, a shorter time interval for deceleration will result in a larger inertial force; a longer time interval will result in a decrease in inertial force. Decreasing an inertial force by prolonging the time interval available for deceleration is called damping. In practical situations, the deformation must be large enough if an appreciable amount of damping is to be achieved. Two examples: If a person jumps off a wall and hits the floor with straight legs, the body's deceleration time will be short and the force between floor and foot will be correspondingly high. If, however, the time interval available for decelerating the body is lengthened, either by bending the knees (deformation of the body) or by a deformable (sprung) gym floor, the magnitude of the inertial force will be smaller. Or, if a shoe has a low heel, the heel can in the nature of things only be slightly deformed upon heel strike. There is therefore little scope for damping the force between shoe and floor, whatever material is used for the heel.

In many biomechanical problems gravitational forces play an important role. The force of gravity is always directed perpendicularly downwards; its magnitude is given by

(1.7) $$F = m \cdot g$$

In this equation, m designates the mass, given in kilograms [kg]. g is a constant, determined from free fall or pendulum experiments; it is called *gravitational acceleration*. The constant g has the numerical value of 9.81 [m/s^2]. It follows that a mass of 1 kg exerts a gravitational force equal to $1 \cdot 9.81$ kg $\cdot$ m/s^2 = 9.81 N. If errors in the order of 2% are deemed to be negligible (as is usually the case in orthopedic biomechanics), the numerical value of g can be rounded off to 10.0 [m/s^2]. Thus, the gravitational force (or *weight*) of a mass of 1 kg amounts (when rounded) to 10.0 N.

To describe the effect of a gravitational force on a body, a specific point, the *center of mass*, can be defined. The mass of the body is thought of as concentrated at this point and the force is thought of as acting on this point. Determination of the location of the center of mass is explained in Chapter 11.

Two remarks on gravitational force:

1. Colloquially, the terms *mass* and *weight* are used synonymously. Strictly speaking, this usage is not correct. The mass of a body is given in kilograms [kg], and its weight in newtons [N]. In everyday life, the imprecise use of the technical terms does not give rise to any misunderstanding. In biomechanical calculations, however, the weight of a mass must always be expressed in newtons (as the product m · g). Otherwise both the dimension and the numerical value of the result will be wrong.

2. g has the dimension of an acceleration. If a body is resting on a table, gravitational force is acting on it. Why don't we see any acceleration? The answer is, of course, that the table is exerting a force on the body in the opposite direction, and the accelerations of the gravitational force and the opposing force cancel each other out to zero (see also **Fig. 1.3**). If the body is allowed to fall freely, by contrast, no opposing force will be acting on it and the acceleration of the body will be clearly visible.

Forces, like all vectors, are described by magnitude and direction. This description does not include the point at which the force is applied to the body: in other words, the point of application is not a property of the force vector. For this reason, force vectors may be shifted at will along or parallel to their direction in graphic representations, as this changes neither the individual forces nor the vector sum. The effect of a force on a body depends of course on the point of application. If, for example, the force is applied such that its line of action (a line drawn to extend the force vector) passes through the center of mass, the body will be linearly accelerated in accordance with Newton's second law. If the line does not pass through the center of mass, the force also effects a moment. In this case the body will also show an accelerated rotation.

1.2 Moment

The moment effected by a force can be defined in different ways, as a number or as a vector (see Chapter 4). If calculations are limited to two-dimensional problems where the axis of rotation is perpendicular to the plane of interest, the moment can be defined for reasons of simplicity as a (positive or negative) number.

(1.8)
$$M = \pm L \cdot F$$

In this equation L is the magnitude of the perpendicular distance of the line of action of the force from a reference point. The line of action is an imagined line in the direction of the force and running through the point of force exertion. F is the magnitude of the force. If one is interested in the moment with respect to a joint, the position of the axis of rotation is chosen as reference point. If one is interested in the bending of a bone or an implant, a point in the bone or the implant is chosen as reference point. In the context of orthopedic biomechanics, the distance L is often called the *moment arm* of the force **F**—for example, the moment arm of a muscular force with respect to the axis of rotation of a joint, or the moment arm of the ground reaction force with respect to a point in the tibia where fracture may occur.

In mathematical notation, where the bars indicate the magnitude (positive value) of distance and force, we can write

(1.9)
$$M = \pm |\mathbf{L}| \cdot |\mathbf{F}|$$

Alternatively, the moment can be given as a product of the distance L_1 of the point of the force exertion from the fulcrum, the sine of the angle φ between the direction of the force and the line connecting the point of force exertion and the fulcrum, and the magnitude of the force:

(1.10)
$$M = \pm L_1 \cdot \sin\varphi \cdot F$$

In this equation, φ is the smaller of the two angles between the direction of the force and the distance line. φ is $\leq 90°$ and the numerical value of $\sin\varphi$ lies between 0 and +1. In the case of a distance line perpendicular to the direction of the force, φ equals 90° and $\sin\varphi$ equals +1; the two definitions of M above are thus identical.

Fig. 1.7 illustrates the definition of moment. The gravitational force $F = m \cdot g$ of the mass m of the body held in the hand exerts a moment M with respect to the axis of rotation in the center of the humeral condyle. Using both definitions stated above

(1.11) $$M = L \cdot F = L_1 \cdot \sin\varphi \cdot F = L \cdot m \cdot g$$

L and L_1 form the side and the base of a right-angled triangle; thus $L = L_1 \cdot \sin\varphi$.

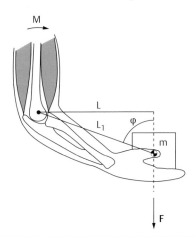

Fig. 1.7 Moment M of the gravitational force of the body held in the hand in relation to the axis of the elbow joint located in the center of the humeral condyle. For the calculation of the moment, either the perpendicular distance L of the axis from the line of action of the force, or the distance L_1 from the axis to the point of force exertion (the center of mass of the body) can be used. In the second case, the product of distance and force has to be multiplied by the sine of the angle φ between L_1 and the direction of the force.

If the moment is defined as a product of the magnitudes of distance and force (and not as a product of vectors; see Chapter 4 on vector algebra), an additional rule has to be followed to obtain the positive or negative sign of the moment. If the force effects a rotation in a clockwise direction, by convention the moment is counted as positive; if the rotation effected is counterclockwise, the moment is given a negative sign. In the example given in **Fig. 1.7**, the force effects a clockwise rotation; this moment is positive. In graphic illustrations, the moments defined as numbers (and not as vectors) are depicted by circular curved arrows with the arrowhead pointing in the direction of the rotation. It should be pointed out that, for historical reasons, the direction of rotation where moments are counted positive (that is, clockwise) does not match the definition of positive angles (angles are defined as positive when rotation is in a counterclockwise direction).

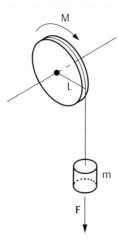

Fig. 1.8 Illustration of the effects of a moment M: accelerated rotation or torsional deformation. Under the influence of the force on the rope slung around the wheel, the wheel will undergo an accelerated rotation. If the wheel were fixed to the axis, the axis would be twisted.

Like forces, moments cannot be observed directly; only their effects can be observed. These effects are the acceleration of a rotational motion and the deformation of a body in torsion or bending. **Fig. 1.8** illustrates these effects: angular acceleration and torsional deformation. If a mass m is attached to the rope around a wheel, the wheel is loaded by a moment of magnitude

(1.12) $$M = L \cdot m \cdot g$$

and the wheel performs an accelerated rotation. If the wheel were fixed (nonrevolving) on the axis, application of the moment would result in a torsional deformation of the axis. For a thin axis of elastic material, the relation between the moment M and the angle of torsion φ is given by

(1.13) $$M = c \cdot \varphi$$

c is a constant which depends on the material properties, the cross section, and the length of the axis. (The equation is analogous to the equation describing the deformation of a spring under a force.)

Fig. 1.9 illustrates a situation where a torsional deformation of the lower extremity occurs. When the ski hits an obstacle, a sideways-directed force of magnitude F applied at a distance L from the long axis of the leg exerts a moment L · F on the leg. The range of rotational motion about the long axis of the leg amounts to approx. 15° in the hip joint while the range in the ankle and knee joint is very small, so once the endpoint of the range of motion is reached, torsional deformation of the leg follows. If the ski is long and the force is high, the resulting moment may be great enough to effect a torsional fracture of the tibia or to rupture the ligaments of the knee.

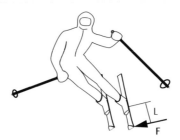

Fig. 1.9 A laterally directed force **F** applied at distance L from the leg exerts a moment of magnitude L · F on the leg. The leg will undergo an accelerated rotation about its longitudinal axis. At the end of the range of motion, the leg will deform in torsion.

The relation between moment and accelerated rotation is given by

(1.14)
$$M = I \cdot \alpha$$

α designates the angular acceleration. Angles are dimensionless quantities; they are measured in degrees (°) or radians (rad). A full rotation of 360° corresponds to an angle of 2π rad ($\pi = 3.14159...$); accordingly 1 rad corresponds to an angle of 57.2958°. Angular velocity ω is the rotational angle covered per second, measured in radians or degrees per second (1/s). Angular acceleration α is the change over time in angular velocity, measured in radians or degrees per second squared ($1/s^2$). By analogy to the definition of the inertial force, the quantity

(1.15)
$$M_i = I \cdot (-\alpha)$$

characterizes resistance of a body against accelerated rotation. M_i opposes the moment that causes the acceleration. I denotes the moment of inertia of the body in relation to the axis of rotation. I depends on the distribution of the body's mass with respect to the axis of rotation. A mass m concentrated at a point located at a distance L from the axis has a moment of inertia equal to $m \cdot L^2$. For the calculation of moments of inertia, see Chapter 11.

In general, a force acting on a body effects a rotation as well as a linear acceleration. According to Newton's second law, the acceleration depends on the force **F** and the mass m of the body. If, by contrast, two forces of equal magnitude but opposing direction act on a body, the forces effect a moment (provided the forces are not applied at the identical point), but the sum of the forces equals zero. In this case, the two forces exert a *pure*

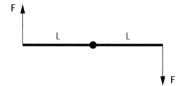

Fig. 1.10 If two forces of equal magnitude but opposite direction act on a body, the sum of the forces equals zero. If the two forces are neither applied at the same point nor act along the same line, the pair of forces effects a moment on the body. In the example shown, the magnitude of the moment in relation to the fulcrum of the beam amounts to $2 \cdot L \cdot F$.

moment. **Fig. 1.10** illustrates this with the example of a pivoted beam loaded by a pair of forces (force couple). Related to the fulcrum, the moment is the sum of the moments exerted by the two forces and amounts to

(1.16) $$M = 2 \cdot L \cdot F$$

The reference point can, however, be chosen arbitrarily. Related to the left end of the beam, the moment would be

(1.17) $$M = 0 \cdot F + 2 \cdot L \cdot F = 2 \cdot L \cdot F$$

Choosing any other reference point would result in the identical moment. Because the moment is independent of the choice of the reference point, it is called a *free* moment. A single force **F** which loads a body at a distance L from the fulcrum (**Fig. 1.11**) can be replaced by a pure moment $2 \cdot (L \cdot 1/2\ F) = L \cdot F$ and a force **F**

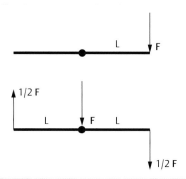

Fig. 1.11 A single force **F** acting at a distance L from the fulcrum can be replaced by a pure moment of the magnitude $L \cdot F$ and a force **F** acting at the fulcrum. In both cases a force **F** and a moment $L \cdot F$ act on the body; the two loading modes are identical.

exerted at the fulcrum. This replacement is advantageous if the linear acceleration of the whole setup and the rotational acceleration are to be investigated separately.

When dealing with objects that are very long in comparison with their cross section (beams or long bones, for example), moments that load the objects in certain directions have specific names. A moment that twists a beam about its long axis is called *torsional moment* or *torque*. A moment that bends the beam is called a *bending moment*. In **Fig. 1.12**, the force **F** on the free end of the angled beam exerts a bending moment on part a and both a bending and a torsional moment on part b of the beam. According to the definition of the moment, the bending moment in part a increases with the distance from the point at which the force is applied. The same is true for part b: the highest bending moment occurs at the location where the beam is fixed to the wall. In contrast to this, the torsional moment is constant throughout the length of part b, because the distance between the point at which the force is applied and the long axis of part b does not change along the length of part b. On the end face A, and on all cross sections that are parallel to A, a shear force acts that is equal to **F**. The beam and wall undergo downward acceleration and accelerated clockwise rotation exerted by force **F**. That the beam and wall remain where they are instead of accelerating away is due to the opposing force and moment exerted by the ground on the wall.

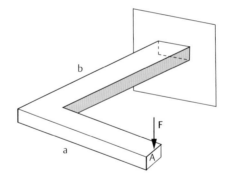

Fig. 1.12 A force **F** on an angulated beam exerts different moments on the different parts of the beam. The force exerts a bending moment on section a, and both a bending and a torsional moment (torque) on section b.

If a force acts on a body, the moment of this force can be stated with respect to any chosen point inside or outside of the body. Which is the best point to choose for reference depends on the problem to be solved. Here are four examples:

1. To obtain information about muscle forces and joint loads, the reference point chosen is the center of rotation. **Fig. 1.13** illustrates this using the example of the elbow joint. In relation to the center of rotation in the humeral condyle, the moment of the load **F** amounts to $L_1 \cdot F$, and the moment of muscular

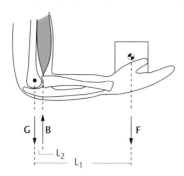

Fig. 1.13 When calculating joint loads, for reasons of simplicity the moments of the load **F** and the muscle force **B** are related to the center of rotation of the joint. The moment of the joint load **G** is then equal to zero and does not contribute to the sum of moments.

force **B** amounts to $-L_2 \cdot B$ (the negative sign is dictated by the sign convention for moments). The moment of joint load **G** is zero, because this force passes through the center of rotation and thus its moment arm is equal to zero. If the precise location of a joint's center of rotation is unknown, a point at the center of the surface of the joint can be chosen as an approximation.

2. To investigate mechanical stress in the bones of the lower arm (**Fig. 1.14**), a reference point is chosen within the bone, for example at a distance L_3 from the force application point. At this point the bones are acted on by a moment $L_3 \cdot F$. This moment bends the humerus and ulna downwards. Equilibrium is established by compressive and tensile stresses in the bones.

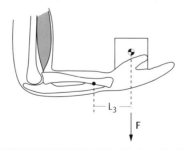

Fig. 1.14 To investigate a bending moment exerted on a bone, the moment is related to a chosen reference point within the bone.

3. To work out how to help transfemoral amputees stop the prosthetic knee from buckling at the moment of heel strike, one focuses on the moment of the ground reaction force **F** with respect to the axis of rotation (**Fig. 1.15**). With respect to the axis of the healthy, anatomical knee (filled circle), force **F** exerts a

flexion moment. To prevent flexion (that is, to keep the leg straight), healthy subjects activate their knee extensors (quadriceps) at heel strike. In an amputee without knee extensors, however, another solution must be found. The answer is to employ, instead of a simple hinge joint, a so-called polycentric knee that deliberately shifts the joint's axis of rotation (open circle in **Fig. 1.15**) to a position posterior to the anatomical axis. The effect of this is that the ground reaction force **F** generates an extension moment at heel strike, thus allowing the amputee to maintain stability. Alternatively, an electronically controlled prosthesis may be employed, which identifies the heel strike phase (extended knee, loaded) and blocks joint flexion during this phase.

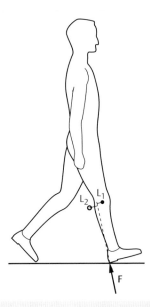

Fig. 1.15 To investigate the moment of the ground reaction force exerted on a knee, the moment is related to the anatomical axis of the knee if this is intact (filled circle) or, in the case of a polycentric prosthesis, on its momentary axis (open circle).

4. Mechanical equilibrium exists when the sum of all forces and moments equals zero (see Chapter 12). In the state of equilibrium (and only in this state), any point can be chosen as the reference in order calculate the sum of moments. This theorem can be used in any given setup to check whether the equilibrium of moments is fulfilled. As an example, **Fig. 1.16** analyzes an exercise designed for isometric activation of the quadriceps muscle. The lower leg is acted on by the force F_2 of the patellar tendon (activated by the quadriceps) and the tibiofemoral force F_1. An external, posteriorly directed force F_3 acting on the lower leg prevents extension of the knee. If the application point of F_3 is chosen such that its line of action runs through point P (the intersection of the lines of action of forces F_1 and F_2), it follows

that the sum of moments equals zero. This is because the moment arms of all three forces in relation to point P equal zero and thus the sum of the moments equals zero. This holds in relation to any other point of reference, including the center of rotation of the knee joint. If, by contrast, the line of action of F_3 did not pass through P, mechanical equilibrium would not exist.

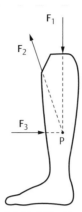

Fig. 1.16 If the lines of action of all forces intersect at a single point, the sum of moments about this point equals zero. This is because all moment arms related to this point equal zero. For mechanical equilibrium, it holds that the sum of moments related to any point equals zero.

1.3 Pressure

Pressure describes in detail how force is transmitted from one object to another via an interface. Pressure is defined as *magnitude of a force perpendicular to an interface, divided by the area of the interface:*

(1.18)
$$p = F / A$$

In this equation force F is expressed in newtons [N] and the area A in square meters [m^2]. The unit of pressure [N/m^2] is called the *pascal* [Pa]. The terms *compressive stress* and *pressure* are synonyms.

In simple cases the pressure on an interface can be calculated directly from the definition. If a rigid body lies with a plane side on a plane surface (**Fig. 1.17**), the pressure may be assumed to be uniform over the whole area A of the interface. When loaded by a force **F** directed perpendicularly to the surface, the pressure is calculated as $p = F/A$. If the force remains constant and the area A is increased, the pressure decreases in proportion to the increase in area. If, however, we imagine a small rock being inserted between the rigid body and the plane, the pattern of force transmission changes completely. Now the force is transmitted only through the rock and some points or lines of contact between the rigid body and the plane. The definition $p = F/A$ remains valid, but the magnitude of the pressure at the contact locations will of course be higher than the value F/A.

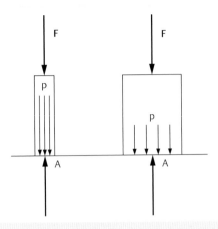

Fig. 1.17 Illustration of the definition of pressure. Pressure p is defined as the magnitude of the force **F** perpendicular to an interface divided by the area A of the interface. In simple cases, the pressure can be directly determined from its definition. In the case of a plane surface between rigid bodies, p = F/A. If the area is increased (with the force kept constant), the pressure decreases.

Plane areas of contact are rarely encountered between the human body and its environment or between articulating bones. And even if the interface is plane, as between the bare foot and the floor (**Fig. 1.18**), or between the camper's thin insulation mat and the ground, experience tells us that the pressure is not of identical magnitude at different points of the contact area. If the pressure is of different magnitudes at different points of a contact area, there is a *pressure distribution*. The fraction d**F** of the total force transmitted

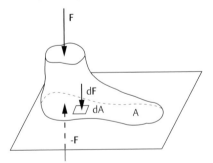

Fig. 1.18 Even in the case of a plane interface between the bare foot and the floor, the pressure p = dF/dA is not uniform over the contact area. A pressure distribution exists. The points of maximum and minimum pressure depend on the architecture of the hard and soft tissues of the foot. The mean pressure over the area of contact is F/A.

by each area element dA of the contact area, the pressure dF/dA on each element of the contact area, varies from place to place. In the case of the foot or the camper's mat it is obvious why the pressure is different at different locations. The local pressure depends on the architecture of the bones and ligaments and on the thickness and mechanical properties of the tissues as well as on the material properties of the ground.

The majority of opposing joint surfaces in the human body are incongruent. When they are loaded, contact occurs only over small areas, and consequently high pressure must be expected in these areas. Inserting a deformable tissue into the joint space increases the area available for force transmission and may bring about an almost uniform pressure distribution. Examples are the menisci between the femur and the tibia, and the intervertebral disks of the lumbar spine.

Calculating the distribution of pressure, for example under the sole of the foot, is a complicated problem and often only an approximate result can be expected. However, a simple formula exists that can be used to get a rough idea of the magnitude of the pressure. The term *mean pressure* denotes the mean value of the pressure, averaged over the pressure distribution on the interface. The mean pressure p_{mean} can be calculated by dividing the magnitude of the force **F** by the projected area A_{proj}:

(1.19) $$p_{mean} = F / A_{proj}$$

The projected area is the area seen by looking at the interface area along the direction of the force. Knowing the mean pressure implies that the actual pressure will in some places be higher and in other places lower than the mean. Furthermore, the formula implies that the mean pressure increases or decreases in proportion to the force. The formula for calculating the mean pressure is of practical importance in biomechanics. If, for example, the force exerted on a joint can be reduced by a change in posture or external loading, it would be expected that the mean pressure on the joint surface would decrease proportionately. (Strictly speaking, this is true only if the shape of the pressure-transmitting joint surface remains unchanged; usually it is, more or less.) Conversely, increasing the area of the force-transmitting interface may be expected to reduce the pressure—an effect made use of when soft, deformable underlayers are used in hospital beds to increase the area the patient is lying on and thus reduce the pressure to which fragile skin regions are exposed.

In the example in **Fig. 1.18**, the projected area equals the area of the foot's contact with the floor. In symmetric stance, F equals one half of the body weight. The mean pressure on the plantar surface then amounts to

(1.20) $$p_{mean} = \frac{1}{2} \cdot \text{body weight} / \text{contact area of the foot}$$

Assuming a body mass of 60 kg and a contact area of 160 cm² one obtains

(1.21) $$p_{mean} = \frac{1}{2} \cdot 60 \cdot 10 / 0.016 \, \text{N} / \text{m}^2 = 18750 \, \text{Pa}$$

Conversion into the conventional unit for blood pressure (division by approx. 133) gives

(1.22) $p_{mean} = 18750/133$ corresponding to 141 mmHg

This pressure is higher than the arterial pressure in the sole of the foot, which in standing ranges between 110 and 130 mmHg.

Fig. 1.19 shows how the formula for the mean pressure can be employed to estimate the pressure on joint surfaces. The figure shows a hip joint, loaded by a force **H**, and the pressure distribution calculated using model assumptions. The mean pressure is obtained by dividing the magnitude of the force **H** by the projected area of the joint. In this case, the projected area is a circle oriented perpendicular to **H** with a diameter equal to the diameter of the femoral head.

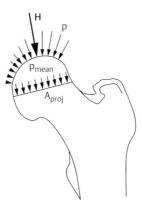

Fig. 1.19 A pressure distribution exists on the surface of the femoral head loaded by a force **H**. The mean pressure is equal to the magnitude of the force **H** divided by the projected area of the joint surface A_{proj}. In the case of the hip joint, the projected area is a circle with the diameter of the femoral head.

If a force **F** acts between two bodies, and if only compressive stress but no tensile or shear stress exists on the contact area, there is a mathematical relation between the force and the pressure distributed over the contact area. If one imagines the area as divided into small elements A_i, for mechanical equilibrium the sum of all the individual forces transmitted by the elements must equal the applied force,

(1.23) $$\mathbf{F} = \sum_i \mathbf{F}_i = \sum_i p_i \cdot \mathbf{A}_i$$

In this formula p_i denotes the pressure on the area element A_i. The notation $p_i \cdot \mathbf{A}_i$ indicates that the forces transmitted by the area elements are vectors. Their magnitude is $p_i \cdot A_i$ and their direction is perpendicular (normal) to the position of the area element. In case of a continuous pressure distribution, the sum is to be replaced by the area integral $\int p \cdot d\mathbf{A}$. In the case of a plane contact area positioned perpendicular to the force $\mathbf{F}$, all force elements $\mathbf{F}_i$ point in the identical direction. For the magnitude of the force $\mathbf{F}$, it then holds that

(1.24) $$F = \sum F_i = \sum p_i \cdot A_i$$

This, for example, holds for the plantar pressure distribution in standing on a pressure sensor mat laid on a plane floor. A pressure sensor mat is a matrix arrangement of small pressure sensors (electronic devices for pressure measurement). Pressure sensor mats employed in gait analysis have the form of a plane rectangle or are shaped to fit into a shoe as an insole. If a pressure distribution is measured by means of such a mat, the sum of the products of the area of the individual pressure sensors times the individual pressure will equal the body weight.

The pressure between an amputee's stump and the prosthesis shaft varies over the contact area: that is, a pressure distribution exists. However, the above relation (Eq. 1.23) between pressure and force is not valid in this case, because the stump not only exerts pressure but also adheres by friction to the inner surface of the shaft. In other words, the force between the stump and the prosthesis is transmitted not just by compressive stress but also by shear stress. The force equals the sum (or the integral) of the compressive and shear forces extended over the contact area. In general, the direction of the force is not perpendicular to the inner surface of the prosthesis.

During gait, in addition to compressive stress, shear stress may exist on the plantar surface of the foot. At heel strike, a force component directed parallel to the floor and against (opposite to) the direction of gait acts on the foot. This force decelerates the body and exerts shear stress in the plantar skin. At toe-off, the force component parallel to the floor (the shear force on the foot) changes direction. While pressure distributions between a foot and the floor or between a stump and a prosthesis shaft can be measured by pressure sensor mats, however, unfortunately no method is available to determine the distribution of shear stresses. Thus, we have very little information about the magnitude of shear stress and its effects on the skin of a stump or of the plantar surface of the foot.

In contrast to solid bodies, the molecules of fluids or gases can move against each other with almost complete freedom. In a given vessel, a fluid may fill part of the volume. A gas will fill the whole volume because of the lack of attraction between its molecules. Because of the unrestricted mobility of the molecules, the direction of the force exerted by fluids or gases at rest is always perpendicular to the wall of the vessel. If a component of the force existed that was parallel to the wall (a shear force), the fluid or gas would move until the shear force disappeared. From the fact that the force exerted by fluids or gases is always directed perpendicular to containing surfaces, it follows that the pressure at any point within a fluid or gas volume is equal in all directions.

In the absence of gravitational force, the pressure in a volume of fluid or gas would be equal at every point. With gravity, the pressure depends on the weight of the volume of fluid or gas perpendicularly above the point of interest. Here are three examples: (1) The pressure of the atmosphere at ground level is equal to the weight of the air contained in a column rising perpendicularly from the ground into completely air-less space, divided by the cross-sectional area of the column. (2) The pressure at the base of a column of mercury is equal to the weight of the column divided by its cross-sectional area. In medical terminology, this pressure is given in units of millimeters of mercury [mmHg]. Strictly speaking, millimeters are not the correct dimension; correctly, the pressure should be stated in pascals (1 mmHg corresponds to roughly 133 Pa). (3) Because of gravity, arterial pressure at the feet of a person standing upright (but not one lying down) is noticeably higher than the pressure measured close to the heart.

If the internal space of a cylinder with a moveable piston is connected to the outside environment by an open tube, the pressure on the walls of the cylinder and on the inner and outer surfaces of the piston is identical. If some air is pumped out of the internal space, the internal pressure will decrease. The magnitude of the force acting on the piston is expressed as

(1.25)
$$F = \Delta p \cdot A$$

where Δp is the pressure difference between the outside and the inside and A is the area of the piston. This force presses the piston into the cylinder. In prosthetics, this effect is put to use to fix a stump into the socket of a prosthesis. The stump is inserted into the socket, driving the air out (or the air is pumped out) through a valve. The resulting negative (below atmospheric) pressure generates a force that pulls the stump into the shaft.

1.3.1 Center of Pressure

Where a pressure distribution exists on a contact surface, as for example between a foot and the floor, for simplicity some biomechanical applications ignore the details of the distribution, relying instead on a quantity derived from it, known as the *center of pressure*. The center of pressure is defined as the point of application of that force F_z that has the same mechanical effect on the body as the totality of the compressive forces exerted by the pressure distribution. The calculation for locating the center of pressure will now be outlined using the example of the pressure distribution between a foot and the floor. Similar formulae hold for locating the center of pressure between the buttocks and a seat (for the investigation of sitting posture control, for example).

Replacing the effect of a pressure distribution by the effect of a single force may always be done in cases where one is not interested in the local effects of the pressure, but only in the effect of the force transmitted through the contact area to the body as a whole. For the mechanical state to remain unchanged, two conditions must be fulfilled: (1) The perpendicular component $\mathbf{F}_z$ of the force $\mathbf{F}$ on the contact area must be equal to the sum of all compressive forces $\mathbf{F}_{zi} = \mathbf{A}_i \cdot p_i$ transmitted via the elements A_i of the contact area. (2) The moment of the force $\mathbf{F}_z$ in relation to the axes of an xy-coordinate system must equal the sum of the moments of the forces $\mathbf{F}_{zi} = \mathbf{A}_i \cdot p_i$ in relation to the same axes (irrespective of the orientation of the xy-coordinate system).

If the pressure distribution is measured using a pressure sensor mat (**Fig. 1.20**), the pressure p_i is exerted on each area element A_i with coordinates x_i, y_i ($I = 1, ..., n$). The magnitude of the force $\mathbf{F}_z$ equals the sum of the forces F_{zi}:

(1.26)
$$F_z = \sum_{i=1}^{n} F_{zi} = \sum_{i=1}^{n} p_i \cdot A_i$$

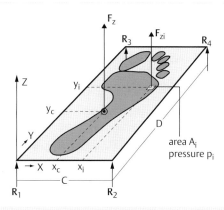

Fig. 1.20 Calculation of the center of pressure x_c, y_c from the pressure distribution on the plantar surface of the foot, or alternatively from the measured force values of transducers R_1 to R_4 of a force platform.

In relation to the x- and y-axes of a coordinate system, the sum of the magnitudes of the moments of the forces $\mathbf{F}_{zi}$ must equal the magnitude of the moment of the force $\mathbf{F}_z$. It holds that

(1.27)
$$F_z \cdot x_c = \sum_{i=1}^{n} F_{zi} \cdot x_i = \sum_{i=1}^{n} p_i \cdot A_i \cdot x_i$$
$$F_z \cdot y_c = \sum_{i=1}^{n} F_{zi} \cdot y_i = \sum_{i=1}^{n} p_i \cdot A_i \cdot y_i$$

Solving these for coordinates x_c, y_c of the application point of force $\mathbf{F}_z$, one obtains

$$x_c = \frac{\sum_{i=1}^{n} p_i \cdot A_i \cdot x_i}{F_z}$$

(1.28)
$$y_c = \frac{\sum_{i=1}^{n} p_i \cdot A_i \cdot y_i}{F_z}$$

Point x_c, y_c is designated the *center of pressure*. In practical applications, areas A_i and their coordinates x_i, y_i are supplied by the manufacturer of the pressure-sensitive mat or insole. The pressure data p_i are read into a computer and a program calculates F_z and x_c, y_c.

Alternatively, a force platform can be used to locate the center of pressure (**Fig. 1.20**). A force platform is a rigid plate mounted on four force transducers (electronic devices for measurement of a force). When a person stands on the platform, the ground reaction force is transmitted from the floor through the force transducers to the feet. The transducers are located at the corners of a rectangle with length D and width C. $\mathbf{R_1}, \mathbf{R_2}, \mathbf{R_3}$, and $\mathbf{R_4}$ are the z-components of the forces measured. Replacing the four forces $\mathbf{R_1}, \mathbf{R_2}, \mathbf{R_3}$, and $\mathbf{R_4}$ by one single force acting at x_c, y_c (the center of pressure) will not change the mechanical state.

The magnitude of the force $\mathbf{F_z}$ equals the sum of the magnitudes of the forces of the four transducers:

(1.29)
$$F_z = R_1 + R_2 + R_3 + R_4$$

In relation to the x- and y-axes of the coordinate system shown in **Fig. 1.20**, the magnitude of the moments of the force $\mathbf{F_z}$ must equal the sum of the magnitude of the moments of forces $\mathbf{R_1}$ to $\mathbf{R_4}$:

(1.30)
$$F_z \cdot x_c = (R_2 + R_4) \cdot C$$
$$F_z \cdot y_c = (R_3 + R_4) \cdot D$$

The moments of $\mathbf{R_1}$ and $\mathbf{R_3}$ in relation to the y-axis and of $\mathbf{R_1}$ and $\mathbf{R_2}$ in relation to the x-axis are zero because their respective moment arms are zero. Thus they do not contribute to the right side of Eq. 1.30. With $F_z = R_1 + R_2 + R_3 + R_4$, the point of application x_c, y_c of the force $\mathbf{F_z}$ can be calculated as

(1.31)
$$x_c = \frac{(R_2 + R_4) \cdot C}{(R_1 + R_2 + R_3 + R_4)}$$
$$y_c = \frac{(R_3 + R_4) \cdot D}{(R_1 + R_2 + R_3 + R_4)}$$

Point x_c, y_c is designated the *center of pressure* despite the fact that it has been defined without reference to any pressure distribution. It physically coincides with the center of pressure that would be determined from Eq. 1.28 if a pressure sensor mat were placed over the force platform. (Anyway, the reader will note that the calculation of the center of pressure from the data of a pressure sensor mat or a force platform is identical. In the first case forces from all pressure sensors are taken into account; in the second case forces from four force transducers are taken into account.)

1.4 Mechanical Stress

When a force acts on a body, a deformation is observed in the direction of the force (**Fig. 1.21**). Compressive or tensile forces shorten or stretch the body; shear forces effect an angular deformation. The deformation changes the relative locations of atoms or molecules within the material. This gives rise to internal forces (repulsion and attraction) of electrical origin, which balance the external forces.

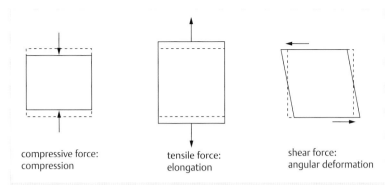

compressive force:
compression

tensile force:
elongation

shear force:
angular deformation

Fig. 1.21 A force effects a deformation of a body; in static equilibrium, internal forces balance the external force. The deformation occurs in the direction of the force, but simultaneous, additional deformations in other directions (not illustrated here) are possible. A tensile force effects elongation, a compressive force results in compression, and a shear force causes an angular deformation.

The mechanical stress on the surface of a small cube-shaped volume element of a loaded body (**Fig. 1.22**) is defined as the fraction dF of the magnitude of the total force transmitted via the surface dA and divided by this surface area.

(1.32)
$$\sigma = dF / dA$$
$$\tau = dF / dA$$

If the force **dF** is directed perpendicular to the surface dA there is compressive or tensile stress σ. If the force **dF** runs parallel to the surface dA, there is shear stress τ. (The definition of compressive stress on an imaginary inner surface is identical with the definition of pressure on an external surface. The terms *pressure* and *compressive stress* are synonymous.)

In static mechanical equilibrium, stresses on opposite sides of a cube-shaped volume element are equal in magnitude but oppositely directed. Different values of compressive, tensile, and shear stress may exist on the three pairs of opposing surfaces of the cube. The state of mechanical stress of a cube-shaped volume element is thus uniquely described by six numbers (three compressive or tensile stresses, three shear stresses). It has to be pointed out that the stress on the surface of a volume element imagined as cut from a body depends on the spatial orientation of the element with respect to the body. If (with the loading mode left unchanged) a different orientation of the volume element in **Fig. 1.22** were chosen, different values of the stress on the surfaces of the cube would be found. The stress values for different orientations are interrelated; conversion formulae (not given here; see textbooks on properties of materials) allow the change in stresses to be calculated in dependence on the change in orientation.

In simple cases it is possible to employ the definition of stress given above to calculate the stress directly. In the example in **Fig. 1.22**, with the body loaded by a compressive force F_1 and a shear force F_2, the stress

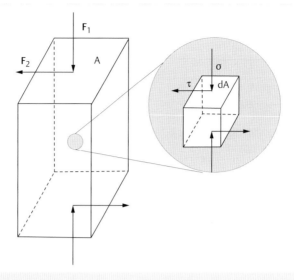

Fig. 1.22 Loading a body effects mechanical stress within the volume of the body. The mechanical stress on the surface of a cube imagined to be cut from the volume of the body is defined as the fraction of the force dF transmitted through the surface dA of the cube. If the force dF is directed perpendicular to the surface dA, the stress is termed compressive or tensile stress; if the force is directed parallel to the surface, the stress is termed shear stress. For reasons of mechanical equilibrium the stresses on opposite sides of a cube are equal and oppositely directed. Stresses on adjacent sides of the cube can be different. In a given loading situation the stresses depend on the spatial orientation of the cube; the stresses in different orientations can be obtained by mathematical conversion.

may be assumed to be uniform over any internal surface parallel to the outer surface A. Under this assumption, the compressive stress σ and the shear stress τ on the surface dA of a cube-shaped volume element oriented parallel to the outer surface A amount to

(1.33)
$$\sigma = F_1 / A$$
$$\tau = F_2 / A$$

Mechanical effects on the tissues of the human body depend ultimately not on the forces but on the pressure on surfaces (skin, articular cartilage), on the internal stresses within the tissues (bone, muscle), and their deformation under load. On the other hand, pressure, mechanical stress, and deformation depend on (1) the magnitude and direction of the force, (2) the architecture of the organs, and (3) the details of the force application. Obviously it makes a considerable difference whether a needle is pressed (with equal force) onto the skin with its blunt end or its sharp end. If pressure or stress are to be influenced, this could in principle be achieved either by altering the load and the mode of application or by altering the geometry and material properties of the organs. In the human body, however, the last two options are rarely available. It is easier to try to influence the external loading and the mode of load transmission to the human body. These considerations have practical relevance when, for example, a patient is in need of temporary or permanent reduction of the pressure on joint surfaces.

1.5   Friction Force

Friction arises between the surfaces of rigid bodies. This so-called *external friction* has a number of causes: electrostatic attraction between the molecules of the materials, small surface irregularities catching on each other, and elastic or plastic deformation of contaminating materials on the surfaces. It follows that friction depends on the materials in contact, on the microscopic architecture of their surfaces, and on the presence of other materials (lubricants, dust) on the surfaces.

Experience shows that the friction force depends on the compressive force between the bodies and on their relative velocity. The friction force is parallel to the contact area and directed opposite to the direction of motion (or impending motion) (**Fig. 1.23**). Static friction is distinguished from kinetic friction. The static friction coefficient μ_s describes the empirical relation between the magnitudes of the friction force $\mathbf{F}_f$ and the *normal* force $\mathbf{F}_n$ (that is, acting perpendicular to the contact area) for the case that the bodies are just at the very point of moving relative to each other.

(1.34)
$$F_f = \mu_s \cdot F_n$$

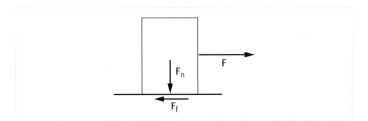

Fig. 1.23 External friction between two solid bodies. The friction force $\mathbf{F}_f$ is oppositely directed to the force $\mathbf{F}$. $\mathbf{F}_f$ depends on the material properties of the two bodies, on the normal force $\mathbf{F}_n$, and on the relative velocity of the bodies.

The kinetic friction coefficient μ_k describes the empirical relation between the magnitudes of the friction force $\mathbf{F}_f$ and the normal force $\mathbf{F}_n$ for the case that the bodies are moving relative to each other.

(1.35)
$$F_f = \mu_k \cdot F_n$$

In general, the kinetic friction coefficient is smaller than the static friction coefficient. At the onset of motion, or when the relative motion is very slow, the value of the actual friction coefficient lies between the values of the static and the kinetic friction coefficients. Motion against a friction force consumes energy. In the end this energy is dissipated as heat.

If a body is moved through a gas or a fluid—for example, the hand is moved through air or water—a force directed opposite to the direction of motion acts on the body. This force is due to *internal* friction. During motion in a fluid, the attraction between the molecules has to be overcome. In addition, during motion in a gas or a fluid, kinetic energy is transmitted to the molecules. Here, too, energy is consumed and dissipated as heat.

Friction in a fluid is described by its viscosity η. In the basic experiment to determine viscosity, a plane plate of area A is moved through the fluid at a constant velocity v in parallel to, and at a distance x from, a wall. The movement requires a force of magnitude F which is proportional to the area A and the velocity v and inversely proportional to the distance x.

(1.36)
$$F = \eta \cdot A \cdot \frac{v}{x}$$

η is a material constant of the fluid. The greater the viscosity of a fluid, the greater the resistance exerted on an object moving through it.

If a fluid flows (with moderate velocity) through a tube with diameter 2R and length l, the following relation exists between the fluid volume flow per unit time and the pressure difference p (Hagen–Poiseuille law):

(1.37)
$$\frac{V}{t} = \frac{\pi \cdot R^4}{8\eta} \frac{p}{l}$$

This relation is extremely important to the functioning of the human blood circulation. Blood flow increases with pressure and (to the fourth power) with the radius of the vessel. Increased viscosity of the blood decreases the flow.

1.6 Mechanical Work, Energy, Momentum, and Power

Mechanical work is defined as *force times distance.* The distance L is measured in the direction of the force.

(1.38)
$$E = F \cdot L$$

In the case of rotation, mechanical work is defined as the product of the moment and the angle of rotation:

(1.39)
$$E = M \cdot \alpha$$

In both cases mechanical work has the dimension newton meter [Nm]. This unit is called the *joule* [J]. For conversion between joules and calories: 1 cal is equivalent to 4.2 J.

Here are some examples of mechanical work: (1) A person lifts a mass m through a height h. The gravitational force $F = m \cdot g$ is constant during the lifting process. The person performs mechanical work $F \cdot h = m \cdot g \cdot h$ [Nm]. (2) An object is moved over a distance d against a (constant) friction force F_f; the mechanical work amounts to $F_f \cdot d$ [Nm]. (3) A person compresses (shortens) an elastic coil spring by a distance x. It must be kept in mind that the resistive force of the spring is not constant but increases proportionately as the spring shortens. The work is given by the integral

(1.40)
$$\int F \cdot dx = \frac{1}{2} c \cdot x^2$$

x is the change in length; c is a constant which depends on the form and material properties of the spring. A similar formula applies for the work required to stretch a tendon.

The kinetic energy (motion energy) E of a body in linear motion is given by

(1.41)
$$E = \frac{1}{2} m \cdot v^2 \text{ [Nm]}$$

In this formula m denotes the mass and v the velocity of the body. In the case of rotational motion, the energy is given by

(1.42)
$$E = \frac{1}{2} I \cdot \omega^2 \text{ [Nm]}$$

In this formula I [kg $\cdot$ m^2] denotes the moment of inertia and ω [1/s] the angular velocity. The dimension of kinetic energy is identical for linear and rotational motion [kg $\cdot$ m^2/s^2]. As the unit newton has the dimension [kg $\cdot$ m/s^2], the dimension of kinetic energy equals the dimension of work [Nm]. Energy and work are mechanically the same. Kinetic energy can be viewed as the amount of work performed for the body to reach its final velocity.

Potential energy is stored energy which can be converted into other forms of energy. For example, a mass lifted by a height h above the ground has the potential energy

(1.43)
$$E = m \cdot g \cdot h \text{ [Nm]}$$

When the mass is dropped, this energy can be converted into kinetic energy or, when it hits the floor, into heat. The analogous case holds for the energy stored in a compressed spring or a stretched tendon.

The energy dissipated by the muscles in working originates from chemical processes. Chemical energy is the energy that is required for the formation of chemical compounds. When a compound is decomposed (that is, broken down into its components), chemical energy is released and can be converted into mechanical energy and/or heat. However, the energy consumption of muscles is not the same as mechanical work performed, because muscles consume energy even when they are not performing mechanical work. For example, when a mass is being held motionless in the hand (**Fig. 1.24**), the muscles are consuming chemical energy although they are not performing any mechanical work. Gravity is acting, but since there is no motion, the product of force and distance, or of moment and angle, is equal to zero. Unlike arm muscles, a table does not need to consume energy to hold a mass at a constant height above the floor. Even when the human body does move, energy can be consumed without the production of mechanical work. When a person walks on a level surface, or pushes the handrim of a wheelchair, his or her muscles consume energy. The mechanical work produced, however (ignoring the deformation of the floor, shoes, or wheelchair tires), is zero, because the body's center of mass is the same height above ground at the end of the travel as it was at the beginning. The fact that holding a mass at a constant height or walking or propelling a wheelchair on level ground consumes energy even though no mechanical work is being produced is not an exclusive property of biological systems. If a piece of iron is suspended at a constant height by an electromagnet, energy is consumed but no work is performed. If a car drives from X to Y on level ground, gasoline is consumed but no mechanical work is performed.

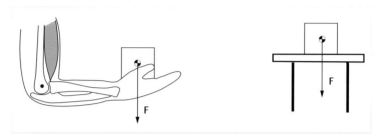

Fig. 1.24 To hold a load in the hand, the muscles consume chemical energy. The muscles perform *internal work*. By contrast, a table does not consume energy to keep a load at a constant height. However, if the load were suspended by an electromagnet, energy would be consumed.

In biomechanics we distinguish between internal and external work of the muscles. External work is performed when objects are moved against a frictional force or lifted against gravity; the latter remains true for the human body itself when it is lifted during uphill walking. Internal work is equal to the energy that is required to move segments of the body. To calculate internal work would require knowing the muscle forces in play. Since at present we have no way of measuring these muscle forces, internal work can only be estimated. Alternatively, internal work can be approximately determined by measuring heat production[3] or oxygen consumption.[4,5] To convert oxygen consumption into energy, the following relation is employed: 1 L of oxygen corresponds to approx. 5 kilocalories [kcal].

The momentum p of a body is the product of mass m and velocity $\mathbf{v}$:

(1.44)
$$\mathbf{p} = m \cdot \mathbf{v}$$

A force acting on the body changes the momentum. In the case of a constant force $\mathbf{F}$ acting over a time interval Δt, the change Δp of the momentum (the *linear impulse*) is equal to $\mathbf{F} \cdot \Delta t$. In the case of a time-dependent force, the change of momentum $\Delta \mathbf{p}$ is equal to the integral

(1.45)
$$\int \mathbf{F}\, dt = \mathbf{p}_2 - \mathbf{p}_1 = \Delta \mathbf{p}$$

In this equation $\mathbf{p}_1$ and $\mathbf{p}_2$ denote the momentum at the beginning and the end of the time interval. $\mathbf{F}$ is the net force acting on the body.

As an example, **Fig. 1.25** shows the force component parallel to the floor which acts on the foot during walking. In the heel strike phase, this force acts in the opposite direction to the gait velocity. The time integral (the area below the curve) is positive. Since the force is directed against the direction of gait, the change $\Delta\mathbf{p}$ in the momentum of the body is negative. The velocity of the body decreases; it is decelerated. In the following toe-off phase, the sign of the force and thus the sign of the change in momentum are reversed; the body is accelerated. In symmetric gait, the changes in momentum in the deceleration and acceleration phases are expected to be equal for the right and left legs. An inequality would be an indication that one leg is under more mechanical stress than the other.

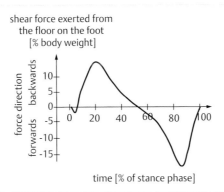

Fig. 1.25 During gait, a shear force directed along the line of progression acts on the foot. The time integral over this force (the area under the force–time curve) equals the change in the body's momentum. At heel strike, the momentum decreases; i.e., the velocity of the body decreases. During the following toe-off, the sign of the momentum changes. The velocity of the body increases. (Adapted from Jahss.[6])

Mechanical power P is defined as work per unit time, measured in newton meters per second [Nm/s]. This unit is called the watt [W]. In the case of linear motion, this definition is identical with the definition of power as the product of force and velocity:

(1.46) $$P = F \cdot v \ [\text{Nm/s}]$$

In rotational motion, power is the product of moment and angular velocity:

(1.47) $$P = M \cdot \omega \ [\text{Nm} \cdot \omega = \text{Nm/s}]$$

The dimensions of power [Nm/s] defined for linear and rotational motion agree. The product of power and time $P \cdot t$ (or, in case of a time-dependent force, the integral $\int P\,dt$) is equal to the energy.

For a joint in the human body, the product of moment and angular velocity describes the power of the muscles that span the joint. **Fig. 1.26** shows an example from gait analysis. The gait cycle starts at the

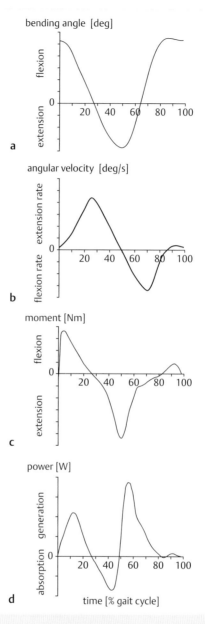

Fig. 1.26a–d Course over time of angular position and angular velocity of the hip joint and moment and power of the muscles that span the joint (qualitatively). (Adapted from Kerrigan et al.[7])

a Bending angle.   **c** Moment.
b Angular velocity.   **d** Power.

moment of heel strike. The angular position of the hip joint (**Fig. 1.26a**) was measured over the course of the gait cycle. The angular velocity (**Fig. 1.26b**) is the change in the angle over time; it is counted as positive when the leg moves in extension. The moment at the hip joint (**Fig. 1.26c**) was determined via a lengthy calculation from the measured ground reaction force and the moments of inertia of the segments of the lower extremity. The power of the hip muscles (**Fig. 1.26d**) is the product of the curves shown in **Figs. 1.26b** and **1.26c**. The power is greatest when the product of moment and angular velocity is greatest. The power is zero when one of the two factors is zero. The power can be positive or negative depending on whether the muscles are generating or absorbing energy (that is, whether the muscle contractions are concentric or eccentric, see Chapter 9).

1.7 Stability and Instability

A mechanical system is called *stable* if a small external perturbation leaves the system fundamentally unchanged. By contrast, the system is called *unstable* if a small perturbation suffices to change it completely. For example, a sphere lying at the deepest point of a bowl is in a mechanically stable state, because on receiving a small push (perturbation) it will roll back and forth, but in the end it will remain in the bowl. A sphere on the top of a mountain will be in an unstable state, because on receiving a small push it will roll down and not return to its initial location.

In physical terms, the stability or instability of a state is characterized by its potential energy. A stable state is characterized by a (relative) minimum of its potential energy. In the example discussed, input of energy is required to displace the sphere out of the deepest point of the bowl. An unstable state is characterized by a (relative) maximum of potential energy. If this state is perturbed—in our example, when the sphere rolls off down the mountain—energy is released. In this sense, the posture of the human body is unstable when standing but stable when lying supine.

Some joints of the human body can be mechanically unstable. In vivo, these joints are kept stable (insensitive to external perturbations) by contraction of the muscles that span them. An example is the shoulder joint, where an inconspicuous movement or a small external force could dislocate the humeral head from the socket if its stability were not maintained by activation of the rotator cuff muscles. This activation, however—especially the co-contraction of agonists and antagonists—results in increased stress and stiffness of the joints—the price paid for maintaining stability. The shape of the spine, composed of vertebrae, disks, and ligaments, is unstable; the stability of its shape is, again, maintained by muscular forces. In the context of medical problems, the term *instability* is sometimes used imprecisely, such as when joints exhibiting a range of motion larger than normal are called *unstable*. The correct term in such cases would be *hypermobile*. For example, motion segments of the spine are (except in trauma cases) mechanically stable, but they can be hypermobile.

A person standing motionless or seated will not fall so long as his or her center of mass is positioned above the base of support. If this person stands on one foot, the base of support is the contact area of the foot (**Fig. 1.27**); if he or she is standing on both feet, the base of support also includes the area between the feet. As soon as the center of mass ceases to be vertically above the base of support (that is, the vertical projection of the center of mass, called the *line of gravity*, moves outside the support base), the reaction force from the floor exerts a moment acting on the center of mass. The higher the center of mass, the greater the moment. In consequence, the body will start to rotate forward, backward, or sideways, depending on where the center of mass has moved to, and the body starts to fall. In everyday language: we lose our balance.

Even during unperturbed erect standing on two legs, it can be seen that the position of the center of mass is not fixed but varies within certain limits. It is not possible to maintain a completely rigid posture. In consequence, the body's neuromuscular control continually generates small corrective movements to keep the line of gravity within the base of support. It follows that the body's ability to avoid falling depends both on the size of the base of support and on the ability to generate corrective movements fast enough. If the person shown in **Fig. 1.27** were to lean over sideways a little further, the line of gravity would shift beyond the end of his foot. In this situation, the other foot would have to move sideways or the person would fall.

Walking or climbing stairs differs from standing to the extent that the line of gravity is only briefly located within the base of support (that is, within the contact area of the loaded foot). For most of the time in walking, the center of mass is shifted to the side of the raised leg, while in climbing stairs it is mostly shifted anteriorly. In both cases a fall is imminent, and to avoid falling, the second foot needs be placed quickly enough in the right place. For this reason, walking and stair climbing are sometimes referred to as *controlled falling*.

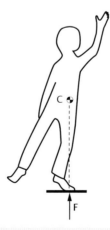

Fig. 1.27 To avoid a fall, the center of mass C must be positioned over the area of support, which in the case shown means over the contact area of the forefoot.

References

1. Alonso M, Finn E. Physics. Harlow: Addison Wesley; 1996

2. Nelson EW, Best CL, McLean WG. Engineering Mechanics. New York: McGraw Hill; 2010

3. Webb P, Saris WHM, Schoffelen PFM, Van Ingen Schenau GJ, Ten Hoor F. The work of walking: a calorimetric study. Med Sci Sports Exerc 1988;20(4):331–337

4. Brockway JM. Derivation of formulae used to calculate energy expenditure in man. Hum Nutr Clin Nutr 1987;41(6):463–471

5. Mansell PI, Macdonald IA. Reappraisal of the Weir equation for calculation of metabolic rate. Am J Physiol 1990;258(6 Pt 2):R1347–R1354

6. Jahss MH, ed. Disorders of the Foot and Ankle. Vol 1. 2nd ed. Philadelphia: Saunders; 1991

7. Kerrigan DC, Todd MK, Della Croce U. Gender differences in joint biomechanics during walking: normative study in young adults. Am J Phys Med Rehabil 1998;77(1):2–7

2 Mechanical Properties of Solid Materials

The mechanical, electrical, magnetic, optical, or chemical properties of materials are determined in standardized experiments. The protocols of such experiments and the description of the material properties are always designed so that the dimensions of the samples under investigation do not influence the result. In other words, the experimentally determined parameters describe the materials as such: for example, the properties of the material *steel* or the material *polyethylene*, or *bone*. The properties of structures fabricated from a material—for example, the mechanical properties of a frame made of steel beams, or those of an orthosis or a femoral bone consisting of cortical and trabecular bone—must be determined in separate experiments. Obviously, the mechanical properties of a steel frame depend on the material properties of steel, but they also depend on the dimensions and joints of the beams.

A material is termed *homogeneous* if its matter is uniformly distributed over its whole volume. Every small volume element of a homogeneous material possesses identical material properties. By contrast, a sample of a material with irregular holes or with other materials or impurities included is described as *inhomogeneous*. A material is termed *isotropic* if its internal structure and/or its elastic properties show no preferred directions. Examples of isotropic materials are rubber or cast iron. Wood and bone, by contrast, are termed *anisotropic* due to the internal alignment of fibers in preferred directions. Semifinished products made of metals or plastics may be anisotropic if they have been pressed or pulled during the production process. The material properties of an anisotropic material depend on the orientation in which the sample was cut, while those of an inhomogeneous material depend on the location from which the sample was cut from a larger block of the material. The material properties of a sample of cortical bone, for example, will depend on the site on the bone from where the sample has been cut. In addition, samples cut longitudinally from a long bone will also exhibit different properties from samples cut transversely from the same bone. Trabecular bone is inhomogeneous because of the voids between the beams and plates, and because the trabeculae align in preferred directions it is (usually) anisotropic as well.

Materials are characterized not by a single parameter but rather by a set of parameters that describe their behavior in different applications and environments. In orthopedic biomechanics, the most important parameters are those describing deformation, failure, friction, and abrasion.

2.1 Elongation and Compression

In a tensile test, a beam-shaped sample of a material is subjected to a tensile force **F** (**Fig. 2.1**). In this test, the change dL in the length of the sample is measured in relation to the tensile force. To ensure that the material property to be determined does not depend on the dimensions (cross-sectional area A, length L)

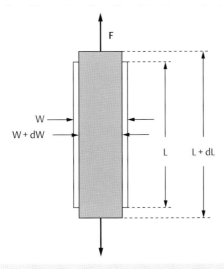

Fig. 2.1 Deformation of a sample of a solid material under the influence of a force **F**. L and W designate the initial length and width of the sample; dL and dW designate the change of length and width. In a tensile test dL is positive and dW negative; in a compression test dL is negative and dW positive.

of the sample tested, it is not the length change dL in relation to the force **F** that is reported, but rather the strain in relation to the mechanical stress (**Fig. 2.2**). The stress σ is defined as the magnitude of the force F divided by the cross-sectional area A of the sample.

(2.1) $$\sigma = F / A$$

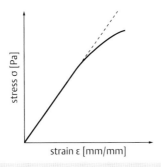

Fig. 2.2 Typical stress–strain diagram of metals. The slope of the graph in its linear part is called the *modulus of elasticity*. In the region of higher stress the graph deviates from a straight line.

Mechanical stress (or, simply, *stress*) has the dimension (is measured in) *newtons per square meter* [N/m²] or *pascals* [Pa]. The strain ε is defined as the length change dL divided by the initial length L.

(2.2)
$$\varepsilon = dL / L$$

As the quotient of two lengths, strain is a dimensionless quantity. For clarity, however, the dimension of strain is sometimes quoted as [mm/mm] or [μm/μm].

In qualitative terms, many materials exhibit similar behavior in a tensile test. Under low values of stress, the strain increases in proportion to the stress. In the region of low stress, the dependence of the stress on the strain can be described by a straight line (**Fig. 2.2**). Above a certain stress value characteristic of the material, the stress–strain graph deviates from a straight line. The quotient of stress and strain in the linear portion of the graph (that is, the slope of the graph in this region) is called the *modulus of elasticity* or *Young's modulus*. The modulus of elasticity is stated in [N/mm²] or [Pa].

In the linear part of the stress–strain graph, Hooke's law is valid.

(2.3)
$$\sigma = E \cdot \varepsilon$$

Hooke's law states that the stress is proportional to the strain. A steep slope of the stress–strain graph indicates that a high stress is necessary to effect a specified strain. The modulus of elasticity of such a material has a high numerical value. A shallow slope of the stress–strain graph indicates that a low stress is sufficient to effect a specified strain. The modulus of elasticity of such a material has a low numerical value. In everyday language, materials with a high modulus of elasticity are termed *hard* and those with a low one, *soft*.

To avoid quoting large numbers, the moduli are usually quoted in units of N/mm², not in units of N/m². **Table 2.1** lists the moduli of elasticity of technical materials that are frequently used in the construction of implants together with, for comparison, the moduli of cortical and trabecular bone. The numbers in **Table 2.1** show that, compared with metals, cortical bone and polyethylene are soft and trabecular bone

Material	Modulus of elasticity E [N/mm²]
Stainless steel	$2 \cdot 10^5$
Titanium alloy	$1 \cdot 10^5$
Polyethylene	$1 \cdot 10^3$
Cortical bone	$18 \cdot 10^3$
Trabecular bone	90

Table 2.1 Moduli of elasticity of materials employed in the construction of implants in relation to the moduli of cortical and trabecular bone

is very soft. The numerical values in **Table 2.1** are only approximate, because the precise value of the modulus of elasticity depends for metals on the details of the production process, for polyethylene on the degree of polymerization, and for cortical and trabecular bone on the location, the orientation, and the bone density of the sample tested.

In a tensile test it is not only a change in the length of a sample that is observed, but also a decrease in the diameter, of magnitude |dW| (**Fig. 2.1**). The quotient of the strains in longitudinal and transverse directions

(2.4)
$$\mu = -(dW \,/\, W) \,/\, (dL \,/\, L)$$

is a parameter characteristic for every material and is termed *Poisson's ratio*. Poisson's ratio typically has values between 0.2 and 0.5.

Some materials, for example soft tissues, exhibit in a tensile test a comparatively large increase in their strain under low values of stress before a region is reached where the stress increases (approximately) in proportion to the strain. If there is a further increase in the stress, a disproportionate increase of the strain may again be observed (**Fig. 2.3**). In such cases the slope of the stress–strain curve and thus the modulus of elasticity depend on the strain. For this reason, if a modulus of elasticity is quoted, the strain value at which the modulus was measured must be specified. For a guide value, the modulus of elasticity derived from the approximately linear portion of the stress–strain curve may be quoted.

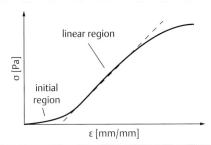

Fig. 2.3 Typical stress–strain diagram of soft tissues. An initial region with a large increase in strain under low stress is followed by a region with an (approximately) linear increase of the strain with the stress. In the region of higher stress, the graph deviates again from a straight line.

Rather than being subjected to a tensile force, a material sample may be subjected to a compressive force and the compressive strain dL/L may be plotted in relation to the compressive stress. In such a test it must, however, be ensured that the sample will not bend under the influence of the compressive force.

A change in length caused by bending (and not by pure compression) would not allow direct comparison with the results of a tensile test. Experiments show that, for many materials in the region of low stress, the dependence of strain on stress in the linear region is virtually identical in tensile and compressive tests. 'Low' stress designates stress much lower than the breaking stress of the sample. In this region, then, the modulus of elasticity characterizes the deformation of a material under tensile as well as under compressive stress.

2.2 Shear

If two parallel and opposite forces of magnitude F act on two sides of a cuboid (**Fig. 2.4**), a shear stress τ is generated.

(2.5) $$\tau = F / A$$

A shear stress does not effect a change in length, but rather a change in the shape of the sample. The initially vertical faces of the cuboid are now seen to be tilted. For small angles of tilt it holds that

(2.6) $$\tau = G \cdot \alpha$$

G is a material constant and is termed the *shear modulus*. The angle α is measured in radians. It can be shown (the proof is not given here) that the modulus of elasticity E, Poisson's ratio μ, and the shear modulus G are related.

(2.7) $$E = 2G \cdot (1 + \mu)$$

Thus the deformation of a homogeneous, isotropic material is fully characterized by two of these three material constants.

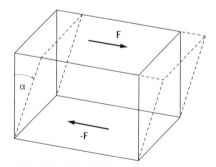

Fig. 2.4 Loading of a sample by a shear force **F** effects no changes in width or length but an angular deformation.

2.3 Elastic, Viscoelastic, and Plastic Deformation

For some materials, if in a tensile test the stress is first increased and then reduced to zero, the stress–strain curves for increasing and for decreasing stress are observed to be superimposed. After completion of the load cycle, a sample of such a material returns to its initial length. This type of deformation is termed *elastic*. If the stress is increased above a certain peak value, which is characteristic for each material, the stress–strain curves for increasing and decreasing stress are observed to be no longer superimposed; deviations from elastic behavior will then be seen. The designation of a deformation or a material as "elastic" must thus be supplemented by information on the maximum stress level involved. Most metals, for example, show elastic deformation, provided the maximum stress is not too close to that leading to destruction of the sample.

If tissues of the human body or plastics are subjected to a tensile test, striking deviations from elastic behavior are observed. The stress–strain curve for increasing stress deviates from the curve for decreasing stress; the two curves form a hysteresis loop (**Fig. 2.5**). At the end of the load cycle (that is, when the load and thus the stress have returned to zero), the sample is not restored to its original length but a strain $d\varepsilon$ remains. If, over time and without any exposure to an external force, this strain $d\varepsilon$ recedes to zero, the deformation is termed *viscoelastic*. If, by contrast, the strain $d\varepsilon$ remains constant, the deformation is termed *plastic*. As an example of a plastic deformation, **Fig. 2.6** shows the measured stress–strain curves of the material PVC. In this material, the plastic deformation increased with increasing peak stress of the four load cycles applied.

If a sample of a viscoelastic material is held under constant stress, the initial strain ε_i is observed to increase with time until it reaches a limiting value ε_l (**Fig. 2.7**). The increase in strain under constant stress is termed *creep*. The decrease in strain under zero stress after completion of a load cycle, mentioned above,

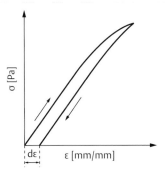

Fig. 2.5 For some materials, the strain under increasing stress is different from that under decreasing stress. The stress–strain diagram forms a *hysteresis loop*. If a deformation remains after the end of a load cycle under zero stress, the material (or the deformation) is designated as *viscoelastic* or *plastic*.

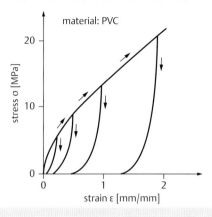

Fig. 2.6 Viscoelastic or plastic deformation depends on the magnitude of the stress previously exerted upon it. This example shows the plastic deformation of PVC in relation to the peak value of the stress. (Adapted from Andrews.[1])

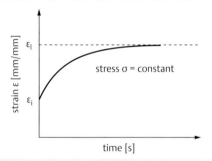

Fig. 2.7 Under constant stress, the strain of a viscoelastic material increases with time. This effect is termed *creep*.

is the reverse event. If a sample of a viscoelastic material is loaded up to a certain strain, and the strain is subsequently kept constant, it is observed that the stress within the material decreases with time from its initial value σ_i to a limiting value σ_l (**Fig. 2.8**). This effect is termed *stress relaxation*.

If a sample of a viscoelastic or plastic material is cyclically elongated and compressed, the stress–strain curve forms a complete hysteresis loop (**Fig. 2.9**). In addition to the hysteresis loop, **Fig. 2.9** shows the stress–strain curve of the first half of the first loading cycle, which starts at the origin of the graph. It should be noted that, due to the viscoelastic or plastic properties of the material, the strain at zero stress varies within a region $d\varepsilon$. The size of this region $d\varepsilon$ depends on the peak values of the tensile and compressive stress. If the peak values are increased, the viscoelastic or plastic deformation of the material increases and thus the region $d\varepsilon$ increases as well. In other words, the deformation seen at zero stress in cyclic loading

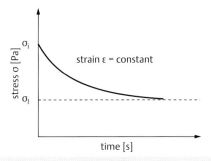

Fig. 2.8 Under constant strain, the stress of a viscoelastic material decreases with time. This effect is termed *stress relaxation*.

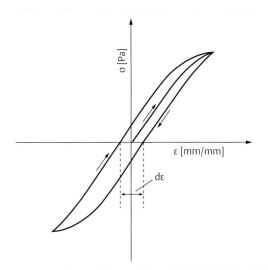

Fig. 2.9 If a viscoelastic or plastic material is cyclically loaded in tension and compression, the stress–strain graph follows a complete hysteresis loop. The magnitude of the region of deformation dε, observed at zero stress, depends on the mechanical history (that is, on the maximum values of the tensile and compressive stresses previously exerted).

tests depends on the mechanical history (that is, the type and magnitude of past loading). Thus, the deformation range dε is not a property of the material, but is dependent on the test conditions.

In 1963, Buehler and coworkers[2] observed a stress–strain dependence very different from other metals for a nickel–titanium alloy. **Fig. 2.10** shows this behavior in relation to the behavior of spring steel. Starting from zero stress, the Ni-Ti alloy (nitinol) shows an increase of stress with strain. This is followed by a region of strain where the stress shows virtually no increase. This property is designated *superelastic*. A considerable number of technical applications, including some in the medical field, make use of this property. For

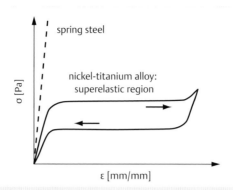

Fig. 2.10 Stress–strain graphs of a superelastic material (nitinol) and of spring steel. In the superelastic region, the material exhibits a large region of strain where the stress remains approximately constant. In addition, the stress–strain graph of the superelastic material forms a hysteresis loop.

example, a superelastic material can be employed to design springs, the spring force of which is virtually independent of their deformation.

2.4 Hardness

In engineering, three procedures are in use to define the hardness of a material. The Mohs qualitative hardness scale groups mineral materials in a scale from 1 to 10, such that a material of greater hardness will scratch those lower on the scale. The Mohs scale begins with talc (no. 1) and ends with diamond (no. 10). Brinell hardness is defined by measuring the area of the impression of a very hard (virtually nondeformable) sphere pressed against a planar surface of the material under investigation. Thus, Brinell hardness characterizes the plastic deformation of a material. Shore hardness is defined by the depth of impression of a standardized test body (for example, pyramid-shaped) under specified loads. Shore hardness thus characterizes the elastic or plastic deformation of a material. The deformation properties of rubber and rubber-like plastics are usually described by their Shore hardness. The hardness of a material according to these tests and the modulus of elasticity of a material are only qualitatively related: the hardness of a material does not equate to the hardness measured in a tensile test (see Section 2.1).

In orthopedic biomechanics, Mohs and Brinell hardness are of interest when selecting materials for the construction of artificial joints, because hardness influences deformation and wear. Examples are the deformation of a plastic socket loaded by a spherical metal head, or the abrasion and wear of small particles of bone cement between the metal head and polyethylene socket of an artificial joint. Shore hardness is frequently used to describe the properties of rubber or plastic foams employed in the construction of artificial limbs, orthoses, or insoles. To characterize the mechanical properties of human tissues, the depth of indentation of an indenter of known shape is employed. The depth of indentation into the surface of articular cartilage specimens, or in vivo into the plantar soft tissue, provides qualitative information on the hardness of these tissues.

Testing the hardness of a muscle or another organ by palpation for diagnostic purposes, although it has a certain similarity with the Shore test, is not identical with any of the engineering hardness tests described above. In the clinical context, hardness does not characterize a material but an organ, which may be made up of several different materials. Furthermore, the hardness determined by palpation usually characterizes the stress in the organ, for example the state of stress of a muscle. In the muscle, the stress varies according to the level of activation. Such effects are not encountered in technical materials.

2.5 Friction

If two bodies are loaded by a force $\mathbf{F}_n$ directed perpendicularly to the plane of contact, a friction force $\mathbf{F}_f$ directed parallel to the plane of contact is generated (see Chapter 1, **Fig. 1.23**). The friction force is directed opposite to the direction of motion or impending motion. It is proportional to the magnitude of the force $\mathbf{F}_n$.

(2.8)
$$|\mathbf{F}_f| = \mu \cdot |\mathbf{F}_n|$$

The factor of proportionality μ has different values depending on whether there is relative motion (μ_k, coefficient of kinetic friction) or no relative motion (μ_s, coefficient of static friction). The coefficient of static friction is larger than the coefficient of kinetic friction. Save for very slow or very large velocities, the coefficient of kinetic friction is virtually independent of the relative velocity. **Table 2.2** lists coefficients of static and kinetic friction for material combinations in the technical domain, of anatomical and artificial joints, and of materials employed for orthoses and prostheses.[3,4] The numbers in **Table 2.2** are approximate values, subject to variation in relation to the surface geometry and finish and the presence of lubricants.

Friction is of great importance in orthopedic biomechanics. For example, the kinetic friction between intact cartilaginous joint surfaces is extremely small; if this were not so, it would be difficult to flex or extend highly loaded joints. Friction between the head and the socket of an artificial hip joint of radius R loaded by a force **F** (**Fig. 2.11**) effects a friction moment of the magnitude

(2.9)
$$M = R \cdot F_f$$

This moment is directed opposite to the motion of the joint: it brakes the joint motion. At the same time this moment loads the anchoring of the socket in the acetabulum. The elastic or plastic deformation of contacting bodies by the normal force $\mathbf{F}_n$ and the shearing deformation by the friction force $\mathbf{F}_f$ cause abrasion from the moving surfaces. Wear debris in turn affects the structure of the surfaces and consequently the friction properties. In the human body, wear debris from artificial joints may cause inflammation leading to joint loosening.

Material combination	μ_s	μ_k
Iron–iron		1.0
Steel–steel	0.4–0.8	0.4–0.7 (dry)
		0.1 (lubricated)
Leather–metal	0.6	0.2 (dry)
		0.1 (lubricated)
Wood–wood	0.4–0.6	0.2–0.4 (dry)
		0.04–0.16 (lubricated)
Steel–ice	0.03	0.014
Ice–ice		0.02
Teflon–Teflon		0.04
Rubber–hard material	1.0–4.0	
Ceramic–ceramic[a]		0.002–0.07
Ceramic–metal[a]		0.002–0.07
UHMWPE–metal[a]		0.06–0.08
Metal–metal[a]		0.25
Cartilage–cartilage[a]		0.001
Skin–silicon	0.61	
Skin–PE foam	0.75	
Skin–wool socks	0.51	

Table 2.2 Approximate values of the coefficients of static (μ_s) and kinetic friction (μ_k)

Abbreviation: UHMWPE, ultra-high-molecular-weight polyethylene.
[a] Lubricated by synovial fluid.

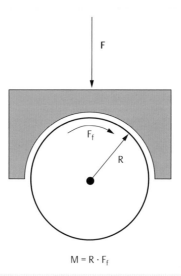

$$M = R \cdot F_f$$

Fig. 2.11 Moment M of the friction force $\mathbf{F}_f$ (symbolically represented by the curved arrow) in a loaded ball-and-socket joint.

During gait, the friction force between a foot and the floor enables deceleration of the body in the heel-strike phase and acceleration in the toe-off phase. Reduced friction between the foot and the floor may cause slipping leading to a fall. A film of water or oil on the floor will considerably increase the risk of a fall, because the first contact that occurs is between shoe and fluid, and the friction coefficient between these two materials is very small.

2.6 Failure

If in a tensile test the stress of the sample exceeds a certain limit characteristic of the material, the sample fails (**Fig. 2.12**). A steep initial slope of the stress–strain graph characterizes a *hard* material. Materials exhibiting a large amount of deformation at low stress values are designated as *soft*. Materials exhibiting only a small amount of strain before failure occurs are termed *brittle*. Examples of brittle materials are glass and cortical bone. Materials that tolerate a larger amount of strain before failure occurs are termed *tough*. Examples of tough materials are stainless steel and polyethylene.

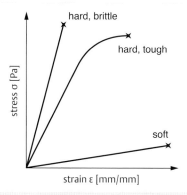

Fig. 2.12 Stress–strain graph of different materials in a tensile test. The endpoints of the curves represent the points at which failure of the samples occurred. A steep slope of the initial part of the graph characterizes a *hard* material; a shallow initial slope characterizes a *soft* material. Materials tolerating a large strain before fracture occurs are termed *tough*; materials tolerating only a small amount of strain before fracture occurs are termed *brittle*.

Quantitatively, the failure properties of a material are characterized by specifying the ultimate stress σ_B (*breaking stress*) and the ultimate strain ε_B (*breaking strain*) at the point of failure (**Fig. 2.13**). The region of stress and strain where the stress–strain curve deviates notably from a straight line is characterized by *stress and strain at the 0.2% limit*. To locate this limit, a straight line is drawn parallel to the linear part of

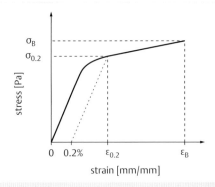

Fig. 2.13 Determination of the so-called 0.2% stress and 0.2% strain from the stress–strain graph. A line at a distance $\varepsilon = 0.2\%$ is drawn parallel to the initial, linear part of the stress–strain curve. The intersection of this line with the actual stress–strain curve defines stress and strain at the 0.2% limit.

the stress–strain curve, at a distance of $\varepsilon = 0.2\%$. The intersection of this line with the stress–strain curve defines stress and strain at the 0.2% limit.

The value of the ultimate compressive stress, where compressive failure occurs, can be determined in a compression test. To permit comparison with the ultimate tensile stress established in a tensile test, the material sample must be guaranteed not to bend under load before destruction of the sample is observed. Whether a given sample under compressive load exhibits pure compression, or bending in addition to compression, depends on the shape of the sample. A long beam will tend to bend under load; a short, squat column will not. If bending occurs, the distribution of stress within the material differs from a uniform compressive stress, and direct comparison with the ultimate tensile stress will not be feasible. The ultimate compressive stress determined in a compression test is usually not equal to the ultimate tensile stress determined in a tensile test. In viscoelastic materials, the ultimate stress also depends on the loading rate (that is, on the load change per unit time) and the duration of loading. Thus, the ultimate stresses quoted in **Table 2.3** must be regarded only as an approximate guide.

Material	Ultimate stress [N/mm²]	Ultimate strain [%]
Stainless steel	700	15
Titanium alloy	1200	6
Polyethylene	20	400–800
Cortical bone	150	1.5
Trabecular bone	2	2.5

Table 2.3 Ultimate tensile stress and ultimate tensile strain (approximate values) of materials employed in the construction of implants, in relation to ultimate stress and ultimate strain of cortical and trabecular bone.

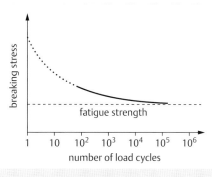

Fig. 2.14 Under cyclic loading, a decrease of the breaking stress (the stress where failure occurs) is observed. This effect is termed *material fatigue*. The breaking stress at high load cycle numbers approaches a lower limit termed *fatigue strength*. If the stress level stays below this value, an arbitrary number of load cycles may be endured without fracture occurring.

If a sample is loaded several times in succession, it is observed that the sample fails at a stress appreciably lower than the ultimate stress observed in a single loading cycle. The decrease in breaking stress with increasing number of loading cycles is termed *material fatigue*. **Fig. 2.14** illustrates qualitatively the relationship between breaking stress and the number of load cycles. In virtually all materials the breaking stress decreases as the number of load cycles increases. In many (but not all) materials the breaking stress at high load cycle numbers approaches a lower limit termed *fatigue strength*. If the stress in a sample stays below this value, an arbitrary number of load cycles may be endured without failure occurring.

Material fatigue occurs because there is no material that has no internal faults. During production it cannot be ruled out that a material may contain irregularities in its crystal lattice, inclusions of other materials or voids even of small dimensions. Under load, small fissures tend to originate first and foremost from such inhomogeneities. Surface irregularities like small scratches or indentations have a similar effect. Under repeated loading the fissures grow in length or several small fissures unite. The microdamage increases until macroscopic failure occurs. In some cases the progressive damage to the sample can be seen when inspecting the fracture surfaces.

When investigated in detail, the fatigue process at high stresses and low load cycles is seen to differ from the fatigue process at low stresses and high cycle numbers. These processes are termed *high cycle* and *low cycle* fatigue. It follows that material fatigue, that is, the relationship between breaking stress and load cycle numbers, cannot be described by one single function. In **Fig. 2.14** this is indicated by dividing the curve into a dashed and a solid portion. In other words: no conclusions on the fatigue behavior between, say, 10^2 and 10^6 cycles can be drawn from the fatigue behavior observed between

1 and 100 cycles (and vice versa). The fatigue properties at low and high cycle numbers must be documented separately.

Bone fractures interpreted as fatigue fractures are observed in vivo in subjects exposed to an activity with many high load cycles without preparatory training. For example, it is hypothesized that fractures of the tibia or the calcaneus seen in young soldiers after marching over longer distances are fatigue fractures of the bone material. Fatigue fractures of lumbar vertebrae also seem possible if the spine undergoes a large number of load cycles within a relatively short time interval at the workplace or in athletic training. In the individual case, however, it is difficult to prove conclusively that a fatigue fracture has occurred, because an inspection of the fractured surfaces is not feasible. In addition, it must be kept in mind that repair processes in living tissues may prevent the accumulation of microdamage. Whether fatigue fractures occur in a living tissue depends on the rate of healing in relation to the time interval where cyclic loading occurs. Fatigue will be evident only if cyclic loading occurs within a time interval that is too short for any significant repair of microdamage.

References

1. Andrews EH. Fracture. In: The Mechanical Properties of Structural Materials. Cambridge: Cambridge University Press; 1980
2. Buehler WJ, Gilfrich JV, Wiley RC. Effect of low-temperature phase changes on the mechanical properties of alloys near composition TiNi. J Appl Phys 1963;34:1475–1477
3. Sanders JE, Greve JM, Mitchell SB, Zachariah SG. Material properties of commonly-used interface materials and their static coefficients of friction with skin and socks. J Rehabil Res Dev 1998;35(2):161–176
4. Zhang M, Mak AFT. In vivo friction properties of human skin. Prosthet Orthot Int 1999;23(2):135–141

Reference Works

Abé H, Hayashi K, Sato M, eds. Data Book on Mechanical Properties of Living Cells, Tissues, and Organs. Tokyo: Springer; 1996

Fung YC. Biomechanics. Mechanical Properties of Living Tissues. 2nd ed. New York: Springer; 1993

Yamada H. Strength of Biological Materials. Baltimore: Williams & Wilkins; 1970

3 Deformation and Strength of Structures

The term *structure* designates an object built from one or more materials in a specific architecture. In this context, the term *architecture* refers to the geometrical shape of the object and the way in which its components are assembled and fixed together. Examples of structures in this sense are a beam made of wood, a vertebral body composed of an outer shell of cortical bone filled with trabecular bone, or a joint of the human body consisting of bone, cartilage, joint capsule, and ligaments. The mechanical properties of a structure depend on its architecture and on the mechanical properties of its building materials.

The deformation of a structure under load depends on several variables:

- *The nature of the load.* The structure may be loaded by a compressive or a tensile force, by a moment, or by a combination of forces and moments. If it is loaded by a force, the deformation is measured in meters [m] or relative units [%] in relation to its initial dimensions. If it is loaded by a moment and torsion is observed, the deformation is measured in degrees [°]; if bending is observed, the deflection is usually measured in meters [m].

- *The architecture of the structure.* The deformation of a beam under bending or torsion depends on its length and cross section. The deformation of a joint depends on the deformation of the bone and on the architecture of the cartilage and the ligaments crossing the joint.

- *The properties of the building materials.* In the case of a wooden beam, the deformation depends on the type of wood used (for example: oak or pine). In the case of a joint, the mechanical properties of the building materials bone, cartilage, and ligament come into play, or in the case of an orthosis, the mechanical properties of steel and plastic materials. The mechanical properties are characterized by the moduli of elasticity and shear and by the elastic, viscoelastic, or plastic properties.

The strength of a structure is defined as that load which effects a destruction of the structure. Destruction occurs if the tensile, compressive, or shear stress in any one component of the structure exceeds its ultimate value, and the structure (or a part of it) is torn, fractured, or irreversibly deformed. Depending on the loading mode, we distinguish between compressive, tensile, or shear strength of a structure. Strength under tensile or compressive load is designated by the force effecting the destruction and is quoted in newtons [N]. Torsional or bending strength is designated by the moment effecting the destruction and designated in newton meters [Nm].

Tensile, compressive, bending, or torsional strengths of a structure are independent of one another and may assume widely different values. A pile of bricks, for example, has high compressive but very low tensile strength. The compressive strength of cortical bone is higher than its tensile strength. A rope, a muscle, or a ligament has high tensile but only low compressive, torsional, or bending strength.

Deformation and strength of structures may be determined experimentally or by calculation. For the experimental determination, the testing methods are similar to those employed when determining properties of materials. The structures are set up in a testing machine and loaded by a tensile or compressive force, or by a moment in bending or torsion. The resulting change in shape (deformation) is recorded in relation to the load. If the load is further increased, the load effecting destruction will eventually be found. Alternatively, a deformation can be imposed on the structure and the reaction force (that is, the resistance to the deformation) or the reaction moment can be recorded. It must be pointed out, however, that interpretation of the results of such experiments differs from interpretation of the results of experiments determining material properties. This is due to the fact that, when testing structures, the architecture as well as the properties of the building materials influence the result. It is obvious that a low-strength structure can be built with high-strength materials. On the other hand, a structure made out of relatively low-strength materials may have a high strength.

For structures composed of one single material and having simple geometrical shapes, formulae are available that allow deformation and strength to be calculated in the case of simple loading modes, provided the material properties are known. Simple geometrical shapes are, for example, beams or tubes with rectangular or circular cross sections. Simple loading modes include, for example, tension or compression or torsion about the axis of such beams. The prerequisite for the validity of these formulae is that the resulting deformations under load remain small. If more than one material is used to build a structure, and in the case of irregular shapes and simultaneous loading by forces and moments, deformation, stress, and strength can be determined by the finite element method.

3.1 Experimental Determination of Deformation and Strength

The relationship between deformation and load may vary within broad limits. In the following, this is illustrated by examples of different tissues and organs. A tensile test provides data on deformation and strength under a tensile force. **Fig. 3.1** shows the tensile force of a ligament in relation to its increase in length. At each point of the force–deformation curve, the slope is approximated by the quotient dF/dL. In this expression dL designates the length change observed under a small change dF of the tensile force applied. dF/dL is termed the *stiffness* of the structure. Stiffness is measured in newtons per meter [N/m] or newtons per millimeter [N/mm]. The numerical value of the stiffness indicates how many newtons are necessary to effect a length change of 1 m or 1 mm respectively. In the case of torsion (see **Figs. 3.5** and **3.7**), *torsional stiffness* is defined as the slope of the moment versus the angle of the torsion curve. Torsional stiffness is measured in newton meters [Nm] (the angle being a dimensionless quantity).

The shape of the curve shown in **Fig. 3.1** is typical of the behavior of soft tissues under tension. In general the force–deformation graph does not follow a straight line; the slope of the curve and thus the stiffness assume different values along the curve. In the example shown, the slope of the curve and hence the stiffness

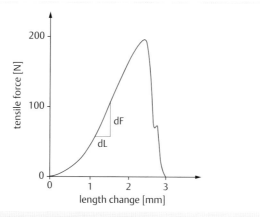

Fig. 3.1 Force–deformation diagram of a ligament under a tensile force. (Adapted from Amiel et al.[1])

have low values under low forces and higher values under higher forces. In ligaments, this property is due to the collagen fibers becoming more and more aligned in the direction of the force as the tensile force increases.

If the magnitude of the tensile force F exceeds the strength of the structure, a partial or total rupture of the ligament is observed. In the example shown in **Fig. 3.1** the first partial rupture occurred at a tensile force of about 200 N. It is a common finding in ligaments that rupture occurs stepwise, because under a given load not all fiber bundles of the ligament undergo the same deformation. In each bundle the ultimate tensile strain is reached at a different elongation of the whole ligament. In the example shown, complete rupture occurred only after an increase in length of about 3 mm. Between the point where the tensile strength of the ligament (about 200 N) was reached and the total rupture, the ligament can still transmit a tensile force, though of restricted magnitude.

Fig. 3.2 shows the force–deformation graph of human skin. In this example the initial region of high elongation under low forces (region of low stiffness) and the adjoining region with a relatively low increase

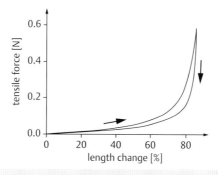

Fig. 3.2 Force–deformation diagram of skin. (Adapted from Lanir and Fung.[2])

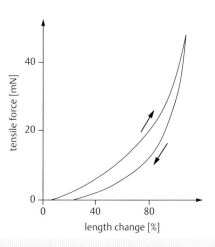

Fig. 3.3 Force–deformation diagram of the passive elongation of a muscle. (Adapted from Sparks and Bohr.[3])

of length under higher forces (region of higher stiffness) can be clearly distinguished. The force–deformation graph forms a hysteresis loop. The deformation is elastic because (at the levels of loading shown) no permanent deformation is observed after completion of the load cycle. The force–deformation curve of skin demonstrates that this structure is highly adapted to its physiological function (that is, enabling large deformations under low forces but only up to a certain limit).

Fig. 3.3 shows the force–deformation graph of passive elongation of a muscle in vitro. As in the preceding example, the stiffness assumes different values at each point of the graph. The graph forms a hysteresis loop. After completion of the loading cycle, the residual deformation subsequently decreases to zero. This structure is viscoelastic. We expect the force–deformation graph of a muscle measured in vivo to assume a different form, because innervation of a muscle will change its stiffness.

Fig. 3.4 illustrates the deflection of bones in a three-point bending experiment. In such an experiment the bone is supported at both ends and loaded in its mid-section by a force **F**. The deflection is measured at the point where the force is applied. All curves shown end at the point where fracture occurred. Force–deflection graphs of different bones are given here in one diagram merely to provide an overview. A quantitative comparison of deflection and strength of different bones, for example of fibula and femur, makes little sense, because deflection and bending strength depend on the bone material, the cross-sectional area, and the length of the bones. If, in contrast, effects of implantation-induced temporary immobilization or instrumentation have to be evaluated, conclusions can be drawn by comparing pairs of bones, for example the right and left femur specimen of a person or an experimental animal.

Fig. 3.5 shows experimental results for torsional deformation and torsional strength of bones. In this type of experiment, the bone is fixed at one end and a moment about the long axis of the bone is applied

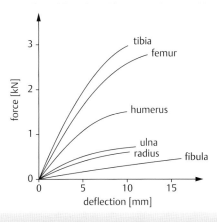

Fig. 3.4 Deflection of human bones under three-point loading. (Adapted from Yamada.[4])

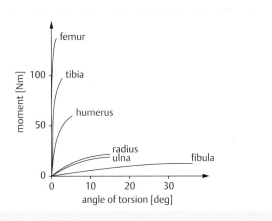

Fig. 3.5 Torsion of human bones by a moment directed along the long axis of the bones. (Adapted from Yamada.[4])

at the other. Deformation and torsional strength depend on the bone material, the length, and the shape of its cross section. It is therefore not surprising that large differences with respect to torsional stiffness (slope of the curves), torsional strength, and maximum deformation (end point of the curves) of the bones are observed.

Fig. 3.6 depicts the compression of a lumbar vertebral body by a force directed perpendicularly to the plane of the vertebral endplates. In this example, the stiffness (slope of the curve) increases with increasing load. The compressive strength of the vertebra shown is approximately 9 kN. After fracture, the ability to support a compressive load is not reduced to zero but is still approximately 5 kN. This is due to the fact that fragments of the trabecular bone may support one another until complete collapse occurs at larger

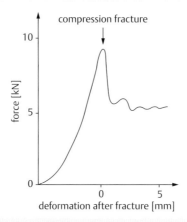

Fig. 3.6 Compressive deformation of a human lumbar vertebral body. In the example shown, the compressive strength amounts to approximately 9 kN. After fracture, a load-bearing capacity of approximately 5 kN remains. (Adapted from Plaue et al.[5])

deformations. In vivo, the ability to support some compressive force in the long run after occurrence of a compression fracture of a vertebra depends on whether and how fast the fractured bone material can be replaced by new bone.

If a structure contains components made out of viscoelastic or plastic materials, or if the components have some play in their connection so that small relative movements are possible, a permanent

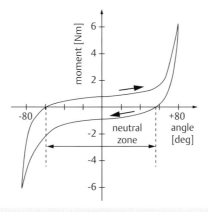

Fig. 3.7 Passive rotation of the cervical spine by an external moment. If rotation is performed to the right and to the left, the moment–deformation graph forms a complete hysteresis loop. The amount of deformation observed at zero moment depends on the magnitude and direction of the previously exerted moment. (Adapted from McClure et al.[6])

deformation is observed after the end of a load cycle. **Fig. 3.7** illustrates this effect using the example of the passive, axial rotation of the cervical spine under the application of an external moment. In the example shown, the range of motion between maximum rotation to the right and to the left is approximately 160°. The angular position of the cervical spine in relation to the moment follows a hysteresis loop. The region of plastic deformation (that is, the deformation at zero moment) extends from +60° to −60°. In this region the angular position depends on the mechanical history, that is, on the magnitude of the previously applied moment.

In the orthopedic and biomechanical literature, the region of plastic deformation of a structure is occasionally termed the *neutral zone*. Doubt may well be cast on the usefulness of this designation, because the well-established term *plastic deformation* already describes this effect. In addition, it must be pointed out that the extent of the plastic deformation is not characteristic of the structure under investigation but rather depends on the magnitude of the previously exerted load. If the load is increased or decreased, the "neutral" zone (plastic deformation) increases or decreases as well. Thus, the designation "neutral" zone is hardly appropriate for describing biomechanical characteristics of the human locomotor system.

Deforming a structure demands energy (work). When loaded by a force, the energy required to deform a structure (deformation energy) is defined as the momentary force multiplied by the momentary change in length. When loaded by a moment, the energy is defined as the momentary moment multiplied by the momentary change in angle. In both cases the dimension of the deformation energy is newton meters [Nm]. The total energy needed to achieve a specific deformation is determined by summation (or integration) of the deformation energy from the initial to the final state of deformation. It can be shown (the proof is not presented here) that the total energy required to effect a certain deformation is represented by the area (the integral) below the load–deformation graph. This is independent of whether the graph follows a straight line or some irregular curve.

Fig. 3.8 shows load–deformation graphs of structures A and B which have been differently deformed. Structure A exhibits a greater stiffness than structure B. However, the deformation energy, which depends on the shape of the load–deformation graph and on the extent of the deformation, is greater in case B than in case A. Practical use is made of this fact when damping impacts by means of a low-stiffness structure permitting a large deformation so that a large amount of energy can be absorbed.

3.2 Deformation and Strength of Beam-like Structures

Structures whose length is large in relation to their cross section are termed *beams*. If the cross-sectional area has a simple geometrical shape (rectangle, hexagon, circle, tube), and in simple loading modes, the stress distribution in the beam can be theoretically deduced. Examples of simple loading modes are the loading of a beam by a longitudinally directed tensile or compressive force or by a moment in bending or

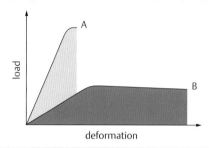

Fig. 3.8 The area under the load–deformation graph is a measure of the energy required for the deformation of the structure. The deformation energies of structures A and B are represented by the areas under the respective curves.

torsion. If the moduli of elasticity and shear of the material from which the beam has been manufactured are known, the resulting deformation can be calculated from the stress distribution. Since the stresses increase in proportion to the loading force or moment, it is also possible to calculate that magnitude of the load where the stress at some volume element of the beam reaches the value of the ultimate stress. The appertaining load designates the tensile, compressive, or torsional strength of the beam.

In the case of beams with irregularly shaped cross sections or of complex (that is, not simple) loading modes, the formulae given below allow deformation and strength values to be calculated, at least approximately. For this purpose geometry and loading mode can be sufficiently simplified. The cross section of a long bone can, for example, be approximated by a tube with the diameter of the bone and a wall thickness equal to the mean thickness of the cortical bone. If a structure is loaded by more than one force and/or moment, only the force or moment with the highest magnitude may be taken into account for an initial approximation.

In the following, the procedure used to calculate deformation and strength is illustrated by the examples of a beam of arbitrary cross section under a tensile or compressive force, a beam with rectangular cross section under a bending moment, and a beam with circular cross section under a torsional moment exerted about its long axis.

3.2.1 Deformation of a Beam under Tension or Compression

If a beam is loaded by a compressive or tensile force directed in its longitudinal direction (**Fig. 3.9**) the stress may be assumed to have equal values at each point of the cross-sectional area A at some distance from the point of force application. The stress σ has the value

(3.1) $$\sigma = F / A$$

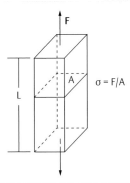

Fig. 3.9 The tensile stress in a beam loaded by a tensile force **F** assumes equal values on each cross section parallel to A (provided that the cross section is located at some distance from the point of application of the force). Its magnitude is given by $\sigma = F/A$.

For the length change dL of the beam of initial length L, we obtain from Hooke's law

(3.2)
$$\sigma = E \cdot dL / L$$
$$dL = \sigma \cdot L / E$$
$$dL = (F \cdot L)/(A \cdot E)$$

The length change is proportional to the initial length L and the magnitude of the force F and inversely proportional to the modulus of elasticity E and the cross-sectional area A.

If the quotient F/A exceeds the value of the ultimate stress σ_u of the material, the beam will fracture. It follows that

(3.3) $$\text{tensile or compressive strength} = \sigma_u \cdot A \text{ [N]}$$

The strength of the beam increases with increasing ultimate stress σ_u and increasing cross-sectional area A. The strength does not depend on the modulus of elasticity E or on the length L of the beam.

3.2.2 Bending of a Beam Fixed at One End

If a beam is fixed at one end and loaded at its free end by a force directed perpendicularly to the long axis of the beam, the beam will be bent (**Fig. 3.10**). The material will be elongated in the upper layers of the beam and compressed in the lower layers. The length of the middle layer (*neutral fiber*) at the border between regions of compression and elongation will remain unchanged. Inside the beam, tensile and compressive stresses σ_t and σ_c are generated. The stresses have their maximum value at the upper and lower beam surfaces and decrease toward the neutral fiber. At each cross section at a distance L_1 from the point of application of force the tensile and compressive stresses generate a moment which equilibrates the external moment $L_1 \cdot F$.

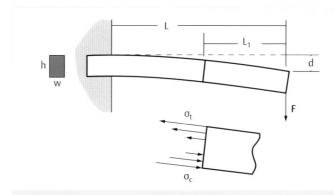

Fig. 3.10 Deflection d of a beam fixed at one end and loaded by a force **F** at its free end.

It can be shown (the proof is not given here) that the deflection d of the beam at its free end is given by

(3.4)
$$d = (F \cdot L^3) / (3 \cdot E \cdot I) \ [m]$$

In this equation, F designates the magnitude of the force, L the length of the beam, E the modulus of elasticity of the beam material; I is called the *moment of inertia* (or *second moment of area*). The moment of inertia (having nothing to do with the moment of a force) is a geometrical quantity determined solely by the shape of the cross section of the beam. For a rectangular cross section of width w and height h it holds that

(3.5)
$$I = w \cdot h^3 / 12 \ [m^4]$$

It can be seen from the above formulae that the length L and the height h of the beam have a great influence on the deflection. The tensile stress at the upper surface of the beam at a distance L_1 from the point of force application is given by

(3.6)
$$\sigma = M / Z \ [N/m^2]$$
$$\sigma = L_1 \cdot F / Z \ [N/m^2]$$

In this formula, M denotes the moment $L_1 \cdot F$. Z is called the *section modulus*. Like the moment of inertia, Z is a purely geometrical quantity and depends on the shape of the beam's cross section. For a beam with a rectangular cross section it holds that

(3.7)
$$Z = w \cdot h^2 / 6 \ [m^3]$$

Since the moment of the external force F, and hence the stress on the surface of the beam, increases with increasing distance from the point of application of the force according to $\sigma = M/Z$, the largest value of the stress is to be expected at the location ($L_1 = L$) where the beam is fixed. If the stress at this location exceeds the ultimate stress σ_u of the beam material, the beam will fracture at the fixation. It follows that the bending strength of a unilaterally fixed beam is given by

(3.8)
$$\text{bending strength} = \sigma_u \cdot Z / L \, [\text{N}]$$

For a beam with a rectangular cross section it follows that

(3.9)
$$\text{bending strength} = \sigma_u \cdot w \cdot h^2 / 6 \cdot L \, [\text{N}]$$

The formula shows that the bending strength of a beam with a rectangular cross section depends more on the height h than on the width w of the beam. The strength decreases with increasing length L.

Formulae for calculating the moment of inertia I and the section modulus Z for other shapes of cross sections (circle, tube, triangle) are listed in reference books on mechanics. In such books the reader can also find formulae to calculate deflection of beams under other simple loading modes such as three-point or four-point bending or uniform distribution of the load along the whole beam. By means of these formulae, deflection and strength can be obtained in the same fashion as in the example set out above.

The bent beam with tensile strain at its convex surface and compressive strain at its concave surface is frequently used as model in the medical context. Where do we expect to see the first signs of failure in a bone loaded in bending, bearing in mind that bone material has high compressive but low tensile strength? On which side does the orthopedic surgeon apply a plate to a fractured bone? Why does the distance between the spinous processes increase with forward bending of the trunk (Schober sign)? In which direction must an adhesive plaster be applied to protect a cut wound from tearing open?

3.2.3   Torsion of a Beam About Its Long Axis

A beam of circular cross section may be fixed at one end and loaded at its free end by a moment exerted around its long axis. To derive the relation between the moment, the properties of the beam material, the shape of the beam, and the angle of torsion, we imagine the beam to be divided into a set of thin-walled cylinders (**Fig. 3.11**). The torsion of a cylinder of radius R and wall thickness dR by an angle β effects a shear of the wall of the cylinder by an angle α. The relation between the two angles is

(3.10)
$$\alpha = \beta \cdot R / L$$

On the cross-sectional area of the cylinder the shear stress

(3.11)
$$\tau = G \cdot \alpha \, [\text{N}/\text{m}^2]$$

is generated. In this formula G denotes the shear modulus. The shear force, given by the product of shear stress τ and cross-sectional area of the cylinder, effects a moment directed opposite to the external moment; the moments of all cylinders together equilibrate the external moment M.

It can be shown (the proof is not given here) that the relation between the angle of torsion β and the external moment is given by

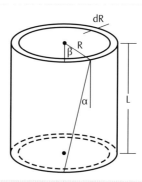

Fig. 3.11 Derivation of the relationship between moment and torsional deformation of a beam of circular cross section. The beam is imagined to be composed of concentric hollow cylinders. The twist of a hollow cylinder by an angle β corresponds to a shear deformation of the lateral area of the cylinder by an angle α caused by a shear stress τ. τ multiplied by the area gives the appertaining shear force. The external moment equals the sum of the moments exerted by all cylinders (that is, of the shear forces multiplied by the relevant radii R).

(3.12)
$$\beta = (M \cdot L)/(G \cdot I_p)$$

In this formula M denotes the external moment, L the length of the beam, G the modulus of shear, and I_p the *polar moment of inertia*. I_p depends only on the geometry of the cross section of the beam. For a beam with a circular cross section and radius R it amounts to

(3.13)
$$I_p = \pi \cdot d^4 / 32 \, [m^4]$$

The shear stress has its maximum value at the surface of the beam. At each point along the beam the stress has the value

(3.14)
$$\tau = M / Z_p$$

In this formula Z_p denotes the *polar section modulus*. Z_p depends (like the polar moment of inertia) only on the geometry of the cross section of the beam. For a beam with a circular cross section it amounts to

(3.15)
$$Z_p = \pi d^3 / 16 \, [m^3]$$

The torsional strength (that is, the maximum moment by which the beam can be loaded) is reached when the shear stress at the beam surface assumes its ultimate value τ_u.

(3.16)
$$\text{torsional strength} = \tau_u \cdot Z_p \, [Nm]$$

Since the shear stress takes equal values along the whole beam between the point of fixation and the point of moment application, no prediction can be made concerning the location at which fracture is to be expected. The location of fracture is determined rather by local deviations from the regular beam geometry or by material inhomogeneities.

Formulae for determining the polar moment of inertia and the polar section modulus for other shapes of cross section (tube, rectangle, triangle) are available in reference books on mechanics. Analogous to the example outlined above, these formulae permit the deformation and strength of such beams under torsional loading to be calculated.

3.3 Decrease of Strength Due to Stress Concentrations

Experience shows that in many cases the strength of structures is considerably lower than the strength value estimated on the basis only of knowledge of the ultimate compressive or tensile strength of the structural materials. To explain this phenomenon, Inglis introduced in 1913 the concept of *stress concentrations*.[7,8] Inglis calculated the stress on the surface of small voids or notches in the surface of a material subjected to compressive or tensile stress. According to Inglis, the stress at the tip of a notch of depth 2d, rounded at its tip with a radius r, is approximately given by

(3.17) $$\sigma_c = \sigma_0 \cdot (1 + 2 \cdot \sqrt{d/r})$$

In this formula σ_0 denotes the stress to be expected under the identical loading mode in the absence of notches or voids. It may be noted that, especially in case of a small radius (a sharp cut into the surface), the stress in the depth of the notch may easily amount to a multiple of the stress σ_0.

If a notch is present on the upper surface of a beam subjected to bending (**Fig. 3.12**), it may happen that in dependence on d, r, and the position of the notch, the stress at the tip of the notch exceeds the stress calculated for the location where the beam is fixed (see Section 3.2.2). Fracture of the beam will then be

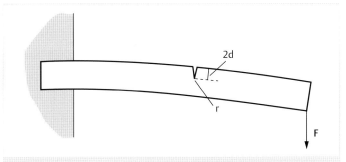

Fig. 3.12 A notch of depth 2d, rounded at its tip with a radius r, effects a stress concentration the magnitude of which is given by the formula of Inglis[7] (Eq. 3.17).

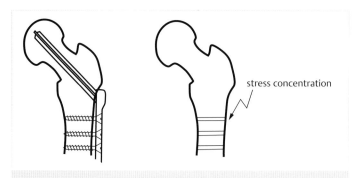

Fig. 3.13 After removal of a plate, the drill holes effect stress concentrations in the cortical bone.

expected to occur at the location of the notch; the strength of the beam is lower than that of a beam with a smooth surface. Use is made of this effect, for example, in cutting glass: the pane fractures precisely along the line where the glass cutter produced a fine, sharp cut into the surface.

Stress concentrations are regularly to be expected at locations where the dimensions of cross sections of structural members undergo a change. The magnitude of these concentrations increases if the change in cross section occurs over a small distance. If, for example, a plate is removed from a healed bone (**Fig. 3.13**), the load capacity of the bone is reduced for a time after surgery. This is due to stress concentrations caused by the open drill holes left behind after the bone screws have been removed. (In addition, the strength of the bone may be compromised as a result of bone resorption in the preceding period of partial weight bearing.) The right design can help to reduce stress concentrations. If, for example, an indentation in the surface of a beam is required for technical reasons (**Fig. 3.14a**), it will be advantageous to round the tip of the indentation. A stress concentration exists in a bone screw at the transition from the cylindrical neck to the thread (**Fig. 3.14b**). The stress concentration is lower when the diameter of the neck is equal to the core diameter of the thread.

Despite considerable progress in the design and construction of highly loadable structures, due to the concept of stress concentrations, some questions remain. Some materials do not fail even in the presence of high stress concentrations. Griffith argued in 1920 that for a fissure to grow within the volume of a material, two conditions must be fulfilled[7,9]: (1) The deformation energy released in the course of the growing fissure must exceed the energy required to fracture the material at the tip of the fissure. (2) The molecular structure of the material must permit transport of the released energy to the tip of the fissure.

Griffith's concept is illustrated in **Fig. 3.15**. Tensile stress exists on the upper surface of the bent beam. A fissure in the surface has the effect that in a certain vicinity the stress decreases: deformation energy is released. According to Griffith, the energy released is proportional to the square of the depth of the fissure.

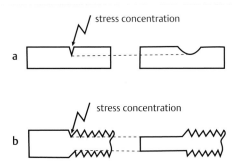

Fig. 3.14a, b Stress concentration at locations where the cross section of a structural member undergoes a change.
a For equal depth of the notch, the stress at the tip decreases if the radius of the tip is increased.
b The stress at the transition from the thread to the cylindrical shape decreases when the diameter of the cylindrical portion is equal to the core diameter of the thread.

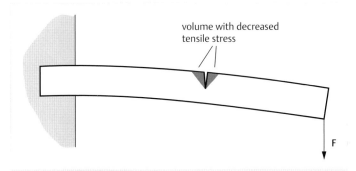

Fig. 3.15 A crack effects a relaxation of stress in its vicinity (shaded volume) and deformation energy is released. If the energy released exceeds the energy required to rip the material, the crack will grow.

A minimum fissure length is required to release enough deformation energy for progression of the crack. According to Griffith, a *critical length* of fissure can be stated for each material.

To summarize, the strength of a structure should be evaluated in three steps. For a given loading mode, it should be checked whether (ignoring possible stress concentrations) there are locations where the ultimate stress of the materials is exceeded. The next step is to examine whether stress concentrations exist that could effectively lower the strength of the structure. If fissures exist within the material, it should be assessed whether they are shorter or longer than Griffith's critical length.

References

1. Amiel D, Woo SLY, Harwood FL, Akeson WH. The effect of immobilization on collagen turnover in connective tissue: a biochemical-biomechanical correlation. Acta Orthop Scand 1982;53(3):325–332

2. Lanir Y, Fung YC. Two-dimensional mechanical properties of rabbit skin. II. Experimental results. J Biomech 1974;7(2):171–182

3. Sparks HV Jr, Bohr DF. Effect of stretch on passive tension and contractility of isolated vascular smooth muscle. Am J Physiol 1962;202:835–840

4. Yamada H. Strength of Biological Materials. Baltimore: Williams & Wilkins; 1970

5. Plaue R, Gerner HJ, Puhl W. Das Frakturverhalten von Brust- und Lendenwirbelkörpern. 4. Mitteilung: Untersuchungen über die Morphologie des Wirbelkompressionsbruches. Z Orthop Ihre Grenzgeb 1973;111(2):139–146

6. McClure P, Siegler S, Nobilini R. Three-dimensional flexibility characteristics of the human cervical spine in vivo. Spine 1998;23(2):216–223

7. Gordon JE, Ball P. The New Science of Strong Materials, or Why You Don't Fall through the Floor. Princeton: Princeton University Press; 2007

8. Inglis CE. Stresses in a plate due to the presence of cracks and sharp corners. Trans Inst Naval Architects 1913;55:219–241

9. Griffith AA. The phenomena of rupture and flow in solids. Philos Trans R Soc Lond 1920;A221:163–197

Part II

Mathematics: Some Basics

4   Vector Algebra

Some physical quantities are comprehensively described by a single number, in some cases in combination with a positive or negative sign. Such quantities are termed *scalars*. Examples are: mass [kg], length or distance [m], volume [m³], or temperature [degree]. There are other physical quantities which are not completely described by quoting their magnitude; a full description requires specification of a direction in a plane or in space. To describe a force unambiguously, for example, it is not sufficient to give the magnitude of the force. The direction of the force must be given as well. Other physical quantities that have to be described by their magnitude as well as by their direction are the location of a point with respect to another point, a velocity, an acceleration, or a moment. Physical quantities that are described by a magnitude and a direction are termed *vectors*. For brevity, it is sometimes stated that "forces, etc., are vectors." What this means is that for addition, subtraction, and (where meaningful) multiplication relating to forces, etc., the mathematical rules that apply are those defined for vectors.

The forces acting on a body or the motion of a body are often illustrated graphically. In such illustrations, the vectors (forces, changes of location, velocities, or accelerations) are depicted by arrows of different lengths and orientations in planes of interest or in three-dimensional space. In the two-dimensional case, where all vectors lie in the same plane, the graphical representation also allows simple operations like addition or subtraction of vectors to be performed by ruler and pencil. For many problems in biomechanics, the limited accuracy of such *graphical illustrations* and *graphical calculations* is adequate.

Alternatively, vectors are represented by their components. The components are vectors in the direction of the x-, y-, and z-coordinate axes. The magnitude and direction of the components are described by positive or negative numbers, depending on whether the component vectors point in the positive or negative direction of the coordinate axes. The representation of vectors by their components must be used if products of vectors are to be calculated; unlike the case for addition or subtraction, there is no simple graphical procedure for the multiplication of vectors. For precise or extensive vector calculations, especially when employing computers, the component representation of vectors is always used. This does not preclude the possibility of results being presented subsequently in graphical format.

To designate vectors, the following convention is adhered to in this book: vectors are designated by bold type. $\mathbf{F}$, for example, designates a force vector. If more than one force is being dealt with, an index 1, 2, etc., may be added, for example $\mathbf{F}_1$ or $\mathbf{F}_2$. A character as index, for example $\mathbf{F}_i$, is used if all forces in a given setup are meant or if the sum of all forces $\mathbf{F}_1, \mathbf{F}_2, \ldots \mathbf{F}_n$ from i = 1 to i = n is to be calculated. The magnitude of a vector is designated by a character in ordinary type; F, for example, designates the magnitude of the force vector $\mathbf{F}$. Alternatively, the magnitude of a vector $\mathbf{F}$ may be designated as $|\mathbf{F}|$; F and $|\mathbf{F}|$ have identical meaning. The components of a vector in relation to a right-handed rectangular xyz-coordinate system are designated by the indices x, y, and z; for example F_x, F_y, and F_z.

4.1   The Trigonometric Functions Sine, Cosine, and Tangent

When decomposing vectors into components or multiplying vectors by vectors, trigonometric functions come into play. This chapter serves to remind the reader of the definition of these functions. Those who remember the meaning of these functions sufficiently well from their schooldays can go straight to the next section.

Sides a and b of a right-angled triangle enclose the 90° angle (**Fig. 4.1**); side c opposite this angle is termed the *hypotenuse*. In relation to the angle α between b and c, side a is termed *opposite* and side b *adjacent*. The trigonometric functions *sine*, *cosine*, and *tangent* describe the quotients of the lengths of the sides of right-angled triangles dependent on the angle α. Using quotients of side lengths makes sense because all right-angled triangles with an angle α between the hypotenuse and the adjacent side are geometrically similar (**Fig. 4.1a**). In other words, for all right-angled triangles with an angle α between the hypotenuse and the adjacent side, the value of the quotient a/b is identical, irrespective of the actual size of the triangles.

The sine of an angle α is defined as

(4.1)
$$\text{sine of } \alpha = \text{opposite} / \text{hypotenuse}$$
$$\sin \alpha = a / c$$

The cosine of an angle α is defined as

(4.2)
$$\text{cosine of } \alpha = \text{adjacent} / \text{hypotenuse}$$
$$\cos \alpha = b / c$$

The tangent of an angle α is defined as

(4.3)
$$\text{tangent of } \alpha = \text{opposite} / \text{adjacent}$$
$$\tan \alpha = a / b$$

Of course the definitions hold for the angle β as well. The sine of angle β in **Fig. 4.1b** is defined as

(4.4)
$$\text{sine of } \beta = \text{opposite} / \text{hypotenuse}$$
$$\sin \beta = b / c$$

Analogous definitions hold for the cosine and the tangent of angle β.

The trigonometric functions are frequently employed because many geometrical problems can be reduced to problems with right-angled triangles. If some elements (side lengths, angles) of a right-angled triangle are known, the remaining elements can be calculated trigonometrically.

Example 1: The length of the hypotenuse c and the angle α between the hypotenuse and one side are known. The trigonometric functions allow the lengths of sides a and b to be calculated. The definitions given above yield

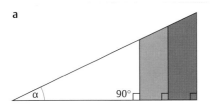 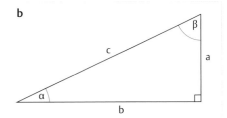

Fig. 4.1a, b Right-angled triangles.

a All right-angled triangles with an angle α between the hypotenuse c and the adjacent side b are geometrically similar.

b The quotients of the adjacent and opposite sides a and b with the hypotenuse c define the trigonometric functions sine and cosine of angle α; the quotient of a and b defines the tangent of angle α.

(4.5)
$$b = c \cdot \cos\alpha$$
$$a = c \cdot \sin\alpha$$

Example 2: Angle α and the length of side b are known. The length of side a is calculated by

(4.6)
$$a = b \cdot \tan\alpha$$

and the length of side c from

(4.7)
$$c = b / \cos\alpha$$

Numerical values of sine, cosine, and tangent can be found in mathematical tables or by means of a pocket calculator. In mathematical formulae the inverse functions of sine, cosine, and tangent are termed asin, acos, and atan. The inverse functions are the angles which correspond to quotients of side lengths of right-angled triangles: asin is the angle α that belongs to a given quotient of the lengths of sides a and c; by analogy, the same applies to acos and atan. Given the length of two sides of a right-angled triangle, the angle between the two sides can be determined using inverse trigonometric functions.

Example 3: The lengths of sides a and b are known. The angle α that belongs to the quotient a/b—that is, the angle between sides c and b—is calculated by

(4.8)
$$\alpha = \text{atan}\,(a / b)$$

Values of the inverse trigonometric functions are also laid down in mathematical tables or stored in pocket calculators. On the buttons of such calculators, the inverse functions asin, acos, and atan are often designated as $\sin^{-1}$, $\cos^{-1}$, and $\tan^{-1}$. (This is an awkward designation, because the symbol "$^{-1}$" is normally used to designate "1.0 divided by ...." The expression $\sin^{-1}\alpha$, however, does not designate $1.0/\sin\alpha$ but the inverse function of the sine, that is, the angle α belonging to a given value of the sine.)

As quotients of lengths of the sides of right-angled triangles, the trigonometric functions are defined only for angles up to 90°. In this domain sine, cosine, and tangent have (as quotients of lengths) positive values. It has proved advantageous, however, to extend the definition of trigonometric functions up to an angle of 360°. The generalized definition relates to quotients of lengths at the *unit circle* (**Fig. 4.2**). The unit circle is a circle whose radius (distance OC) is equal to 1. The magnitude of the sine of an angle is equal to distance BC, the magnitude of the cosine is equal to distance OB, and the magnitude of the tangent is equal to distance AD. The functions, however, bear different positive or negative signs depending on the quadrant in which OC is located. Quadrants I to IV are parts of the plane as partitioned by a rectangular coordinate system. The signs for trigonometric functions are listed in **Table 4.1**.

Quadrant	Angular range	Sine	Cosine	Tangent
I	0° to 90°	+	+	+
II	90° to 180°	+	–	–
III	180° to 270°	–	–	+
IV	270° to 360°	–	+	–

Table 4.1 Signs for sine, cosine, and tangent for angles between 0° and 360°

In the example shown in **Fig. 4.2** (α = 125°), the sine of the angle α = 125° is positive; the cosine and the tangent are negative. The reader might like to confirm that, for angles up to 90°, defining trigonometric functions based on quotients of sides of right-angled triangles is identical to basing them on lengths at the unit circle.

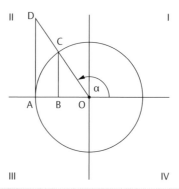

Fig. 4.2 Definition of the trigonometric functions by distances at the unit circle (circle with radius OC = 1). For a given angle α (counted counter-clockwise), the length of BC equals the magnitude of the sine, the length of OB equals the magnitude of the cosine, and the length of AD equals the magnitude of the tangent. Sine, cosine, and tangent have positive or negative signs depending on which of the four quadrants I to IV the radius OC is located in.

Angles are quoted in different units, in degrees or radians. Expressed in degrees, a full rotation corresponds to 360°; expressed in radians, a full rotation corresponds to $2 \cdot \pi = 6.2831$ radians (correct to four decimal places). It follows that 1 radian corresponds to 57.2958°. The degree measure is preferred in practice; computerized calculation programs usually use the radian.

4.2 Representation of Vectors

In graphical illustrations, a vector is represented by an arrow (**Fig. 4.3**). The length of the arrow indicates the magnitude of the vector. The magnitude of a vector is a positive quantity (there are no arrows with a negative length). In order to infer the magnitude of a vector from a graphical representation, the scale factor of the representation must be known. If, for example, the arrow represents a force, it must be known how many centimeters of its length correspond to 1 N. The direction of the vector is given by the direction of the arrow with its arrowhead. In a plane, the direction of a vector can be given by the angle α between the arrow and the x-axis of a rectangular xy-coordinate system and in addition by its arrowhead (**Fig. 4.4**). In a plane, a vector is fully described by its magnitude and its direction. In three-dimensional space, an additional angle has to be given; this is usually the angle between the vector and the z-axis of a rectangular xyz-coordinate system.

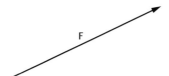

Fig. 4.3 Graphical representation of a vector **F**: the length of the arrow designates the magnitude of the vector. The direction of the arrow and the arrowhead denote the direction of vector **F**.

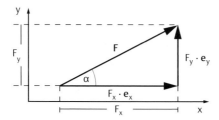

Fig. 4.4 In a plane the direction of a vector can be specified by the angle α with respect to the x-axis of an xy-coordinate system. Alternatively, the vector may be specified by its component vectors $F_x \cdot \mathbf{e}_x$ and $F_y \cdot \mathbf{e}_y$. In this notation, $\mathbf{e}_x$ and $\mathbf{e}_y$ are vectors of length 1 (unit vectors) pointing in the direction of the coordinate axes; F_x and F_y are numbers which may be positive or negative.

Alternatively, a vector can be represented by its components in relation to an xyz-coordinate system. A vector **F** is then given by the vector sum of its components

(4.9) $$\mathbf{F} = F_x \cdot \mathbf{e}_x + F_y \cdot \mathbf{e}_y + F_z \cdot \mathbf{e}_z$$

In this formula $\mathbf{e}_x$, $\mathbf{e}_y$, and $\mathbf{e}_z$ designate unit vectors. Unit vectors are vectors of length 1 in the direction of the coordinate axes. F_x, F_y, and F_z are numbers which may be positive or negative. The x-component $F_x \cdot \mathbf{e}_x$ of the vector **F** is a vector in the direction of the x-axis (**Fig. 4.4**). The length of this vector equals the magnitude (the positive value) of F_x; the direction of this vector (the direction in which the arrow points) is given by the sign of F_x. For example, $5.0 \cdot \mathbf{e}_x$ designates a vector of length 5.0 pointing in the positive x-direction; $-2.0 \cdot \mathbf{e}_x$ designates a vector of length 2.0 pointing in the negative x-direction. The same applies analogously to the other components of **F**.

In commonly used symbolic notation the component representation of a vector **F** is given by

(4.10) $$\mathbf{F} = \begin{bmatrix} F_x \\ F_y \\ F_z \end{bmatrix}$$

In this notation, the unit vectors do not appear explicitly. The brackets indicate that the components of the vector **F** are calculated by multiplying the numbers F_x, F_y, and F_z by the unit vectors. If only vectors in the xy-plane are being dealt with, the z-component is always equal to zero. In this case, the third component can be omitted and the vector may be represented just by the two numbers F_x and F_y.

The numbers F_x, F_y, and F_z are known as the *coordinates* of the vector **F**. It has become usual to refer to F_x, F_y, and F_z as *components* of the vector **F** as well. Strictly speaking, this is not correct, because the components of a vector are vectors and not numbers. However, occasionally this somewhat loose use of the term *component* helps to prevent confusion when the *coordinates* of a point relative to a coordinate system are also being referred to.

Fig. 4.5 and Eqs. 4.11 and 4.12 illustrate the symbolic representation of vectors using the example of the two vectors $\mathbf{F}_1$ and $\mathbf{F}_2$ in the xy-plane. The axes of the rectangular coordinate system are scaled. The components of the vectors are the projections of the vectors on the axes; the signs of the coordinates give the direction of the components (the z-components in this example equal to zero).

(4.11) $$\mathbf{F}_1 = \begin{bmatrix} +5.0 \\ +3.0 \\ 0.0 \end{bmatrix}$$

(4.12) $$\mathbf{F}_2 = \begin{bmatrix} +3.0 \\ -4.0 \\ 0.0 \end{bmatrix}$$

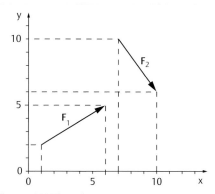

Fig. 4.5 Representation of vectors by specification of their coordinates. The coordinates of vectors $\mathbf{F}_1$ and $\mathbf{F}_2$ equal the lengths of their projections on the x- and y-axis. The signs are given by their direction. In the example shown, $F_{1x} = +5$, $F_{1y} = +3$, $F_{2x} = +3$, $F_{2y} = -4$.

Of course, this representation is valid for all vectors, not only for forces. A distance vector $\mathbf{L}_1$ in the xy-plane, pointing from the point $(x = +1, y = +2)$ to the point $(x = +6, y = +5)$ is represented by

(4.13)
$$\mathbf{L}_1 = \begin{bmatrix} +5.0 \\ +3.0 \\ 0.0 \end{bmatrix}$$

The coordinates of a vector can be calculated from its magnitude and its direction. In the two-dimensional case (**Fig. 4.4**) it holds that

(4.14)
$$F_x = |\mathbf{F}| \cdot \cos\alpha$$
$$F_y = |\mathbf{F}| \cdot \sin\alpha$$

Conversely, the angle α can be determined when the coordinates F_x and F_y are known

(4.15)
$$\alpha = \mathrm{atan}(F_y/F_x)$$

The relation between the coordinates and the magnitude of a vector is given by

(4.16)
$$|\mathbf{F}| = \sqrt{F_x^2 + F_y^2}$$

This formula derives from Pythagoras' theorem. The components $\mathbf{F}_x$ and $\mathbf{F}_y$, together with the vector $\mathbf{F}$, form a right-angled triangle. In a right-angled triangle

$$\text{hypotenuse}^2 = \text{adjacent side}^2 + \text{opposite side}^2$$

(4.17)
$$c^2 = a^2 + b^2$$

(4.18)
$$c = \sqrt{a^2 + b^2}$$

It must be pointed out that the location of the origin of a vector (the starting point of the arrow) is not specified by the vector's magnitude and direction. The three vectors depicted in **Fig. 4.6** have the same magnitude (length) and the same direction; they represent the identical vector. It follows that, when drawn, a vector may be shifted parallel to, or along, its direction. Since magnitude and direction remain unchanged by this procedure, it remains the identical vector. On the other hand, a mechanical state may well be altered when a vector is shifted. We expect different effects when the identical force vector is applied at different points of a body. The force might induce a linear translation and/or a rotation. To describe the effect of a force on a body it is not sufficient merely to communicate the force vector (magnitude and direction); the point of force application must be given as well.

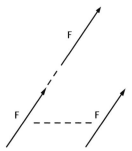

Fig. 4.6 A vector is fully described by specifying its magnitude and direction. The origin of the vector (in the case of a force vector: the point of force application) is not covered by this description. Thus, the three arrows shown, all of identical length and identical direction, represent the same vector.

4.3   Addition of Vectors: Graphical Procedure in the Two-Dimensional Case

A specific rule, differing from the usual one for adding pure numbers, is required for adding physical quantities characterized by magnitude and direction (that is, vectors). **Fig. 4.7** illustrates the graphic procedure for adding vectors—the parallelogram law of vector addition, exemplified by the addition of two forces.

Two coplanar forces of different magnitude and direction act on an object. The resultant force (that is, the sum of the two forces) is to be determined. **Fig. 4.7a** shows an "anatomical" setup. A simplified model of this (**Fig. 4.7b**) has to be agreed on before the problem can be solved. The directions of the forces are inferred from the outlines of the human bodies. The contact areas of the hands, by which the forces are actually transmitted, are replaced by the points of application of the forces. If no further details of the force transmission are known, the points of force application are located centrally between the contact areas of

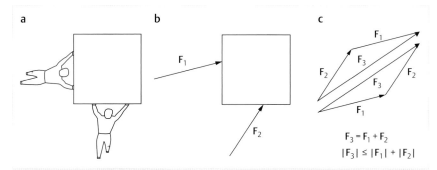

Fig. 4.7a–c Illustration of the addition of two vectors in the two-dimensional case, employing the parallelogram law of vector addition.

the hands. In later chapters of this book the direction of muscle forces in biomechanical models are inferred in identical fashion from the anatomical direction of the muscles. Areas of insertion of muscles and tendons are represented by single points, usually by the center of their area of insertion.

To obtain the vector sum (**Fig. 4.7c**), F_2 is shifted parallel to itself and along its own direction until the origin of F_2 coincides with the tip of F_1. The base in the triangle formed by F_1 and (the shifted) F_2 is the vector sum (also termed the *resultant*) F_3. The identical result is obtained if F_1 is shifted until its origin coincides with the tip of F_2. Again, the vector sum is given by the base of the triangle formed by F_2 and (the shifted) F_1. The two triangles form what is called the *parallelogram of forces*. It is clear that the direction of the resultant F_3 (the diagonal of the parallelogram) coincides neither with the direction of F_1 nor with the direction of F_2. The magnitude of the resultant (length of the arrow) F_3 is always smaller than or, at most, equal to the sum of the magnitudes of the vectors F_1 and F_2.

In the case of two parallel vectors, the construction of the vector sum is very simple. **Fig. 4.8a** shows the "anatomical" setup, **Fig. 4.8b** the simplified model in which the forces exerted are represented by vectors

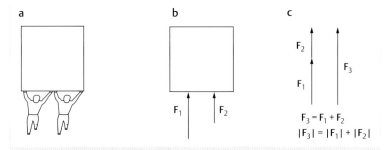

Fig. 4.8a–c In the special case of two parallel vectors F_1 and F_2 the magnitude of the sum vector F_3 is equal to the sum of the magnitudes of the addends (F_1 and F_2). The direction of F_3 equals the direction of the addends.

$\mathbf{F}_1$ and $\mathbf{F}_2$, and **Fig. 4.8c** the addition of these vectors according to the rule given above. In the case of two parallel vectors, the parallelogram of forces shrinks to a straight line. The diagonal in this "parallelogram" is obtained simply by joining vectors $\mathbf{F}_1$ and $\mathbf{F}_2$. In this special case the direction of the vector sum $\mathbf{F}_3$ is seen to equal the direction of the two vectors; the magnitude of the vector sum $\mathbf{F}_3$ is given by the sum of the magnitudes of the two vectors $\mathbf{F}_1$ and $\mathbf{F}_2$. In the special case of parallel vectors (but only in this case), the magnitudes of vectors may be added arithmetically to provide the magnitude of the vector sum.

If more than two vectors are to be added, the parallelogram law of vector addition is repeatedly applied (**Fig. 4.9**). To add $\mathbf{F}_1$, $\mathbf{F}_2$, and $\mathbf{F}_3$, $\mathbf{F}_1$ and $\mathbf{F}_2$ are added first; in a second step $\mathbf{F}_3$ is added to the sum vector $\mathbf{F}_1 + \mathbf{F}_2$. The resultant vector is designated by $\mathbf{F}_4$. It should be noted that it is not necessary to draw $\mathbf{F}_1 + \mathbf{F}_2$ explicitly. To add vectors $\mathbf{F}_1$, $\mathbf{F}_2$, and $\mathbf{F}_3$ it is sufficient to join the three vectors to form a polygon. The sum vector $\mathbf{F}_4$ then points from the origin of $\mathbf{F}_1$ to the tip of $\mathbf{F}_3$.

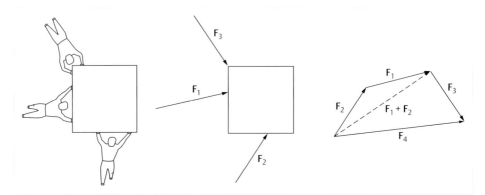

Fig. 4.9 To add vectors $\mathbf{F}_1$, $\mathbf{F}_2$, and $\mathbf{F}_3$, the parallelogram law is applied twice. The vector sum of $\mathbf{F}_1$ and $\mathbf{F}_2$ does not have to be drawn explicitly. Vector $\mathbf{F}_4$ can be determined by joining $\mathbf{F}_1$, $\mathbf{F}_2$, and $\mathbf{F}_3$ to form a polygon.

If vectors to be added form a closed polygon, this is the same as saying that the vector sum equals zero. **Fig. 4.10** illustrates this for vectors $\mathbf{F}_1$, $\mathbf{F}_2$, and $\mathbf{F}_3$. Between the arrowhead of $\mathbf{F}_3$ and the origin of $\mathbf{F}_1$ there is "nothing left"—no space. The resultant is a vector of zero length. A situation where the sum of all forces equals zero is met in static equilibrium. On a drawing this is shown by the fact that the vectors of all forces applied form a closed polygon.

Subtracting one vector from another requires no new rule. Let us assume that the difference

(4.19)
$$\mathbf{F}_7 = \mathbf{F}_6 - \mathbf{F}_5$$

is to be calculated. This difference can also be written as the sum

(4.20)
$$\mathbf{F}_7 = \mathbf{F}_6 + (-\mathbf{F}_5)$$

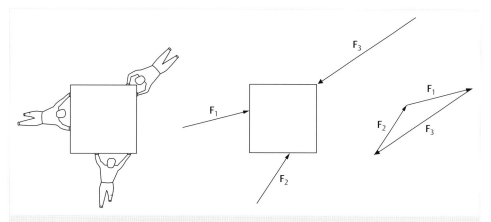

Fig. 4.10 If vectors to be added form a closed polygon, this indicates that the vector sum equals zero. Here it holds that $\mathbf{F}_1 + \mathbf{F}_2 + \mathbf{F}_3 = \mathbf{0}$. The symbol $\mathbf{0}$ designates the so-called null vector, that is, a vector of zero length.

In this formula $-\mathbf{F}_5$ designates a vector having the identical magnitude but the opposite direction of $\mathbf{F}_5$. To show this graphically, we have to draw the arrowhead on the opposite end of the vector. (In the numerical representation, this means that the vector coordinates change their sign, see Section 4.4). Vectors $\mathbf{F}_6$ and $-\mathbf{F}_5$ may now be added according to the scheme shown in **Fig. 4.7**.

4.4 Addition of Vectors: Numerical Procedure

The numerical rule for adding two vectors is based on the addition of the coordinates. The x-, y-, and (in the three-dimensional case) z-coordinates of the sum vector are obtained by adding the respective x-, y-, and z-coordinates of the two vectors to be added. In the case of vectors $\mathbf{F}_1$ and $\mathbf{F}_2$ being added, the coordinates of the sum vector $\mathbf{F}_3$ are obtained from

(4.21)
$$\begin{aligned} F_{3x} &= F_{1x} + F_{2x} \\ F_{3y} &= F_{1y} + F_{2y} \\ F_{3z} &= F_{1z} + F_{2z} \end{aligned}$$

Fig. 4.11 illustrates this rule for the two-dimensional situation (and also shows the graphical procedure for addition). In the example given, the coordinates of vectors $\mathbf{F}_1$ and $\mathbf{F}_2$ are

(4.22)
$$\begin{aligned} F_{1x} &= 4 \\ F_{1y} &= 1 \\ F_{2x} &= 2 \\ F_{2y} &= 3 \\ F_{1z} &= 0 \\ F_{2z} &= 0 \end{aligned}$$

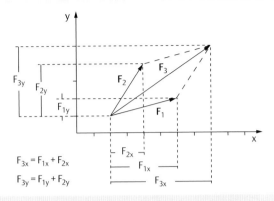

Fig. 4.11 To add vectors $\mathbf{F}_1$ and $\mathbf{F}_2$ numerically, the x- and y-coordinates are added separately to give the x- and y-coordinates of the sum vector $\mathbf{F}_3$. The same rule applies to the z-coordinates in the three-dimensional situation.

For the sum vector $\mathbf{F}_3$ it holds that

(4.23)
$$F_{3x} = F_{1x} + F_{2x} = 4 + 2 = 6$$
$$F_{3y} = F_{1y} + F_{2y} = 1 + 3 = 4$$
$$F_{3z} = F_{1z} + F_{2z} = 0 + 0 = 0$$

or, in symbolic notation

(4.24)
$$\mathbf{F}_3 = \begin{bmatrix} 4.0 \\ 1.0 \\ 0.0 \end{bmatrix} + \begin{bmatrix} 2.0 \\ 3.0 \\ 0.0 \end{bmatrix} = \begin{bmatrix} 6.0 \\ 4.0 \\ 0.0 \end{bmatrix}$$

As described above (Section 4.2), the magnitude and direction of $\mathbf{F}_3$ can be calculated from its coordinates.

4.5 Decomposition of a Vector into Vector Addends

In the same way that a number can be broken down into addends (for example, the number 10 into the addends 4 and 6), a vector can be decomposed into two or more vector addends. The prerequisite is that the vector sum of the addends equals the original vector (in the same sense as the sum of 4 and 6 equals 10). The representation of a vector by components, that is, by vectors in the direction of the coordinate axes, is one example of decomposition. In general, vectors pointing in arbitrary directions can be broken down. In **Fig. 4.9**, vector $\mathbf{F}_4$ can be imagined to be decomposed into vectors $\mathbf{F}_1$, $\mathbf{F}_2$, and $\mathbf{F}_3$.

It should be pointed out that the decomposition of a vector is, in principle, totally arbitrary. Like breaking down a number arbitrarily into addends (for example, the number 10 into $1 + 9$, $3 + 5 + 2$, and so on), a vector may also be decomposed into arbitrary addends. Decomposition makes sense only if specific problems have to be dealt with. **Fig. 4.12** gives an example where the problem of interest is the deformation

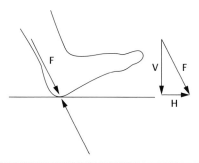

Fig. 4.12 Decomposition of a vector **F** into its components **H** and **V**. Addition of vectors **H** and **V** gives vector **F**.

of the floor and the risk of slipping. For this purpose, the force **F** exerted by the foot on the floor is decomposed into the addends **V** and **H** (the vector sum of **V** and **H** being equal to **F**). The downward bend of the floor depends on the vertically directed force **V**. The risk of slipping on the floor depends on the relation between the horizontally directed force **H** and the coefficient of friction between the foot and the floor.

4.6 Multiplication of Vectors: Scalar Product and Vector Product

For multiplication, unlike addition, no graphic procedures exist. The rules for multiplying vectors always employ the coordinates of the vectors. While there is only one type of multiplication between numbers, vectors **A** and **B** can be multiplied in two different ways, by the *scalar* product ("A times B")

(4.25) $$C = \mathbf{A} \cdot \mathbf{B}$$

and the *vector* product, or *cross* product ("A cross B")

(4.26) $$C = \mathbf{A} \times \mathbf{B}$$

The result of the scalar product of two vectors **A** and **B** is a number C. C is calculated from the coordinates of the two vectors as

(4.27) $$C = A_x \cdot B_x + A_y \cdot B_y + A_z \cdot B_z$$

It can be shown (proof is not presented here) that C amounts to

(4.28) $$C = |\mathbf{A}| \cdot |\mathbf{B}| \cdot \cos\varphi$$

φ being the angle between vectors **A** and **B**. Depending on the relative directions of **A** and **B**, $\cos\varphi$ may assume positive or negative values; thus the scalar product may be positive or negative. If the two vectors are oriented perpendicular to each other, the scalar product equals zero.

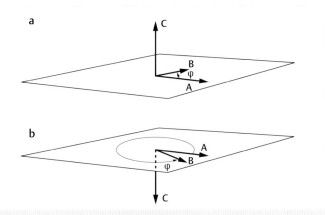

Fig. 4.13a, b Representation of the vector product (cross product) **C** of vectors **A** and **B**. **C** is perpendicular to the plane spanned by **A** and **B**. The direction of **C** is given by the sign of sinφ. The angle φ is counted counterclockwise from **A** to **B**. For angles smaller than or equal to 180° sinφ is positive (**a**). For angles above 180° sinφ is negative (**b**). For this reason the vectors **C** in diagrams **a** and **b** point in opposite directions.

The result of the vector product (cross product) of two vectors **A** and **B** is a vector **C**. The coordinates of **C** are calculated from the coordinates of **A** and **B** as

(4.29)
$$C_x = A_y \cdot B_z - A_z \cdot B_y$$
$$C_y = A_z \cdot B_x - A_x \cdot B_z$$
$$C_z = A_x \cdot B_y - A_y \cdot B_x$$

It can be shown (the proof is not presented here) that vector **C** is perpendicular to the plane spanned by vectors **A** and **B**. The magnitude of **C** is given by

(4.30)
$$|\mathbf{C}| = |\mathbf{A}| \cdot |\mathbf{B}| \cdot |\sin\varphi|$$

φ is the angle through which vector **A** is to be rotated in the direction of vector **B**. The direction of **C** is given by the sign of sinφ. **Fig. 4.13** illustrates this for the case where the angle φ between **A** and **B** is smaller than 180°, and also for the case where the angle φ is larger than 180°. For angles larger than 180° sinφ is negative; for this reason the direction of vector **C** in **Fig. 4.13b** is downwards.

The direction of **C** can be visualized by the *right hand rule* (**Fig. 4.14**). If thumb and forefinger point in the directions of vectors **A** and **B** (not necessarily running perpendicularly to each other), the middle finger of the right hand running perpendicularly to the plane of the thumb and forefinger points in the direction of **C**. This right hand rule also serves to define a right-handed xyz-coordinate system. If **A** points in x-direction and **B** in y-direction, **C** points in the direction of the z-axis of the right-handed xyz-system.

Alternatively, the direction of **C** can be visualized by the rule illustrated in **Fig. 4.15**. Vector **C** runs perpendicular to the plane spanned by vectors **A** and **B**. The direction of **C** is given by the direction of the

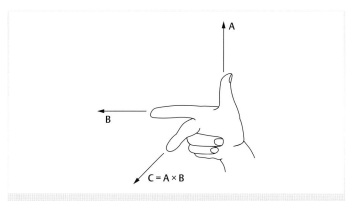

Fig. 4.14 Right hand rule. If thumb and forefinger of the right hand point in the direction of **A** and **B**, the middle finger held at an angle of 90° with respect to the plane of **A** and **B** points in the direction of **C**.

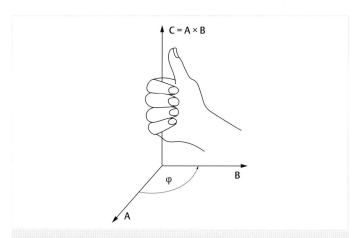

Fig. 4.15 Right hand rule, alternative version. **C** points in the direction of the thumb if the fingers of the right hand are bent around **C** in the direction of the angle φ between **A** and **B**.

thumb if the fingers are bent in the direction of rotation of the angle φ from **A** to **B** around **C**. The reader may (at the risk of a slight contortion of the right hand) convince himself that both rules give the identical result.

The moment, which was defined in Chapter 1 in simplified form as *force times perpendicular distance of the line of force action from the fulcrum*, is really a vector, the vector product of the distance vector L_1 and the force vector **F** (**Fig. 4.16**):

(4.31)
$$M = L_1 \times F$$

The vector L_1 gives the distance and direction from the fulcrum to the point of application of the force. The vector **M** is perpendicular to the plane spanned by L_1 and **F**. Its magnitude amounts to

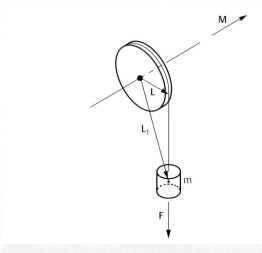

Fig. 4.16 Illustration of the moment vector **M**. Gravity exerts a force on the body of mass m hung on the rope slung around the wheel. The gravitational force **F** of the magnitude m · g is applied at the center of mass of the body. The distance vector L_1 points from the axis to the point of force application. The moment **M** is a vector, given by the vector product (cross product) of the distance vector and the force vector: $M = L_1 \times F$. **M** is oriented perpendicular to the plane spanned by L_1 and **F**. The direction of **M** can be determined by the right hand rule. In the diagram **M** is depicted by an arrow in the direction of the axis. Alternatively, **M** can be expressed by the vector **L** pointing perpendicularly from the axis to the line of force action and the force **F**: $M = L \times F$.

(4.32) $$|M| = |L_1| \cdot |F| \cdot |\sin\varphi|$$

In the illustration shown in **Fig. 4.16**, the distance vector L_1 points from the axis to the center of mass of the body hung on the rope slung around the wheel. Alternatively, the moment can be defined by employing the perpendicular distance vector **L** from the fulcrum to the line of action of the force

(4.33) $$M = L \times F$$

Both definitions yield the same result. For φ equal to 90° and $\sin\varphi$ equal to 1, the first formula merges into the second formula. The magnitude of the moment vector is identical to the value of the moment in its simplified version as defined in Chapter 1

(4.34) $$M = L \cdot F$$

where L and F have to be inserted as positive numbers.

To compare the two definitions, vector **M** is shown in **Fig. 4.16**. As determined by the right hand rule, **M** points in the direction of the axis of rotation. If the rope were suspended from the other side of the wheel, the moment vector would point in the opposite direction. By contrast, in the simplified definition (see **Fig. 1.8**) the moment is visualized by a bent arrow pointing in the direction of rotation. The reader is reminded again that, when calculating vector products, counterclockwise angles are positive. However, in the simplified definition a moment is counted positive if the rotation caused by the moment occurs in a clockwise direction.

Those readers who are familiar with the rules of vector multiplication will always prefer to define a moment as the vector product of a distance vector and a force vector. If the rules for vector multiplication are adhered to, no separate sign conventions have to be kept in mind (as with the simplified definition). The correct positive or negative signs result "automatically." As the distance vector, vector L_1 from the fulcrum to the point of force application is used. It is not necessary to determine vector **L** pointing from the fulcrum perpendicular to the line of action of the force, because by definition the angle φ between L_1 and **F** is taken into account by the vector product.

5 Matrix Notation

Some problems in mechanics require for their description: in the two-dimensional case a set of four numbers (or expressions), in the three-dimensional case a set of nine numbers, or, in the nine-dimensional case, a set of 36 numbers. Examples are the orientation or motion of a rigid body in a plane or in space (transformation matrix) or the description of the stress–strain properties of an inhomogeneous, anisotropic material, for example bone (stiffness matrix). To formulate the relevant equations clearly, matrix notation is employed. Use also can be made of established theorems regarding mathematical properties of matrices. The following introduction to matrix notation covers only the arithmetic operations using matrices that are employed later on in this book.

5.1 Definition of a Matrix

Quadratic matrices are sets of four (for the two-dimensional case) or nine numbers or expressions (for the three-dimensional case), ordered in rows and columns. Like the symbolic notation of a three-dimensional vector $\mathbf{v}$ in the form of a column

(5.1)
$$\mathbf{v} = \begin{bmatrix} v_1 \\ v_2 \\ v_3 \end{bmatrix}$$

a 2×2 matrix $\mathbf{M}$ is written

(5.2)
$$\mathbf{M} = \begin{bmatrix} M_{11} & M_{12} \\ M_{21} & M_{22} \end{bmatrix}$$

and a 3×3 matrix $\mathbf{M}$

(5.3)
$$\mathbf{M} = \begin{bmatrix} M_{11} & M_{12} & M_{13} \\ M_{21} & M_{22} & M_{23} \\ M_{31} & M_{32} & M_{33} \end{bmatrix}$$

The position of each element is designated by two indices. The matrix element M_{23} (spoken as "M sub two three") denotes the element in the second row and the third column.

5.2 Multiplication of a Matrix by a Vector or a Matrix

The multiplication of a matrix $\mathbf{M}$ by a vector $\mathbf{v}$ results in a vector $\mathbf{v'}$. The coordinates of the vector $\mathbf{v'}$ are obtained by multiplication of the elements of the rows of the matrix $\mathbf{M}$ with the coordinates of the vector $\mathbf{v}$ and subsequent addition of the products. In the case of a 3×3 matrix $\mathbf{M}$ it holds that

(5.4)
$$\begin{bmatrix} M_{11} & M_{12} & M_{13} \\ M_{21} & M_{22} & M_{23} \\ M_{31} & M_{32} & M_{33} \end{bmatrix} \cdot \begin{bmatrix} v_1 \\ v_2 \\ v_3 \end{bmatrix} = \begin{bmatrix} M_{11} \cdot v_1 + M_{12} \cdot v_2 + M_{13} \cdot v_3 \\ M_{21} \cdot v_1 + M_{22} \cdot v_2 + M_{23} \cdot v_3 \\ M_{31} \cdot v_1 + M_{32} \cdot v_2 + M_{33} \cdot v_3 \end{bmatrix} = \begin{bmatrix} v'_1 \\ v'_2 \\ v'_3 \end{bmatrix}$$

The new vector $\mathbf{v'}$ is designated the *image* of the vector $\mathbf{v}$, the imaging being mediated by the matrix $\mathbf{M}$.

The product of two matrices **A** and **B** is a matrix **M**

(5.5) $$M = A \cdot B$$

For a calculation of the matrix product, the rows of matrix **A** are to be multiplied by the columns of matrix **B**.

For example, the matrix element M_{13} in the first row and third column of the matrix $M = A \cdot B$

(5.6)
$$
\begin{bmatrix} M_{11} & M_{12} & M_{13} \\ M_{21} & M_{22} & M_{23} \\ M_{31} & M_{32} & M_{33} \end{bmatrix} = \begin{bmatrix} A_{11} & A_{12} & A_{13} \\ A_{21} & A_{22} & A_{23} \\ A_{31} & A_{32} & A_{33} \end{bmatrix} \cdot \begin{bmatrix} B_{11} & B_{12} & B_{13} \\ B_{21} & B_{22} & B_{23} \\ B_{31} & B_{32} & B_{33} \end{bmatrix}
$$

is calculated as

(5.7) $$M_{13} = A_{11} \cdot B_{13} + A_{12} \cdot B_{23} + A_{13} \cdot B_{33}$$

The general rule for the calculation of the elements of the matrix product $M = A \cdot B$ is

(5.8) $$M_{ik} = \sum_{s} A_{is} B_{sk}$$

The Greek letter Σ (capital sigma) symbolizes summation. For each i and k between 1 and n summation is extended over the index s: in the case of 2×2 matrices $(n = 2)$ from 1 to 2, and in the case of 3×3 matrices $(n = 3)$ from 1 to 3. Matrix multiplication is not commutative, that is, in general (and unlike the multiplication of normal numbers), the result depends on the sequence of factors in the matrix product, for example

(5.9) $$A \cdot B \neq B \cdot A$$

This property is of importance in the context of the description of rotation in three-dimensional space.

6 Translation and Rotation in a Plane

Describing body movements is a frequently occurring problem in orthopedic biomechanics. An example of such a motion is the forward bending of the trunk to grasp an object from the floor. At the beginning, the trunk is erect (initial state); at the end it is bent forward (final state). Other examples of movements are the relative motion of adjacent vertebrae while bending forward or the motion of the lower leg in relation to the upper leg when walking. The description of position and orientation is a geometrical problem, and beyond the simple level such problems are solved algebraically. Indeed, for measurements and calculations, especially in three dimensions, algebraic methods must be used. Initially, however, algebra can be dispensed with by analyzing the motion occurring in a plane graphically, using a pair of compasses and a ruler. This is the content of this chapter.

6.1 Graphical Description of Translation and Rotation

In two dimensions we are dealing with plane objects moving in a plane. It is assumed that the objects are rigid (that is, not deformable). This means that their shape and size (internal distances, angles) does not change under the influence of forces. The assumptions of bodies being rigid and movement being confined to a plane are model assumptions frequently used in orthopedic biomechanics. For example, the motion of the lower leg and thigh in walking can be described in the sagittal plane with these two assumptions in mind. In reality, however, the lower leg and thigh are not rigid bodies like the limbs of a puppet; they change their shape noticeably when moving.

To describe the motion of a rigid body in a plane it is not necessary to describe the motion of all points of the body; it is sufficient to describe the motion of two specific points on the body. In what follows, these points will be termed *landmarks*. This term is used because, in many practical applications, markers are affixed to the bodies to be observed. The markers are constructed so as to be clearly visible in film, video, or radiographic images. If two markers are fixed on a rigid body, a reference system is created. The location of all points of the body can be unequivocally specified in relation to this reference system. It follows that, if the location of the landmarks is known, the location of all other points of the body is known as well. For this reason, the description of plane motion of a rigid body may be confined to describing the motion of two landmarks.

6.1.1 Translation

A motion that moves all points of a body on straight lines over identical distances is termed *linear movement* or *translation*. In **Fig. 6.1** two markers P and Q are fixed to a body. The body is moved along a straight line. At the end of the motion the location of the markers is designated by P′ and Q′. Since, by definition, all points of the body have been moved along straight lines and over identical distances, the lines PP′ and QQ′ are parallel

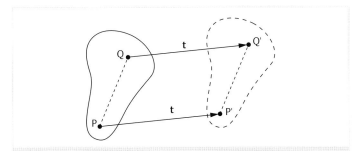

Fig. 6.1 Linear motion (translation) in a plane. To determine location and orientation of a body in a plane, knowledge of the location of at least two landmarks on the body is required. In this and the following figures, the solid outline designates the initial state of the body, and the dashed outline the final state. **t** is the translation vector.

and of equal length. Since the body was assumed to be rigid (that is, not deformable), the lines PQ and P'Q' are of equal length as well. It follows that the points P, P', Q', Q form the corners of a parallelogram. In other words, if the initial and the final state of the motion are known, and if the points P, P', Q', Q (in that order) form the corners of a parallelogram, the movement can be interpreted as a translation. **Fig. 6.1** shows the identical vectors PP' = **t** and QQ' = **t**. The magnitude and direction of **t** characterize the translation.

6.1.2 Rotation

A rotation is characterized by the fact that all points of a body move on concentric circles with the identical angle of rotation around a center of rotation. In **Fig. 6.2** the landmarks P and Q move along arcs of circles to P' and Q'. In **Fig. 6.2a** the center of rotation C is located within the boundary and in **Fig. 6.2b** it is located

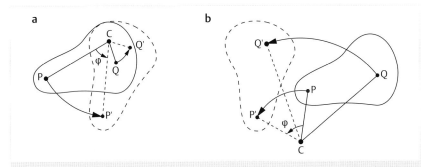

Fig. 6.2a, b Rotation in a plane. All points are rotated about the identical center of rotation C by the angle of rotation φ; the points move on arcs of concentric circles around the center of rotation.

a The center of rotation is located within the boundary of the body.

b The center of rotation is located outside the boundary of the body.

outside the boundary of the rotating body. In both cases the angle between the lines PQ and P′Q′ equals φ. The rotation has a direction; accordingly the angle of rotation may be positive or negative. A positive angle characterizes a counterclockwise rotation, a negative angle characterizes a clockwise rotation. A plane rotation is unequivocally specified by the location of the center of rotation and the angle of rotation.

If the initial and final states of the body are known, the position of the center of rotation and the angle of rotation may be reconstructed (**Fig. 6.3**). Points P and P′ and points Q and Q′ lie on arcs of circles around the (as yet unknown) center of rotation C. If lines PP′ and QQ′ are bisected perpendicularly, the center of rotation C is located at the intersection of these perpendicular bisectors (**Fig. 6.3a**). The assumption underlying this construction is that the perpendicular bisectors are differently orientated (they are not parallel). In the special case when they are orientated identically (they are parallel) (**Fig. 6.3b**), points P, Q, and the center of rotation C lie on a straight line. In this case the center of rotation C is given by the intersection of the lines PQ and P′Q′. In both cases the angle of rotation is given by the angle between the lines PQ and P′Q′.

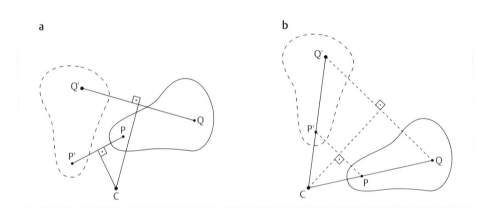

Fig. 6.3a, b Construction of the location of the center of rotation of a plane rotation.
a Standard case (nonparallel bisectors).
b Special case (parallel bisectors).

6.1.3 Combined Translation and Rotation

In general, a motion may combine translation and rotation. In the example given in **Fig. 6.4** the body is rotated in a first step around C by an angle φ in counterclockwise direction. Through this rotation, points P and Q are moved on arcs of circles to P′ and Q′. In a second step the body is moved along a straight line. The final locations of the landmarks are P″ and Q″. The translation is characterized by the translation vector $\mathbf{t} = Q'Q''$.

If the initial and final state of the motion are known, the angle of rotation φ can be obtained by rotating the body in the final state around an arbitrarily chosen center of rotation until the lines connecting the landmarks are parallel. In a second step a translation may be performed until the landmarks coincide.

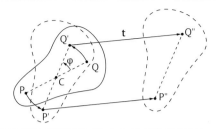

Fig. 6.4 Plane motion combining rotation and translation. In a first step the body is rotated through an angle φ around the center of rotation C; in a second step the body is translated as indicated by the translation vector **t**.

The translation vector thus obtained depends on the preceding choice of the location of the center of rotation; in general it is not identical with **t**. In other words: when describing a motion that combines rotation and translation, only the angle of rotation is unequivocally determined; the contribution of translational motion depends on the choice of the center of rotation.

For plane motions the following noteworthy theorem holds. Any motion resulting from a combination of translation and rotation can be described by a single rotation. This "substitute" rotation occurs around a center of rotation differing from the original center of rotation but with the identical angle of rotation φ. **Fig. 6.5** shows the body in the same initial and final state as in **Fig. 6.4**. The construction of the substitute center of rotation C_s is performed using the same rule as illustrated in **Fig. 6.3.**

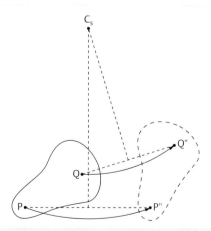

Fig. 6.5 Location of the substitute center of rotation C_s for the combined motion illustrated in **Fig. 6.4**. The location of the substitute center of rotation is constructed according to the rule illustrated in **Fig. 6.3a**.

The fact that an identical change of location of a body may be described either by a pure rotation or by a combination of translation and rotation emphasizes that the description of a motion provides no information about the actual path of the motion between the initial and the final state. In other words, if only the initial and the final location of a body are known, the actual motion between these locations may have varied considerably. Which description to choose in a given situation—a pure translation or a combination of translation and rotation—depends on the biomechanical model adopted. If, for example, a body is known to move around an axis (for example, the lower leg around the axis of the knee joint), the motion is likely to be described as a pure rotation. If translational or rotational movements are suspected to occur simultaneously or in sequence over time (for example, dorsoventral shift and rotation of a lumbar vertebra when bending forward), one can try to decompose the observed motion into a translational and a rotational part.

6.1.4 Error Influences when Describing a Motion

With small angles of rotation and increasing distance of the center of rotation from the body it becomes increasingly difficult to distinguish a rotation from a translational motion. In **Fig. 6.6** the translational motion is depicted by the vector $\mathbf{t}$ pointing from P to P'_t and the rotational motion by the arc b of the circle from P to P'_r. If the vector $\mathbf{t}$ is kept constant and the center of rotation C moves away from P, the radius r of the arc increases and the angle φ decreases. At the same time, arc b tends to coincide with the translation vector $\mathbf{t}$ and the distance d between the points P'_t and P'_r becomes smaller and smaller. If the center of rotation moves away to infinity, there will be no difference between rotational motion along the arc of the circle and translational motion.

The very small difference between translation and rotation in a case where the radius is large and the angle of rotation small dictates that caution must be used in interpreting measured data. Because measurement errors can never be avoided, a translation may be wrongly interpreted as a rotation. In general, therefore, it holds that the interpretation of a motion as rotation is reliable only if the center of rotation is located fairly close the body.

Inevitable measurement errors for the coordinates of landmarks, and the difficulty of discriminating between translation and rotation where angles of rotation are small, result in complications if an attempt is made to trace a motion very precisely by dividing its path into many small segments. Let us imagine a body that in reality moves along a smooth curve. Repeated measurement of the body's location at short intervals splits the path into segments. On average the direction of the segments follows the true curve, but due to measurement errors the direction of individual segments may deviate irregularly from the true (unknown) value. If an attempt were made to describe the motion in each segment of the path by a center and an angle of rotation, a large scatter would probably be found for the location of these centers. Since a zigzag curve

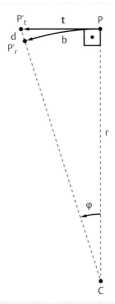

Fig. 6.6 Translation as limiting case of a rotation with the center of rotation shifted to infinity. Point P is shifted by the translation vector **t** to P'_t. b is the arc of a circle through P about the center of rotation C. The endpoint P'_r of the arc b is located together with point P'_t and C on a radius of the circle. With constant **t** and increasing r and decreasing φ, b adapts more and more to the translation vector **t** and the distance d between points P'_t and P'_r becomes smaller and smaller.

of an instantaneous center of rotation cannot be interpreted meaningfully, it is necessary in such cases to smooth the curve mathematically before describing the motion. However, one is now confronted with the problem of selecting a smoothing algorithm (that is, an appropriate mathematical procedure) that leaves the underlying, original curve unchanged.

6.2 Mathematical Description of Translation and Rotation in a Plane

6.2.1 Cartesian Coordinates

So far in this chapter, translation and rotation in a plane have been described in graphical mode, employing a pair of compasses and a ruler. This had allowed the basic concepts to come across vividly without the need to perform any calculations. If, however, the motion of more than a single object is to be monitored, or if high precision is required, it is advisable to use a coordinate-based calculation instead of attempting a graphic solution. This section introduces a simple concept (one that does not use vectors and matrices) for the mathematical description of motion in a plane. The last part of this chapter shows how all equations can be also formulated in matrix notation. Matrix notation is shorter and more to the point than coordinate notation.

If the motion of an object is documented, for example by a series of photographic images, geometric information extracted from the images has to be mathematically processed. Relations between each single image and the recording device (camera) on the one hand and between consecutive images on the other have to be established. For this purpose, coordinate systems are introduced. Within each image the location of an image point can be unequivocally described, for example by an (ordered) pair of numbers designating the distance of the point from the lower and left edges of the image. In this case the edges of the image represent the coordinate system; the distances are the relevant point coordinates.

To introduce a geometric reference system into what is, in principle, an infinitely extended plane, we draw a horizontal and a vertical line (**Fig. 6.7**). The intersecting lines form the xy-coordinate system. The horizontal axis (x-axis) is termed the *abscissa*; the vertical axis (y-axis) is termed the *ordinate*. The point of intersection is termed the *origin* of the coordinate system. The axes bear scales whose zero point coincides with the origin of the coordinate system. Positive values of the scales are plotted to the right or upwards, negative values are plotted to the left or downwards. The location of a point is described by its coordinates x,y. The coordinates are those scale values where a perpendicular from the point intersects the coordinate axes. In **Fig. 6.7** point P has the coordinates x = 2.3 and y = 3.7 (in units of the scales on the axes).

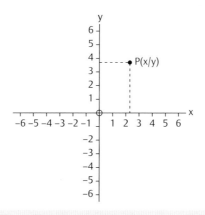

Fig. 6.7 Cartesian coordinate system in a plane.

6.2.2 Translation

A point P(x/y) is translated (**Fig. 6.8**). The shifted point is designated P′(x′/y′). In general, point P′ is designated the (geometric) *image* of point P; x′ and y′ are the image coordinates. Imaging is described by the

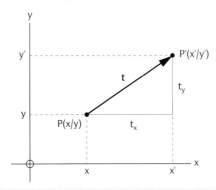

Fig. 6.8 Plane translation. A point P with coordinates x,y is linearly shifted by t_x in the x-direction, and by t_y in the y-direction, to its final location with coordinates x′,y′. P′(x′/y′) is termed the *image* of point P(x/y).

mathematical relation between the initial and the image coordinates. In the case of a translation the shifts t_x and t_y are to be added to the initial coordinates:

(6.1)
$$x' = x + t_x$$
$$y' = y + t_y$$

The shifts t_x and t_y may bear positive or negative signs. Conversely, with known coordinates for the initial point P(x/y) and the shifted point P′(x′/y′), the shifts t_x and t_y can be calculated:

(6.2)
$$t_x = x' - x$$
$$t_y = y' - y$$

6.2.3 Rotation

To describe a rotation, a center of rotation and an angle of rotation have to be specified. In the simplest case a rotation can occur around the origin of the coordinate system (**Fig. 6.9**). Let us consider point P(x/y). Its distance from the origin amounts to $r = \sqrt{x^2 + y^2}$. The line OP is inclined by an angle α with respect to the x-axis. For the coordinates of P it holds that

(6.3)
$$x = r \cdot \cos\alpha$$
$$y = r \cdot \sin\alpha$$

Angles are counted from −180° to +180°, or alternatively from 0° to +360°.

If point P is rotated by an angle φ, the image point P′ (x′/y′) is obtained. The line OP′ is inclined by an angle $\alpha + \varphi$ with respect to the x-axis. Similarly to Eq. 6.3, the coordinates x′,y′ of the image point are obtained from

(6.4)
$$x' = r \cdot \cos(\alpha + \varphi)$$
$$y' = r \cdot \sin(\alpha + \varphi)$$

95

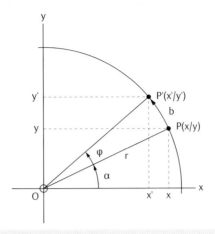

Fig. 6.9 Plane rotation of a point P(x/y) about the origin of the coordinate system. In the initial state the line OP is inclined by an angle α with respect to the x-axis. During the rotational motion the point moves along a circle with radius r = OP by an angle φ. After the rotation along the arc b to the final location P', the line OP' is inclined at an angle (α + φ) with respect to the x-axis. In this diagram as well as in the following ones, the arrowheads on the circular arcs show the direction of rotation. In the example shown, both α and φ are positive.

Using the addition formulae for sine and cosine functions

(6.5)
$$\cos(\alpha + \varphi) = \cos\alpha \cdot \cos\varphi - \sin\alpha \cdot \sin\varphi$$
$$\sin(\alpha + \varphi) = \sin\alpha \cdot \cos\varphi + \cos\alpha \cdot \sin\varphi$$

and employing Eq. 6.3, we obtain for the coordinates of the image point

(6.6)
$$x' = x \cdot \cos\varphi - y \cdot \sin\varphi$$
$$y' = x \cdot \sin\varphi + y \cdot \cos\varphi$$

In the general case a rotation is performed about a center of rotation $C(x_m/y_m)$ (**Fig. 6.10**). The general case can be reduced to that of a rotation about the origin (described above) by introducing an additional uv-coordinate system at point C. This coordinate system is shifted parallel with respect to the xy-coordinate system by x_m in x-direction and by y_m in y-direction. The coordinates u and v are given by the differences

(6.7)
$$u = x - x_m$$
$$v = y - y_m$$

If a rotation is performed in the uv-system, the coordinates of the image point P' read

(6.8)
$$u' = u \cdot \cos\varphi - v \cdot \sin\varphi$$
$$v' = u \cdot \sin\varphi + v \cdot \cos\varphi$$

In a last step a return is made to the xy-system by replacing the u,v with the x,y-based Eq. 6.7 and thus obtaining the image coordinates

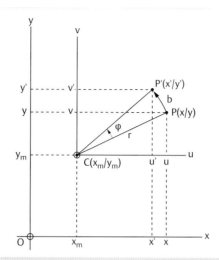

Fig. 6.10 Plane rotation of a point P(x/y) about an arbitrary center of rotation $C(x_m/y_m)$. The point moves along a circle with radius $r = CP$ about an angle φ. By introducing relative coordinates $u = x-x_m$, $v = y-y_m$, this case is reduced to the case illustrated in **Fig. 6.9**.

(6.9)
$$x' = x_m + (x - x_m) \cdot \cos\varphi - (y - y_m) \cdot \sin\varphi$$
$$y' = y_m + (x - x_m) \cdot \sin\varphi + (y - y_m) \cdot \cos\varphi$$

6.2.4 Combined Translation and Rotation

With a given center of rotation $C(x_m/y_m)$, point P is rotated in a first step by an angle φ (**Fig. 6.11**). The intermediate image, calculated using Eq. 6.9, is designated P′(x′/y′). In a second step P′ is shifted to the final location P″(x″/y″). The coordinates of the final image (both steps combined) are

(6.10)
$$x'' = x_m + (x - x_m) \cdot \cos\varphi - (y - y_m) \cdot \sin\varphi + t_x$$
$$y'' = y_m + (x - x_m) \cdot \sin\varphi + (y - y_m) \cdot \cos\varphi + t_y$$

The formulae in Eq. 6.10 can be rewritten as

(6.11)
$$x'' = x \cdot \cos\varphi - y \cdot \sin\varphi + a_x$$
$$y'' = x \cdot \sin\varphi + y \cdot \cos\varphi + a_y$$

with

(6.12)
$$a_x = x_m - x_m \cdot \cos\varphi + y_m \cdot \sin\varphi + t_x$$
$$a_y = y_m - x_m \cdot \sin\varphi - y_m \cdot \cos\varphi + t_y$$

Eq. 6.11 describes the general case of plane motion, that is, rotation about an arbitrary center of rotation $C(x_m/y_m)$ by an angle φ and translation by t_x, t_y, algebraically in the simplest fashion. From a formal point

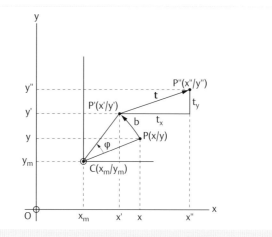

Fig. 6.11 Motion combining translation and rotation. Point P(x/y) is rotated about the center of rotation $C(x_m/y_m)$ by an angle φ to point P'(x'/y'). P' is then shifted by t_x, t_y to point P''(x''/y''). t_x and t_y define the translation vector **t**.

of view, Eq. 6.11 can also be interpreted as a description of a rotation about the origin of the coordinate system and a subsequent translation by a_x, a_y. Eqs. 6.11 and 6.12 comprise the special cases of pure translation and pure rotation.

According to the theorem mentioned above (see Section 6.1.3), that a motion combining rotation and translation can always also be represented by a pure rotation (that is, by a motion without a translation component), the parameters of this rotation should be deducible from Eq. 6.11. Unlike the graphical solution to this problem, the algebraic determination of the location of the center of rotation is not based on the construction of the perpendicular bisectors. Another algorithm (path of calculation) is better suited which makes use of the knowledge that, in a pure rotation, the center of rotation is the only point which does not move. Such a point is termed the *fixed point* of the image. Its coordinates may be denoted x_F and y_F. As the coordinates of the fixed point are not changed (that is, they remain identical after the imaging procedure to what they were before), it holds that

(6.13)
$$x_F = x_F \cdot \cos\varphi - y_F \cdot \sin\varphi + a_x$$
$$y_F = x_F \cdot \sin\varphi + y_F \cdot \cos\varphi + a_y$$

With a known angle of rotation φ, center of rotation x_m, y_m, and translation t_x, t_y, the coordinates x_F, y_F of the fixed point can be determined from Eq. 6.13. The intermediate steps of the simple but somewhat lengthy conversion are omitted here; only the final outcome is stated

(6.14)
$$x_F = (a_x - a_y \cdot \cot(\varphi/2))/2$$
$$y_F = (a_y + a_x \cdot \cot(\varphi/2))/2$$

6.2.5 Determining the Imaging Parameters from Two Points and Their Images

We assume the coordinates of two points (x,y) and (x'',y'') to be known. The task is to determine the imaging parameters. For this purpose, Eq. 6.11 is employed. The imaging parameters are the angle of rotation φ and the translations a_x, a_y. (The information on the intermediate image in the uv-coordinate system [see Eqs. 6.8 and 6.9] is lost and cannot be retrieved in retrospect.)

The three parameters cannot be determined from one single point and its image because only two equations are available. If, however, coordinates of two points and their images are available, the number of equations suffices to determine three unknowns. The calculation starts by inserting the coordinates of points $P(x_1/y_1)$, $Q(x_2/y_2)$ and their images $P'(x'_1/y'_1)$, $Q'(x'_2/y'_2)$ into Eq. 6.11, thus obtaining four equations:

(6.15)
$$x'_1 = x_1 \cdot \cos\varphi - y_1 \cdot \sin\varphi + a_x$$
$$y'_1 = x_1 \cdot \sin\varphi + y_1 \cdot \cos\varphi + a_y$$
$$x'_2 = x_2 \cdot \cos\varphi - y_2 \cdot \sin\varphi + a_x$$
$$y'_2 = x_2 \cdot \sin\varphi + y_2 \cdot \cos\varphi + a_y$$

(The double prime marks in Eq. 6.11 are replaced by single prime marks.) In a first step the angle of rotation is determined by calculating the differences between the coordinates:

(6.16)
$$x'_2 - x'_1 = (x_2 - x_1) \cdot \cos\varphi - (y_2 - y_1) \cdot \sin\varphi$$
$$y'_2 - y'_1 = (x_2 - x_1) \cdot \sin\varphi + (y_2 - y_1) \cdot \cos\varphi$$

This yields an equation for the tangent of the angle of rotation:

(6.17)
$$\tan\varphi = Z/N$$
$$\varphi = \text{atan}(Z/N)$$

with

(6.18)
$$Z = (x_2 - x_1) \cdot (y'_2 - y'_1) - (y_2 - y_1) \cdot (x'_2 - x'_1)$$
$$N = (x_2 - x_1) \cdot (x'_2 - x'_1) + (y_2 - y_1) \cdot (y'_2 - y'_1)$$

If the angle φ equals zero, the motion is considered a pure translation. In this case it holds (as both points translate by the same amount) that

(6.19)
$$x'_1 - x_1 = x'_2 - x_2$$
$$y'_1 - y_1 = y'_2 - y_2$$

In a second step, with a known angle of rotation, parameters a_x and a_y can be determined from Eq. 6.11. For this purpose we insert the coordinates of one point (either of the two points) into this equation. By choosing point P and its image P' we obtain

(6.20)
$$a_x = x'_1 - x_1 \cdot \cos\varphi + y_1 \cdot \sin\varphi$$
$$a_y = y'_1 - x_1 \cdot \sin\varphi - y_1 \cdot \cos\varphi$$

As a result, all parameters of the motion (the imaging) are known from Eqs. 6.17 and 6.20. If the motion is to be represented by a pure rotation, the coordinates of the relevant center of rotation can be calculated from Eq. 6.14, the angle of rotation φ being identical in each case.

The following example may serve to illustrate the relation between calculation and geometrical interpretation. In the case of a combined translational and rotational motion, calculating the center and radius of the substitute rotation using the coordinates of the "fixed point" is not always required. If the initial and final points P and P' as well as the magnitude and sign of the angle of rotation of a motion are known, the radius and center of rotation may be obtained by an elementary calculation (**Fig. 6.12**). The distance between P and P' (that is, the length of the chord) is designated s. With M being the center of the circle and T the midpoint of the chord s, it holds for the distance h between them that

(6.21)
$$h = s / (2 \cdot |\cot(\varphi/2)|)$$

The radius of the circle (that is, the distance MP) is calculated from

(6.22)
$$R = s / (2 \cdot |\sin(\varphi/2)|)$$

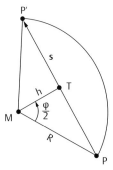

Fig. 6.12 Determination of the midpoint of a circle from the rotation of a point P to P' and the angle of rotation φ. If the angle φ is positive, the midpoint of the circle is located to the left of the chord vector **s** (directed from P to P') at a distance h from its midpoint.

The position of the center M of the circle depends on the direction in which the chord s is constructed and on the direction of rotation of the angle φ. With **s** as the vector of the chord pointing from P to P′ and a positive (counterclockwise) angle of rotation, the center of rotation M is positioned to the left of the vector **s** (**Fig. 6.12**); with a negative angle of rotation it is positioned to the right of the vector **s** (**Fig. 6.13**).

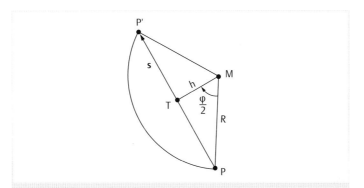

Fig. 6.13 Determination of the midpoint of a circle from the rotation of a point P to P′ and the angle of rotation φ. If the angle φ is negative, the midpoint of the circle is located to the right of the chord vector **s** at a distance h from its midpoint (the magnitude of φ and the lengths are as in **Fig. 6.12**).

6.2.6 Matrix Notation

Matrix and vector notation is frequently employed for a simplified, symbolic description of translation and rotation. Points are represented by their radius vectors. In this notation a translation (Eq. 6.1) is described by

(6.23)
$$\begin{bmatrix} x' \\ y' \end{bmatrix} = \begin{bmatrix} x \\ y \end{bmatrix} + \begin{bmatrix} t_x \\ t_y \end{bmatrix} = \begin{bmatrix} x+t_x \\ y+t_y \end{bmatrix}$$

In this notation the two equations presented as Eq. 6.1 are symbolically combined into one. A rotation about the origin of the coordinate system (Eq. 6.6) is described in matrix notation by

(6.24)
$$\begin{bmatrix} x' \\ y' \end{bmatrix} = \begin{bmatrix} \cos\varphi & -\sin\varphi \\ \sin\varphi & \cos\varphi \end{bmatrix} \cdot \begin{bmatrix} x \\ y \end{bmatrix}$$

In this notation the columns represent the radius vectors before and after the rotation. The matrix describing a rotation in a plane is composed of the matrix elements $M_{11} = \cos\varphi$, $M_{12} = -\sin\varphi$, $M_{21} = -M_{12}$, $M_{22} = M_{11}$. In the following this matrix is designated by the bold letter **D**:

(6.25)
$$\mathbf{D} = \begin{bmatrix} \cos\varphi & -\sin\varphi \\ \sin\varphi & \cos\varphi \end{bmatrix}$$

The description of a rotation about a center of rotation x_m, y_m (Eq. 6.9) reads in matrix notation

(6.26)
$$\begin{bmatrix} x' \\ y' \end{bmatrix} = \begin{bmatrix} x_m \\ y_m \end{bmatrix} + \begin{bmatrix} \cos\varphi & -\sin\varphi \\ \sin\varphi & \cos\varphi \end{bmatrix} \cdot \begin{bmatrix} x - x_m \\ y - y_m \end{bmatrix}$$

The description of a motion composed of rotation and translation (Eq. 6.10) reads

(6.27)
$$\begin{bmatrix} x' \\ y' \end{bmatrix} = \begin{bmatrix} x_m \\ y_m \end{bmatrix} + \begin{bmatrix} \cos\varphi & -\sin\varphi \\ \sin\varphi & \cos\varphi \end{bmatrix} \cdot \begin{bmatrix} x - x_m \\ y - y_m \end{bmatrix} + \begin{bmatrix} t_x \\ t_y \end{bmatrix}$$

Using the abbreviations

(6.28)
$$\mathbf{r} = \begin{bmatrix} x \\ y \end{bmatrix}, \quad \mathbf{r}' = \begin{bmatrix} x' \\ y' \end{bmatrix}, \quad \mathbf{r}'' = \begin{bmatrix} x'' \\ y'' \end{bmatrix}, \quad \mathbf{r}_m = \begin{bmatrix} x_m \\ y_m \end{bmatrix}, \quad \mathbf{t} = \begin{bmatrix} t_x \\ t_y \end{bmatrix}$$

the above equations can be written in an even more condensed format:

Translation:

(6.29)
$$\mathbf{r}' = \mathbf{r} + \mathbf{t}$$

Rotation about the origin:

(6.30)
$$\mathbf{r}' = \mathbf{D} \cdot \mathbf{r}$$

Rotation about a center $\mathbf{r}_m$:

(6.31)
$$\mathbf{r}' = \mathbf{r}_m + \mathbf{D} \cdot (\mathbf{r} - \mathbf{r}_m)$$

Rotation about a center $\mathbf{r}_m$ plus translation:

(6.32)
$$\mathbf{r}'' = \mathbf{r}_m + \mathbf{D} \cdot (\mathbf{r} - \mathbf{r}_m) + \mathbf{t}$$

7 Mathematical Description of Translation and Rotation in Three-Dimensional Space

Describing translation and rotation in three-dimensional space poses mathematical difficulties, and visualizing it is certainly anything but straightforward. In some parts of orthopedic biomechanics, especially in the field of research, we cannot (unfortunately) talk our way around these difficulties. Here are three examples:

Example 1: We wish to document the motion of the upper arm in relation to the trunk. This can be achieved using a commercially available device in which a sensor receives the magnetic field emitted by a spatially fixed transmitter located in the laboratory. The sensor is attached to a person's upper arm (**Fig. 7.1**). From the data received, the position and orientation of the $x_a y_a z_a$-coordinate system of the arm is determined relative to the $x_s y_s z_s$-coordinate system (*space-fixed coordinate system*) of the fixed transmitter. A second sensor is fixed on the trunk such that its orientation coincides with the $x_b y_b z_b$-coordinate system, which relates to the body (*body-fixed coordinate system*). To obtain a description of the motion, the data measured in the $x_s y_s z_s$-coordinate system have to be transformed into the translated and rotated $x_b y_b z_b$ system.

Example 2: In the context of developing artificial joint replacements for the ankle joint, the question to be considered is which rotations actually determine the observed motion of the hind foot. The ankle joint and the subtalar joint are assumed to function like hinged joints with fixed axes. The axes of these joints are, however, not parallel (**Fig. 7.2**). While the axis of the ankle joint in erect stance is approximately horizontal, the axis of the subtalar joint runs obliquely from dorsally downwards to ventrally upwards. The question that arises is whether the rotation of the hind foot about the long axis of the foot can be explained by rotations about these two axes. The theory of three-dimensional rotations states that, in general, unlimited rotational motion can be achieved by combined rotations about three differently oriented axes, or by a single rotation about an axis with unrestricted orientation. If, as is the case here, the directions of two axes are fixed, it follows that rotations about these two axes will not enable all movements to take place.

In fact, the rotation of the hindfoot discussed here requires, in addition to rotation about the ankle and subtalar axes, simultaneous rotation about the long axis of the tibia. This rotation can be effected by rotating the whole tibia or by a "loose fit" of the ankle joint. Combined rotations about these three axes now permit all rotations, as in a ball-and-socket joint. The range of motion in different directions is, however, limited because the participating joints have only small ranges of motion. In addition, due to the muscle attachments and ligamentous connections, rotations about the individual axes cannot be performed independently. The resulting composite motion thus bears some analogy to the motion of a gear box.

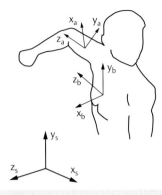

Fig. 7.1 Position and orientation of the $x_a y_a z_a$-coordinate system are measured in the space-fixed $x_s y_s z_s$ system. To describe the movement of the upper arm, the data are transformed into the body-fixed $x_b y_b z_b$ system.

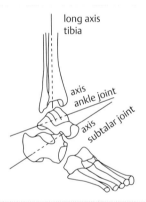

Fig. 7.2 Axes of rotation contributing to the motion of the hindfoot: axis of the ankle joint, axis of the subtalar joint, and long axis of the tibia. (Adapted from Debrunner and Jacob.[1])

Example 3: Fig. 7.3a shows a lumbar vertebra with a body-fixed xyz-coordinate system. In schematic fashion, **Fig. 7.3b** shows the contours of the vertebra as seen in an anteroposterior radiographic view, with the normally shaped vertebra in its physiologic position and orientation. The contours of the vertebral body and the outlines of the insertion of the pedicles are clearly visible. **Fig. 7.3c** shows, again schematically, the contours of a vertebra of a scoliotic spine in the anteroposterior radiographic view. With the three-dimensional shape of a vertebra in mind, we recognize qualitatively that, in relation to **Fig. 7.3b**, the vertebra is now tilted sideways and forwards. In addition, it appears to be axially rotated. We conclude this from the asymmetric location of the pedicle outlines with respect to the contours of the vertebral body.

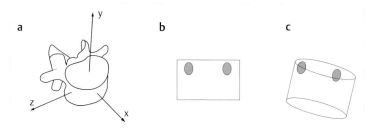

Fig. 7.3a–c Rotation about body-fixed axes illustrated by the example of a vertebra. (Adapted from Drerup.[2])

a Body-fixed xyz-coordinate system of a lumbar vertebra.

b Schematic drawing of a vertebral body in normal, anatomical orientation in an anteroposterior radiograph.

c Schematic drawing of a vertebral body of a scoliotic spine in an anteroposterior radiograph.

How can we best characterize this pathologic deviation from the normal orientation? To achieve a clear picture, it is an advantage to agree on a sequence of the rotations about the three body-fixed axes. For this purpose, it is assumed that the vertebra is rotated first about its x-axis (tilted sideways). It is then rotated about its z-axis (tilted forwards).[2] Finally, it is rotated about its y-axis. This last rotation, the one known as *vertebral rotation*, is the parameter of primary medical interest, because the deformation of the trunk of scoliosis patients seems to be due essentially to vertebral rotation.

It is pointed out that not only is this description based on three rotations on body-fixed axes (that is, axes which move with the rotated body), but the sequence of the rotations is of importance as well. For small angles, the effect of changing the sequence is only minor (this is also true mathematically), but for larger angles the effect will be noticeable. We suggest that the reader might like to make a paper model of the upper endplate of a vertebra, rotate this model through 90° about the z- and x-axes, and then in reverse order about the x- and z-axes, and observe the difference in the outcome.

If a rotation sequence differing from that proposed above were chosen—for example, first the vertebral rotation and then the forward and sideways tilt—a different set of angles of rotation would be required to move the vertebra from its position in **Fig. 7.3b** to the final position in **Fig. 7.3c**. Specifically, the vertebral rotation would assume a different value. The same holds for other possible sequences of the three rotations. Which one, then, is the true value of the vertebral rotation?[3] The answer is that all values are equally true (with respect to the rotation sequence selected). To make a choice, we should rather ask, "Which sequence of rotations is the most sensible?" Here the answer definitely has to be, "That proposed above." Any other sequence would result in the magnitude of the vertebral rotation measured from the radiograph depending on the forward and lateral tilt of the vertebra. This would probably not be a sensible way to describe the geometry of the scoliotic spine.

The above examples include coordinate transformations, combined rotations, the theorem of the sequence dependence of three-dimensional rotations, and criteria for the choice of rotation sequences. The aim of this chapter is to give the reader an overview of the mathematical description of changes of position and orientation in space. It is intended as an aid to understanding biomechanical research papers, but it cannot replace studying a textbook of analytical geometry. Introductory sections on coordinates, vectors, coordinate transformations, translations, and rotations are followed by an explanation of how (in principle) the parameters describing a motion are obtained from the measured position of reference points in the initial and final state. Calculation of the motion of bodies under the influence of forces and moments is not treated here; it lies outside the scope of this book and readers are referred to textbooks on theoretical mechanics.

7.1 Coordinates and Vectors

To describe the location of points in space, a three-dimensional, right-handed coordinate system is introduced. Its axes are in pairs perpendicular to each other; the axes are designated according to the right hand rule (Chapter 4, **Fig. 4.14**) as x (in the direction of the thumb), y (direction of the index finger), and z (direction of the middle finger of the right hand). The intersection of the axes is termed the *origin* of the coordinate system. To describe the location of a point A, three numbers (coordinates) x_A, y_A, z_A must be specified: $A(x_A / y_A / z_A)$. The spatial location of the point can be illustrated by a rectangular parallelepiped with side lengths x_A, y_A, z_A measured from the origin of the coordinate system. The point A is located on the spatial diagonal of the parallelepiped opposite the origin O (**Fig. 7.4**). For a point B, an auxiliary point with coordinates $x_B, y_B, 0$ is constructed in the xy-plane. The point $B(x_B / y_B / z_B)$ is located above this point at a distance z_B. There is a close relation between pairs of points and vectors. It holds that for each pair of points A and B there exists exactly one vector **v**. This vector is illustrated by an arrow beginning at A and ending with its arrowhead at B (**Fig. 7.4**). The vector from B to A is in the opposite direction to that of the vector from A to B and is designated by −**v**.

Unit vectors in the direction of the coordinate axes (**Fig. 7.5**) are defined as follows

(7.1)
$$\begin{aligned} \mathbf{e}_x &= \text{vector, directed from } O(0/0/0) \text{ to } P_1 \ (1/0/0) \\ \mathbf{e}_y &= \text{vector, directed from } O(0/0/0) \text{ to } P_2 \ (0/1/0) \\ \mathbf{e}_z &= \text{vector, directed from } O(0/0/0) \text{ to } P_3 \ (0/0/1) \end{aligned}$$

$O(0/0/0)$ designates the origin of the coordinate system. The length of the unit vectors is one. The unit vectors are in pairs, oriented perpendicular to each other. Any vector **v** can be represented by

(7.2)
$$\mathbf{v} = \mathbf{v}_x + \mathbf{v}_y + \mathbf{v}_z = v_x \cdot \mathbf{e}_x + v_y \cdot \mathbf{e}_y + v_z \cdot \mathbf{e}_z$$

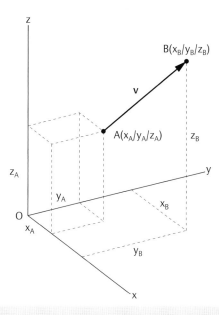

Fig. 7.4 Location of points and related vectors in a Cartesian coordinate system. Points are specified by three coordinates. Illustration of the location of a point by a rectangular parallelepiped (point A) or by three specified edges of a parallelepiped (point B). A vector **v** is assigned to a pair of points A,B (in this order) and depicted as an arrow pointing from A to B.

The reader should note the different notation in Eq. 7.2. $\mathbf{v}_x$ is a component of vector **v** (that is, a vector); v_x is its coordinate with respect to $\mathbf{e}_x$ (that is, a number). The same holds for the y- and z-components. The numbers v_x, v_y, v_z apply only with respect to the base $\mathbf{e}_x, \mathbf{e}_y, \mathbf{e}_z$. If the coordinate system is changed, these numbers will change as well. Using the three unit vectors, it is possible according to Eq. 7.2 to reach any point in three-dimensional space. In mathematical terms, the three unit vectors form a base and span the three-dimensional space. As unit vectors have length one and are perpendicular to each other (in mathematical terms, orthogonal to each other), such a base is termed *orthonormal*. The scalar product of two vectors **a** and **b** is written as

(7.3)
$$\mathbf{a} \cdot \mathbf{b} = a_x \cdot b_x + a_y \cdot b_y + a_z \cdot b_z$$

Using unit vectors, the vector product is written as

(7.4)
$$\mathbf{a} \times \mathbf{b} = (a_y b_z - b_y \cdot a_z) \cdot \mathbf{e}_x + (a_z \cdot b_x - b_z \cdot a_x) \cdot \mathbf{e}_y + (a_x \cdot b_y - b_x \cdot a_y) \cdot \mathbf{e}_z$$

To illustrate the relation between point coordinates and vectors, we observe a point P(x/y/z) and a vector **r** pointing from the origin of the coordinate system O(0/0/0) to the point P. Vectors originating from the

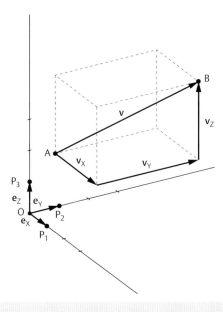

Fig. 7.5 Unit vectors in the direction of the coordinate axes and representation of a vector by the sum of its components. Unit vectors $\mathbf{e}_x, \mathbf{e}_y, \mathbf{e}_z$ are vectors of length 1 pointing from the origin O of the coordinate system in the direction of the coordinate axes. Using the unit vectors, a vector $\mathbf{v}$ is decomposed into three components $\mathbf{v}_x, \mathbf{v}_y, \mathbf{v}_z$ parallel to the coordinate axes. For the purpose of illustration, the vector $\mathbf{v}$ (pointing from A to B) is depicted as a spatial diagonal of a rectangular parallelepiped with side lengths v_x, v_y, v_z. The vector components $\mathbf{v}_x = v_x \cdot \mathbf{e}_x, \mathbf{v}_y = v_y \cdot \mathbf{e}_y, \mathbf{v}_z = v_z \cdot \mathbf{e}_z$ of vector $\mathbf{v}$ point along the edges of the parallelepiped.

origin of the coordinate system are designated *radius vectors*. In the following, such vectors are (usually) designated by the symbol $\mathbf{r}$. A radius vector $\mathbf{r}$ can be decomposed (**Fig. 7.6**)

(7.5) $$\mathbf{r} = x \cdot \mathbf{e}_x + y \cdot \mathbf{e}_y + z \cdot \mathbf{e}_z$$

It can be seen that the coordinates x,y,z of a radius vector are identical with the point coordinates of its end point. Conversely, the coordinates of a radius vector are obtained by scalar multiplication by the unit vectors (for example: $x = \mathbf{r} \cdot \mathbf{e}_x$).

7.2 Coordinate Transformations

The transformation of point coordinates from one coordinate system to another is a frequent task when evaluating experimental data. In gait analysis, for example, the coordinates of reference points measured in the laboratory system by means of film or video sequences must be converted to a reference system

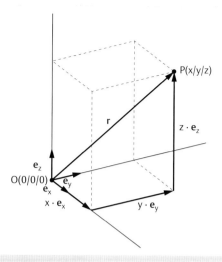

Fig. 7.6 Definition of the radius vector **r**. A vector pointing from the coordinate origin O(0/0/0) to a point P(x/y/z) is called a radius vector. There is an unequivocal relation between point coordinates x,y,z and vector components: $v_x = x \cdot e_x$, $v_y = y \cdot e_y$, $v_z = z \cdot e_z$.

imagined to be fixed to the skeleton of the test person. The laboratory system may be designated by xyz and the body reference system by uvw. The location of a point P(u/v/w) in the body reference system is described by the radius vector $\mathbf{p} = u \cdot \mathbf{e}_u + v \cdot \mathbf{e}_v + w \cdot \mathbf{e}_w$ (**Fig. 7.7**). We imagine the body reference system to be embedded into the laboratory system. In the laboratory system the origin of the reference system is given by the radius vector $\mathbf{r}_m = x_m \cdot \mathbf{e}_x + y_m \cdot \mathbf{e}_y + z_m \cdot \mathbf{e}_z$. The location of P(x/y/z) is to be expressed by the coordinates u,v,w. In the laboratory system the radius vector belonging to point P is given by the vector equation $\mathbf{r} = \mathbf{r}_m + \mathbf{p}$. In full

$$(7.6) \qquad \mathbf{r} = (x \cdot \mathbf{e}_x + y \cdot \mathbf{e}_y + z \cdot \mathbf{e}_z) = (x_m \cdot \mathbf{e}_x + y_m \cdot \mathbf{e}_y + z_m \cdot \mathbf{e}_z) + (u \cdot \mathbf{e}_u + v \cdot \mathbf{e}_v + w \cdot \mathbf{e}_w)$$

After some intermediate calculation (not detailed here) a set of transformation equations is obtained for the coordinates:

$$(7.7) \qquad \begin{aligned} x &= x_m + C_{11} \cdot u + C_{12} \cdot v + C_{13} \cdot w \\ y &= y_m + C_{21} \cdot u + C_{22} \cdot v + C_{23} \cdot w \\ z &= z_m + C_{31} \cdot u + C_{32} \cdot v + C_{33} \cdot w \end{aligned}$$

The coefficients C_{ik} in these equations are the scalar products of the unit vectors in the xyz and uvw systems. The value of the scalar products corresponds to the cosine of the angle between the coordinate axes of the two systems. For example, the coefficient C_{31} equals the cosine of the angle between the unit vectors $\mathbf{e}_z$ and $\mathbf{e}_u$: $C_{31} = \mathbf{e}_z \cdot \mathbf{e}_u$. The orientation of each unit vector in one system is defined by three *direction cosines* with respect to the three unit vectors of the other system. Due to the unit length and orthogonality of the

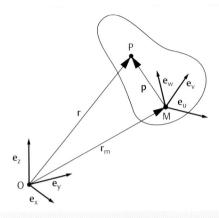

Fig. 7.7 Changing the coordinate system. A point P may be defined in the xyz-coordinate system (origin O; unit vectors e_x, e_y, e_z) or in the uvw-coordinate system (origin M; unit vectors e_u, e_v, e_w). The relative location of the coordinate systems is described by the vector $\mathbf{r}_m$ (pointing from O to M). The relative orientation is given by the set of direction cosines. The location of a point P may be described either by the vector $\mathbf{p}$ (in the uvw system) or by the vector $\mathbf{r}$ (in the xyz system). The (vector-) relation $\mathbf{r} = \mathbf{r}_m + \mathbf{p}$ exists between these vectors. If the u,v,w-coordinates of point P are to be transformed to x,y,z-coordinates, the uvw-unit vectors in the vector equation $\mathbf{p} = u \cdot \mathbf{e}_u + v \cdot \mathbf{e}_v + w \cdot \mathbf{e}_w$ have to be expressed by the xyz-unit vectors using the set of direction cosines.

unit vectors, there are six constraints on the nine direction cosines. Thus, we are left with three independent parameters describing the transformation. The transformation equation (Eq. 7.7) can be written in column and matrix notation:

$$(7.8) \qquad \begin{bmatrix} x \\ y \\ z \end{bmatrix} = \begin{bmatrix} x_m \\ y_m \\ z_m \end{bmatrix} + \begin{bmatrix} C_{11} & C_{12} & C_{13} \\ C_{21} & C_{22} & C_{23} \\ C_{31} & C_{32} & C_{33} \end{bmatrix} \cdot \begin{bmatrix} u \\ v \\ w \end{bmatrix}$$

The following description of rotations in space reveals a close relationship between rotations and coordinate transformations. Coordinate transformations leave the objects unchanged but describe their location and orientation in a rotated (and possibly translated) coordinate system. Conversely, if the relative spatial location and orientation of two coordinate systems is known, for example from a measurement, the relative translation of the two systems and the nine coefficients C_{ik} in Eq. 7.8 can be calculated. The coefficients C_{ik} contain all the information on the relative rotation between the two coordinate systems.

If the vector **p** is to be represented in the uvw system, the equation corresponding to Eq. 7.8 reads

(7.9)
$$\begin{bmatrix} u \\ v \\ w \end{bmatrix} = \begin{bmatrix} F_{11} & F_{12} & F_{13} \\ F_{21} & F_{22} & F_{23} \\ F_{31} & F_{32} & F_{33} \end{bmatrix} \cdot \begin{bmatrix} x - x_m \\ y - y_m \\ z - z_m \end{bmatrix}$$

There is a close relation between matrices **F** and **C**. **F** is derived from **C** by interchanging rows and columns: $F_{ik} = C_{ki}$. **F** is designated the *transpose* of **C**.

(7.10)
$$\mathbf{F} = \mathbf{C}^t \quad (\text{also}: \mathbf{C}^T, \mathbf{C}', \mathbf{C}^+)$$

If the vector

(7.11)
$$\begin{bmatrix} x - x_m \\ y - y_m \\ z - z_m \end{bmatrix}$$

from Eq. 7.8 is substituted in Eq. 7.9, it holds that

(7.12)
$$\begin{bmatrix} u \\ v \\ w \end{bmatrix} = \mathbf{F} \cdot \mathbf{C} \cdot \begin{bmatrix} u \\ v \\ w \end{bmatrix}$$

This is an identity. It means that the matrix product must equal the unit matrix **E** (also designated in the literature by **I**, the *identity matrix*).

(7.13)
$$\mathbf{F} \cdot \mathbf{C} = \mathbf{C}^t \cdot \mathbf{C} = \mathbf{E}$$

A matrix for which the relation $\mathbf{C}^t \cdot \mathbf{C} = \mathbf{E}$ is fulfilled is designated *orthogonal*. This means that the scalar product of two columns of the matrix **C** equals zero (orthogonality of column vectors) and the scalar product of a column with itself equals one (scaling of column vectors). The geometrical implication of orthogonal matrices is that coordinate transformations with orthogonal matrices leave the lengths of vectors and the angles between them unchanged. In other words, such transformations preserve the size and shape of the objects.

7.3 Translation in Three-Dimensional Space

The motion of a point in a given coordinate system is considered here. A translation (motion along a straight line) shifts a point P(x/y/z) by the translation vector **t** to point P′(x′/y′/z′). The radius vectors from O to P and from O to P′ are designated by **r** and **r′** (**Fig. 7.8**). It holds that

(7.14)
$$\mathbf{r}' = \mathbf{r} + \mathbf{t}$$

or in column notation

(7.15)
$$\begin{bmatrix} x' \\ y' \\ z' \end{bmatrix} = \begin{bmatrix} x \\ y \\ z \end{bmatrix} + \begin{bmatrix} t_x \\ t_y \\ t_z \end{bmatrix}$$

111

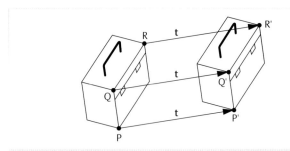

Fig. 7.8 Translation in three dimensions. A rigid body (suitcase) moves parallel to itself. A point P of the body moves to the point P' (difference vector **t**). The movement is a (pure) translation if the difference vectors PP', QQ', RR' of three points P, Q, R, which are not aligned on a line, are equal and identical with **t**. (Coordinate origin and radius vectors are not shown in this diagram.)

A translation in a plane, like translation in three-dimensional space, leaves the orientation of a body unchanged. All points are shifted by an identical distance along parallel lines. If two or more translations are performed consecutively, the result does not depend on the sequence of the translations.

7.4 Rotation in Three-Dimensional Space

While translations in three-dimensional space are, in principle, quite similar to translations in a plane, rotations in three dimensions exhibit new, unexpected properties. One such property is that, if several rotations are performed consecutively, the sequence of the rotations is of importance: that is, identical rotations performed one after the other will yield different results depending on the order in which they are performed.

7.4.1 Single Rotations About the Coordinate Axes

A rotation in three-dimensional space is described by specifying an axis and an angle of rotation. An axis is described by its three-dimensional orientation and location. According to the direction of rotation, the angle of rotation is counted as positive (counterclockwise) or negative (clockwise). A rotation leaves all points on the axis unchanged; all other points move on circular arcs in planes oriented perpendicular to the axis. **Fig. 7.9** illustrates this with a rotation about the z-axis of the coordinate system. This rotation moves an arbitrary point P(x/y/z) in a plane located at a distance z from the xy-plane. The point moves along an arc with radius $R = \sqrt{x^2 + y^2}$ and angle γ. The center of the circle is located on the z-axis. This rotation changes the x- and y-coordinates; the z-coordinate is left unchanged. This permits the formulae describing rotation in a plane to be adopted for x and y.

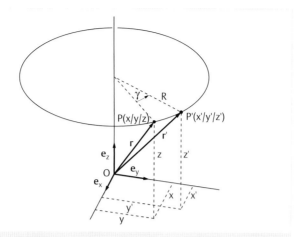

Fig. 7.9 Rotation of a point about the z-axis. The point P(x/y/z) moves, in a plane parallel to and located at a distance z from the xy-plane, along a circular arc through an angle of rotation γ to P'(x'/y'/z'). The related radius vector **r** moves on the surface of a cone with its tip at O, height = z, and radius $R = \sqrt{x^2 + y^2}$.

(7.16)
$$x' = \cos\gamma \cdot x - \sin\gamma \cdot y$$
$$y' = \sin\gamma \cdot x + \cos\gamma \cdot y$$
$$z' = z$$

These equations can also be written as

(7.17)
$$\mathbf{r}' = \begin{bmatrix} x' \\ y' \\ z' \end{bmatrix} = \begin{bmatrix} \cos\gamma & -\sin\gamma & 0 \\ \sin\gamma & \cos\gamma & 0 \\ 0 & 0 & 1 \end{bmatrix} \cdot \begin{bmatrix} x \\ y \\ z \end{bmatrix} = \mathbf{D}_z(\gamma) \cdot \mathbf{r}$$

The matrix describing a rotation about the z-axis is designated $\mathbf{D}_z(\gamma)$. The matrices describing a rotation about the y-axis through angle β and about the x-axis through angle α are similar.

(7.18)
$$\mathbf{r}' = \begin{bmatrix} x' \\ y' \\ z' \end{bmatrix} = \begin{bmatrix} \cos\beta & 0 & \sin\beta \\ 0 & 1 & 0 \\ -\sin\beta & 0 & \cos\beta \end{bmatrix} \cdot \begin{bmatrix} x \\ y \\ z \end{bmatrix} = \mathbf{D}_y(\beta) \cdot \mathbf{r}$$

(7.19)
$$\mathbf{r}' = \begin{bmatrix} x' \\ y' \\ z' \end{bmatrix} = \begin{bmatrix} 1 & 0 & 0 \\ 0 & \cos\alpha & -\sin\alpha \\ 0 & \sin\alpha & \cos\alpha \end{bmatrix} \cdot \begin{bmatrix} x \\ y \\ z \end{bmatrix} = \mathbf{D}_x(\alpha) \cdot \mathbf{r}$$

7.4.2 Rotations Made Up of a Sequence of Rotations

To illustrate the problems associated with combined rotations about body-fixed axes, we consider the example of two consecutive rotations of a suitcase. An xyz system of coordinate axes is imagined to be fixed

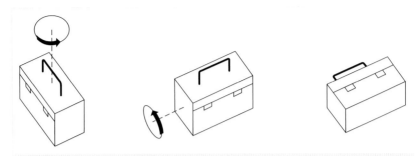

Fig. 7.10 Two consecutive 90° rotations of a rigid body (suitcase) about its vertical and longitudinal axis. In step 1 the body is rotated about its vertical axis; in step 2 the body is rotated about its longitudinal axis. In the final state, the suitcase is lying on its back.

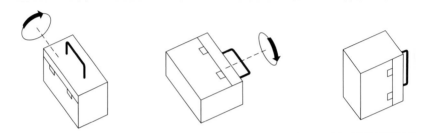

Fig. 7.11 Two consecutive 90° rotations of a rigid body (suitcase) about its longitudinal and vertical axes. The axes and directions of rotation are identical with those in **Fig. 7.10**, but the sequence of the rotations has been changed. The first rotation is about the longitudinal axis, the second about the vertical axis. In the final state the suitcase is lying on its side.

on the suitcase. We rotate the suitcase, first through +90° about its vertical axis and then through +90° about its longitudinal axis. After these two consecutive rotations the suitcase is lying on its back (**Fig. 7.10**). Now, if we perform the same rotations, but in the reverse order, in the final state the suitcase is lying on one side (**Fig. 7.11**). This example illustrates the importance of the sequence of rotations. If the order is changed, the result changes as well.

The rotations in **Figs. 7.10** and **7.11** will now be analyzed mathematically. In the first case the first rotation occurs about the z-axis of the suitcase. The rotation matrix related to the unit vectors $\mathbf{e}_x, \mathbf{e}_y, \mathbf{e}_z$ (compare Eq. 7.17) is

(7.20)
$$\mathbf{D}_z(\gamma = 90°) = \begin{bmatrix} 0 & -1 & 0 \\ 1 & 0 & 0 \\ 0 & 0 & 1 \end{bmatrix}$$

The second rotation occurs about the x′-axis, that is, about a body-fixed axis of the suitcase (previously rotated about its z-axis). The rotation matrix related to the unit vectors $\mathbf{e}'_x, \mathbf{e}'_y, \mathbf{e}'_z$ (compare Eq. 7.19) is

(7.21)
$$\mathbf{D}_{x'}(\alpha = 90°) = \begin{bmatrix} 1 & 0 & 0 \\ 0 & 0 & -1 \\ 0 & 1 & 0 \end{bmatrix}$$

Some intermediate calculation (not presented here) provides for the combined rotation

(7.22)
$$\mathbf{r}'' = \mathbf{D}_z \cdot \mathbf{D}_{x'} \cdot \mathbf{r}$$

In this result, the sequence of the matrices deserves our attention, especially as this sequence differs from what one might expect: the matrix of the second partial rotation is the *first* to act on the vector $\mathbf{r}$; the matrix of the first partial rotation acts *second*. If the sequence of the two partial rotations is switched, the combined rotation is described by

(7.23)
$$\mathbf{r}'' = \mathbf{D}_x \cdot \mathbf{D}_{z'} \cdot \mathbf{r}$$

For rotations about body-fixed axes, it holds in general that the matrix of the last rotation in the sequence of rotations is the first one to be multiplied by the vector to be rotated. The matrix $\mathbf{M}$ describing the image resulting from n partial rotations about body-fixed axes is composed according to the rule

(7.24)
$$\mathbf{M}_{\text{body fixed}} = \mathbf{D}_1 \cdot \mathbf{D}_2 \cdot ... \mathbf{D}_{n-1} \cdot \mathbf{D}_n$$

In this as well as in the following formulae, the indices of the rotation matrices designate the sequence of the rotations: $\mathbf{D}_1$ is the first rotation, $\mathbf{D}_2$ the second rotation, and $\mathbf{D}_n$ the n-th rotation.

If, on the other hand, n rotations were to be performed about axes fixed in space (that is, fixed in the laboratory) and not about body-fixed axes, the sequence of the matrices in the matrix product would be different (the proof of this theorem is not detailed here):

(7.25)
$$\mathbf{M}_{\text{space fixed}} = \mathbf{D}_n \cdot \mathbf{D}_{n-1} \cdot ... \mathbf{D}_2 \cdot \mathbf{D}_1$$

For many applications in biomechanics, it is appropriate to interpret motion as rotations about body-fixed axes. Rotations about body-fixed axes are also easier to visualize. For an illustration, consider the spatial orientation of the vertebra of a scoliotic spine discussed above (see **Fig. 7.3**). It agrees with our visual perception to assume that the vertebra is first rotated about its x-axis (sideways tilt), then rotated about its z-axis (forward tilt), and finally roated about its y-axis oriented perpendicularly on its endplates (axial rotation). If an investigator communicates these three angles, we can clearly visualize how rotation of the vertebra occurred. It would be difficult, if not impossible, to achieve the same visualization on the basis of three reported angles of rotation, together with the sequence in which they occurred, about space-fixed axes defined by an X-ray apparatus in the laboratory. For this reason, the remainder of this chapter deals exclusively with rotations about body-fixed axes.

7.4.3 Euler Angles and Bryan–Cardan Angles

Any desired orientation of a body can be obtained by performing rotations about three axes in sequence. There is, however, a multitude of possible ways of performing three such rotations. In principle, a choice from this multitude can be made at random, but two conventions are frequently used in the literature: Euler rotations and Bryan–Cardan rotations.

According to Euler, the general rotation is composed of three rotations about body-fixed axes as follows (**Fig. 7.12**):

Rotation 1: about the z-axis through the angle ϕ; rotation matrix $\mathbf{D}_z(\phi)$
Rotation 2: about the x′-axis through the angle θ; rotation matrix $\mathbf{D}_{x'}(\theta)$
Rotation 3: about the z″-axis through the angle ψ; rotation matrix $\mathbf{D}_{z''}(\psi)$

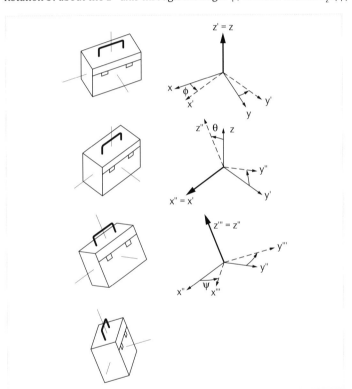

Fig. 7.12 General rotation composed of three partial rotations. Selection of the axes and angles of rotation according to Euler. The coordinates of the initial state are designated x, y, z, those after the first rotation x′, y′, z′, those after the second rotation x″, y″, z″, and those after the third rotation x‴, y‴, z‴. The first rotation takes place about the z-axis (vertical axis of the suitcase) through an angle $\phi = 20°$. The second rotation takes place about the x′-axis (longitudinal axis of the suitcase) through an angle $\theta = 30°$. The third rotation takes place about the z″-axis (vertical axis of the suitcase) through the angle $\psi = 40°$.

The matrix describing Euler's combined rotation is given by the matrix product

(7.26) $$\mathbf{M} = \mathbf{D}_z(\phi) \cdot \mathbf{D}_{x'}(\theta) \cdot \mathbf{D}_{z''}(\psi) \quad \text{(Euler)}$$

According to both Bryan and Cardan, the general rotation is composed of three rotations about body-fixed axes as follows (**Fig. 7.13**):

Rotation 1: about the x-axis through the angle ϕ_1; rotation matrix $\mathbf{D}_x(\phi_1)$
Rotation 2: about the y'-axis through the angle ϕ_2; rotation matrix $\mathbf{D}_{y'}(\phi_2)$
Rotation 3: about the z''-axis through the angle ϕ_3; rotation matrix $\mathbf{D}_{z''}(\phi_3)$

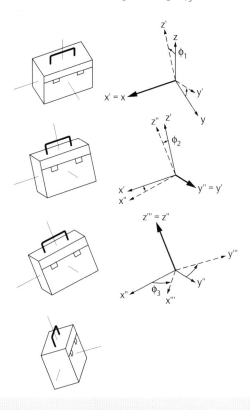

Fig. 7.13 General rotation composed of three partial rotations. Selection of the axes and angles of rotation according to Bryan–Cardan. The coordinates of the initial state are designated x, y, z, those after the first rotation x', y', z', those after the second rotation x'', y'', z'', and those after the third rotation x''', y''', z'''. The first rotation takes place about the x-axis (longitudinal axis of the suitcase) through an angle $\phi_1 = 28.5°$. The second rotation takes place about the y'-axis (transverse axis of the suitcase) through an angle $\phi_2 = 9.8°$. The third rotation takes place about the z''-axis (vertical axis of the suitcase) through the angle $\phi_3 = 57.5°$. The angles of rotation in this diagram are selected in such a way that, when starting from an initial state identical with that of **Fig. 7.12**, the identical final state is reached. For this reason, the angles ϕ_1, ϕ_2, ϕ_3 are not integers.

The matrix describing the combined rotation is given by the matrix product

(7.27) $$\mathbf{M} = \mathbf{D}_x(\phi_1) \cdot \mathbf{D}_{y'}(\phi_2) \cdot \mathbf{D}_{z''}(\phi_3) \quad \text{(Bryan – Cardan)}$$

We recognize that both conventions are based on three angles and a specified sequence of rotations to define the rotation matrix $\mathbf{M}$. This bears some similarity to the transformation between two coordinate systems, where the relative orientation of the unit vectors was likewise described by three parameters.

The above calculations are to be regarded as examples. Any sequence of rotations where the first and the third partial rotations occur about the same axis is designated an Euler rotation. Any sequence of rotations where the partial rotations occur about different axes is designated a Bryan–Cardan rotation.

7.4.4 Rotation About an Arbitrary Axis

For reasons of simplicity, we have dealt with single or combined rotations about coordinate axes up to this point. The concept is now to be generalized as we deal with rotations about arbitrary axes. For the moment, however, the discussion is confined to axes passing through the origin of the coordinate system. In **Fig. 7.14** the axis of rotation is represented by the unit vector $\mathbf{n}$. The radius vector of an arbitrary point P in space is designated by $\mathbf{r}$. When rotated by an angle φ, P moves along a circular arc to P'. The related radius vector is termed $\mathbf{r}'$. The relation between $\mathbf{r}'$ and $\mathbf{r}$ depends on the angle φ as well as on the axis $\mathbf{n}$ of rotation (the proof is not detailed here)

(7.28) $$\mathbf{r}' = \cos\varphi \cdot \mathbf{r} + (1 - \cos\varphi) \cdot \mathbf{n} \cdot (\mathbf{n} \cdot \mathbf{r}) + \sin\varphi \cdot (\mathbf{n} \times \mathbf{r})$$

The relation between $\mathbf{r}'$ and $\mathbf{r}$ can also be expressed in matrix notation. The coordinates of the unit vector $\mathbf{n}$ are designated u,v,w

(7.29) $$\mathbf{n} = \begin{bmatrix} u \\ v \\ w \end{bmatrix}$$

With the abbreviations

(7.30) $$\begin{aligned} C &= \cos\varphi \\ F &= 1 - \cos\varphi \\ S &= \sin\varphi \end{aligned}$$

the imaging equation can be written as

(7.31) $$\mathbf{r}' = \mathbf{D}_n(\varphi) \cdot \mathbf{r} = \begin{bmatrix} C + F \cdot u^2 & F \cdot u \cdot v - S \cdot w & F \cdot u \cdot w + S \cdot v \\ F \cdot v \cdot u + S \cdot w & C + F \cdot v^2 & F \cdot v \cdot w - S \cdot u \\ F \cdot w \cdot u - S \cdot v & F \cdot w \cdot v + S \cdot u & C + F \cdot w^2 \end{bmatrix} \cdot \mathbf{r}$$

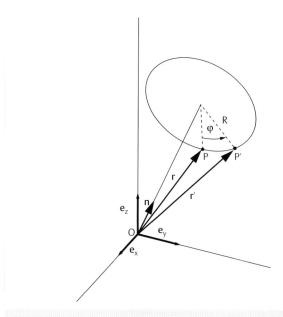

Fig. 7.14 Rotation about an arbitrary axis passing through the coordinate origin. Rotation takes place about an arbitrarily oriented axis (unit vector **n**) through an angle φ. The radius vector OP = **r** moves on the surface of a cone with its tip at the origin of the coordinate system to OP′ = **r′**. The radius R of the base of the cone is equal to R = |**n** × **r**| (magnitude of the vector product).

If we insert for **r** the vector **n**, we obtain

(7.32) $$\mathbf{n}' = \mathbf{D}_n(\varphi) \cdot \mathbf{n} = \mathbf{n}$$

This means that the image vector **n′** is identical with the original vector **n** in respect of direction and magnitude. Points on the axis of rotation do not change their location (as is generally true of rotations). In mathematical terms, the vector **n** is called the *eigenvector* of the matrix $\mathbf{D}_n$. In general it holds that, if for a matrix **M** a vector **m** exists with the property $\mathbf{M} \cdot \mathbf{m} = \lambda \cdot \mathbf{m}$, **m** is the eigenvector of **M** and λ is the *eigenvalue* of **M**. Eq. 7.32 states **n** to be an eigenvector of $\mathbf{D}_n$ with an eigenvalue equal to one.

The theorem holds that "any rotation resulting from a series of consecutive rotations can also be described by one single rotation." In other words, the product of rotation matrices is again a rotation matrix. The proof of this theorem, which is far from obvious, is not detailed here; it is furnished in the context of the theory of orthogonal matrices. The importance of this theorem in the context of biomechanics is that any arbitrary sequence of consecutive rotations can be described by one single (combined) rotation about the Euler or Bryan–Cardan angles or as a rotation about one specific axis through one specific angle of rotation.

7.4.5 Motion Combined from Translation and Rotation; Chasles' Theorem

Rotation and translation are now to be integrated into one single motion. To start with, the restriction that the axis of rotation runs through the coordinate origin is still maintained. In a first step the vector **r** is rotated about **n** through the angle φ. Its image **r′** is

(7.33)
$$\mathbf{r'} = \mathbf{D_n}(\varphi) \cdot \mathbf{r}$$

In a second step the image vector is translated by the translation vector **t**

(7.34)
$$\mathbf{r''} = \mathbf{r'} + \mathbf{t} = \mathbf{D_n}(\varphi) \cdot \mathbf{r} + \mathbf{t}$$

We wish to discuss three special cases of this imaging. In the first case **t** is parallel to **n** ($\mathbf{t} = \mathbf{t_p}$). We consider a point P with radius vector **r** at a distance R from the axis of rotation **n** (**Fig. 7.15**). When being rotated, the point P moves along a circle with radius R, in a plane perpendicular to **n**, to its intermediate image P′. Subsequently,

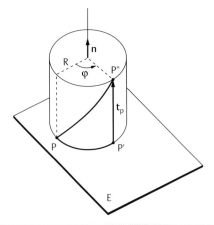

Fig. 7.15 Motion combined from rotation and translation. Special case 1: Translation parallel to the axis of rotation. Rotation is performed through an angle φ about an arbitrarily oriented and located axis of rotation (unit vector **n**). For each given point P in space, there exists a plane E perpendicular to the axis of rotation **n**. The motion occurs on the (imagined) surface of a cylinder. The axis of the cylinder coincides with the axis of rotation, the base of the cylinder lies in plane E, and the radius R of the cylinder is given by the length of the perpendicular from P onto the axis of rotation. The first partial motion is a rotation where the point P moves along a circular arc (periphery of the cylinder base) to point P′. The second partial motion is a translation with translation vector $\mathbf{t_p}$ parallel to **n**, by which the point P′ moves to P″ on a straight surface line (*generatrix*) of the cylinder. In addition to the actual path P–P′–P″, the helix from P to P″ is shown in the diagram

it is translated from P′, by the vector $\mathbf{t}_p$ parallel to the axis of rotation, to P″. If we imagine a cylinder with radius R constructed around the axis of rotation, P, P′, and P″ are located on the surface of that cylinder. The curve on which the point moves from its initial to its final position exhibits a sharp bend at P′. The alternative path, along a helix, would have been a smooth curve from P to P″. Despite the fact that Eq. 7.34 was formulated under the condition of consecutive rotation and translation, the motion is nevertheless termed *helical motion*.

A motion that really does follow a helix is described similarly to Eq. 7.34. Along the helix, rotation and translation take place simultaneously. For this purpose, both angle and translation depend linearly and continuously on a parameter λ

(7.35)
$$\mathbf{r}'(\lambda) = \mathbf{D}_n(\lambda \cdot \varphi) \cdot \mathbf{r} + \lambda \cdot \mathbf{t}_p \quad (0 \le \lambda \le 1)$$

The initial and final location of the point are given by $\lambda = 0$ and $\lambda = 1$, respectively. Any intermediate position on the helix is described by $0 < \lambda < 1$. In the final location, Eq. 7.35 is identical with Eq. 7.34.

In the second special case $\mathbf{t}$ is perpendicular to $\mathbf{n}$ ($\mathbf{t} = \mathbf{t}_q$). P is a point with radius vector $\mathbf{r}$, at a distance R from the axis of rotation $\mathbf{n}$ (**Fig. 7.16**). Starting from P this point moves on a circular arc with radius R to

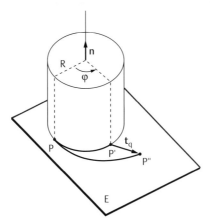

Fig. 7.16 Motion combined from rotation and translation. Special case 2: Translation perpendicular to the axis of rotation. Rotation is performed through an angle φ about an arbitrarily oriented and located axis of rotation (unit vector $\mathbf{n}$). For comparison purposes, a cylinder identical to that in **Fig. 7.15** is shown. The first partial motion is a rotation where the point P moves along a circular arc (periphery of the cylinder base) to point P′. The second partial motion is a translation with translation vector $\mathbf{t}_q$ perpendicular to $\mathbf{n}$, by which the point P′ is moved to P″ in plane E. Thus the combined motion occurs in a plane. As demonstrated in the two-dimensional case, one can also move from P to P′ on a circular arc about the substitute center of rotation with the identical angle of rotation φ.

the intermediate image P′. (The radius of the arc equals the magnitude of the perpendicular from P to the axis of rotation. As shown in **Fig. 7.14**, the radius equals the magnitude of **r** multiplied by the sine of the angle between **n** and **r**, that is R = |**n** × **r**|.) P′ is then translated by the vector $\mathbf{t}_q$ (in the identical plane) to P″.

(7.36)
$$\mathbf{r}'' = \mathbf{D_n}(\varphi) \cdot \mathbf{r} + \mathbf{t}_q$$

This situation is quite similar to the two-dimensional case. In two dimensions, there is a common movement of all points in the xy-plane. In the three-dimensional case discussed here, each point moves in a plane perpendicular to the axis of rotation and passing through the intersection of the perpendicular from the point with the axis. It has been shown in Chapter 6 that translation and rotation in a plane can be substituted by one single rotation about the fixed point of the imaging. We thus suspect that in three dimensions there might be a *substitute* axis of rotation parallel to **n** with the properties of a fixed point (or, better, a *fixed line*). We imagine the parallel planes appertaining to the points **r** projected on top of each other. The fixed point determined in this plane is the point where the substitute axis intersects this plane. It can be shown (not detailed here) that a fixed line really does exist. If translation and rotation are performed consecutively, a sharp bend exists at P′. Alternatively, one could travel on a smooth curve from P to P″ on the circular arc of the substitute rotation through the angle φ about the fixed point of the motion.

In the third special case the translation **t** is thought of as composed of components parallel and perpendicular to the axis of rotation **n**: $\mathbf{t} = \mathbf{t}_p + \mathbf{t}_q$. We imagine the motion to be performed in two steps (**Fig. 7.17**). The motion in plane E is described by

(7.37)
$$\mathbf{r}' = \mathbf{D_n}(\varphi) \cdot \mathbf{r} + \mathbf{t}_q$$

The motion perpendicular to plane E is described by

(7.38)
$$\mathbf{r}'' = \mathbf{r}' + \mathbf{t}_p$$

The first step is equal to that in special case 2, discussed above. The point moves on a circular arc from P to P′, and after a sharp bend it moves in a straight line to Q. If the fixed point of the (plane) motion is known, the midpoint and radius of the substitute circular path from P to Q are known. This circular arc defines a cylinder; the translation $\mathbf{t}_p$ on a line from Q to P″ lies on the surface of this cylinder. Now we substitute (as in special case 1) the path that is sharply bent at Q by a helix on the surface of the (substitute) cylinder running from P to P″. From the geometrical point of view, the three special cases discussed above comprise all the phenomena of motion in three dimensions. For calculation, however, some peculiarities have to be taken into consideration, as will be outlined in the section dealing with Chasles' theorem (below).

The discussion is now to be broadened as the rotation is performed through the angle φ about an axis of rotation with direction parallel to **n** and running through point $\mathbf{r}_0$. The image is then given by

(7.39)
$$\mathbf{r}' = \mathbf{r}_0 + \mathbf{D_n}(\varphi) \cdot (\mathbf{r} - \mathbf{r}_0)$$

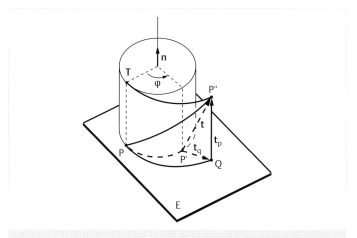

Fig. 7.17 Motion combined from rotation and translation. Special case 3: Translation perpendicular and parallel to the axis of rotation. Rotation is performed through an angle φ about an arbitrarily oriented and located axis of rotation (unit vector **n**). For comparison purposes, a cylinder identical to that in **Figs. 7.15 and 7.16** is shown. The first partial motion is a rotation where point P moves on a circular arc (periphery of the cylinder base) to point P'. The translation vector from P to P" (vector **t**) is further decomposed into the motion from P' to Q (vector **t**$_q$, perpendicular to **n**) and from Q to P" (vector **t**$_p$, parallel to **n**). As in **Fig. 7.16**, the motion PP'Q is replaced by motion along a circular arc, again the periphery of a cylinder base. The axis of this cylinder is the fixed line of the special case 2. The third partial motion from Q to P" occurs along a straight surface line (*generatrix*) of the cylinder. The surface defined by points P, Q, P", and T is a part of the surface of this cylinder (height PT = QP" = |**t**$_p$|). The helix from P to P" is drawn on this surface.

This equation tells us that the origin of the coordinate system has been shifted to $\mathbf{r}_0$. The point $\mathbf{r}$ is rotated with respect to $\mathbf{r}_0$; that is, the rotation is performed on the vector $\mathbf{p} = (\mathbf{r} - \mathbf{r}_0)$. After the rotation the vector $\mathbf{r}_0$ is added to the image $\mathbf{p}' = \mathbf{D}_n(\varphi) \cdot \mathbf{p}$. To combine translation and rotation, the (already rotated) point is shifted by the translation vector $\mathbf{t}$

$$(7.40) \qquad \mathbf{r}'' = \mathbf{r}' + \mathbf{t} = \mathbf{r}_0 + \mathbf{D}_n(\varphi) \cdot (\mathbf{r} - \mathbf{r}_0) + \mathbf{t}$$

If no restrictions are imposed on the direction of $\mathbf{t}$, Eq. 7.40 describes the general motion in three-dimensional space. Eq. 7.40 can be re-formulated as

$$(7.41) \qquad \mathbf{r}' = \mathbf{D} \cdot \mathbf{r} + \mathbf{a}$$

and with **a** defined as (**r″** being replaced by **r′**)

(7.42) $$\mathbf{a} = \mathbf{r}_0 - \mathbf{D}_n(\varphi) \cdot \mathbf{r}_0 + \mathbf{t}$$

Chasles' theorem states that the general motion in three-dimensional space is helical motion, or alternatively, the basic type of motion adapted to describe any change of location and orientation in three-dimensional space is helical motion. The relevant axis of rotation is designated the *helical* or *screw axis*. Chasles' theorem is also known as the *helical axis theorem*.

A possible path for proving this theorem may be outlined as follows. In the case of a rotation about a coordinate axis, for example through the angle φ about the z-axis, the situation is readily comprehensible. We proceed as in the above discussed special case 3. The motion

(7.43) $$\mathbf{r}'' = \mathbf{D}_z(\varphi) \cdot \mathbf{r} + \mathbf{t}$$

is expressed in coordinates

(7.44) $$\begin{aligned} x'' &= \cos\varphi \cdot x - \sin\varphi \cdot y + 0 \cdot z + t_x \\ y'' &= \sin\varphi \cdot x + \cos\varphi \cdot y + 0 \cdot z + t_y \\ z'' &= \quad 0 \cdot x + \quad 0 \cdot y + 1 \cdot z + t_z \end{aligned}$$

It can be seen that the first two equations can be treated independently from the third and, vice versa, the third equation can be treated independently from the first two. This so-called decoupling provides a significant simplification. The motion is performed in two steps

(7.45) $$\begin{aligned} \mathbf{r}' &= \mathbf{D}_z(\varphi) \cdot \mathbf{r} + \mathbf{t}_q \\ \mathbf{r}'' &= \mathbf{r}' + \mathbf{t}_p \end{aligned}$$

with **t** broken down into the components

(7.46) $$\mathbf{t}_q = \begin{bmatrix} t_x \\ t_y \\ 0 \end{bmatrix}$$

(7.47) $$\mathbf{t}_p = \begin{bmatrix} 0 \\ 0 \\ t_z \end{bmatrix}$$

The examination of the first partial motion permits the fixed line (the axis of the helix) to be computed. The second partial motion provides the magnitude of the translation parallel to the axis of the helix. (The reason for breaking down the translation into $\mathbf{t}_q$ and $\mathbf{t}_p$ is that in the three-dimensional case fixed elements exist only for translations perpendicular to the axis of rotation.) The general case, rotation through an angle φ about an arbitrarily directed axis **n** in arbitrary location, can be simplified by accepting the axis of rotation **n** as the ζ-axis of a ξηζ-coordinate system. Instead of the complicated matrix $\mathbf{D}_n(\varphi)$ in the xyz-coordinate system, one has to deal only with the simple rotation matrix $\mathbf{D}_\zeta(\varphi)$. Finally, only the vectors **r**, **r′**, and **t** have to be transformed into the ξηζ system. By doing this, the general case is reduced to the special case.

7.5 Calculation of the Parameters of Rotation and Translation in Three-Dimensional Space from the Coordinates of Reference Points and Their Images

If the parameters of the motion (rotation and translation) and of the initial location and orientation of a body are known, the formulae given in the previous section permit its final location and orientation to be calculated. In biomechanics, however, one is quite often confronted with the inverse problem. The coordinates of reference points on a body are known in the initial and final state and the parameters of the motion (the imaging) have to be determined. In the following, the solution to this problem is outlined under the assumption that measurement of the coordinates is performed with no experimental error (a condition never met in reality).

7.5.1 Parameters of the Motion of a Body Observed in a Laboratory Coordinate System

To reconstruct the parameters of the motion of a rigid body in a laboratory coordinate system, the coordinates of three reference points fixed on the body but not lying on a straight line have to be known in the initial state and the final state (**Fig. 7.18**). To fit the parameters, the following ansatz is made (compare Eq. 7.40):

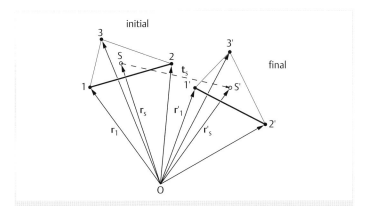

Fig. 7.18 Motion of a rigid body: minimum configuration of three reference points to determine the parameters describing the spatial motion. Three reference points, which must not be aligned along a straight line, are fixed on the rigid body. In this diagram the body itself is not shown; instead, we imagine the body to be replaced by the triangle formed by the three reference points. In addition to the corners of the triangle 1–3, their geometric center S is shown. The spatial motion can be described as a rotation of the triangle about an axis passing through S and a subsequent translation of the rotated triangle by the translation vector $\mathbf{t}_s$. Points and vectors in the final state are designated by symbols with primes.

(7.48)
$$\mathbf{r}' = \mathbf{r}_S + \mathbf{D} \cdot (\mathbf{r} - \mathbf{r}_S) + \mathbf{t}_S$$

In this ansatz, $\mathbf{r}$ designates the locations of the reference points and $\mathbf{r}_S$ the location of the geometric center of the reference points in the initial state. $\mathbf{r}'$ and $\mathbf{r}'_S$ designate the locations of the reference points and their geometric centers in the final state. The steps of the calculation are then: (1) calculation of the translation vector $\mathbf{t}_S$ from the initial to the final state and reversal of the translation; (2) determination of the rotation matrix $\mathbf{D}$; (3) with $\mathbf{D}$ and the translation vector already determined in step 1 being known, the motion can be interpreted according to Chasles as helical motion; (4) alternatively, it is possible to select another interpretation for the rotation matrix, that is, one based on Euler or Bryan–Cardan.

Step 1: Translation of the Geometric Centers

The geometric centers referred to in the following are the geometric centers of the reference points. From three reference points with radius vectors $\mathbf{r}_1, \mathbf{r}_2, \mathbf{r}_3$ the radius vector of their geometric center $\mathbf{r}_S$ is calculated as

(7.49)
$$\mathbf{r}_S = 1/3 \cdot (\mathbf{r}_1 + \mathbf{r}_2 + \mathbf{r}_3)$$

The translation vector $\mathbf{t}_S$ points from the geometric center in its initial location to its final location. Reversal of the translation

(7.50)
$$\bar{\mathbf{r}}_i = \mathbf{r}'_i - \mathbf{t}_S \quad (i = 1, 2, 3)$$

means that the geometric centers of the reference points are superimposed. We are now left with a difference in orientation (a rotation) of the body.

Step 2: Determination of the Rotation Matrix

After the translation has been reversed the following ansatz is made to obtain the rotation matrix:

(7.51)
$$\bar{\mathbf{r}}_i - \mathbf{r}_S = \mathbf{D} \cdot (\mathbf{r}_i - \mathbf{r}_S) \quad (i = 1, 2, 3)$$

The most commonly employed procedure for solving this equation for the rotation matrix $\mathbf{D}$ is trial and error by iteration. For example, we could insert Eq. 7.31 for the matrix $\mathbf{D}$ and, starting from rough estimates for the direction of the axis of rotation $\mathbf{n}$ and the angle of rotation φ, change both parameters in small steps until we finally arrive at a parameter set which satisfies Eq. 7.51. If the coordinates of the reference points are not known exactly, but only within certain error limits, it is not possible to find a set of parameters that satisfy Eq. 7.51 exactly, but only a solution that satisfies this equation as nearly as possible (a *best possible fit*). Algorithms of iterative procedures have been adapted for use on computers; for details the reader is referred to textbooks on numerical methods. Alternatively, for $\mathbf{D}$ we could make the ansatz of the Euler or

Bryan–Cardan angles (Eqs. 7.26 or 7.27) and solve these equations for the set of angles, again by stepwise iteration.

Step 3: Interpretation of the Motion as Helical Motion

When the direction of the axis of rotation $\mathbf{n}$, the angle of rotation φ, and the translation vector $\mathbf{t}_S = \mathbf{r}'_S - \mathbf{r}_S = \mathbf{r}_{S'} - \mathbf{r}_S$ are known, the motion is comprehensively described. In this description, the axis of rotation passes through the geometric center of the reference points on the body. The direction of the axis, the geometric center of the reference points, and the translation vector are given in the laboratory coordinate system. If we wish to interpret the motion as helical motion, we conclude from Chasles' theorem that this is always possible. The description as helical motion requires specification of the direction of the axis, of a point in space through which the axis passes, and of a translation vector along this axis. A point in space $\mathbf{r}_A$, through which the axis passes, is calculated from

(7.52)
$$\mathbf{r}_A = \frac{\mathbf{r}_S + \mathbf{r}'_S}{2} + \frac{1}{2} \cdot \cot(\frac{\varphi}{2}) \cdot \mathbf{n} \times (\mathbf{r}'_S - \mathbf{r}_S)$$

The translation vector $\mathbf{t}_p$ is obtained from the projection of the translation vector $\mathbf{t}_S$ onto the direction of the helical axis.

(7.53)
$$\mathbf{t}_p = (\mathbf{t}_S \cdot \mathbf{n}) \cdot \mathbf{n}$$

Because of its importance in the interpretation of biomechanical measurements, the content of Eqs. 7.52 and 7.53 is illustrated in **Fig. 7.19**. As we have said, comprehensive description of a helical motion requires specification of a point in space through which the axis of rotation passes. We recognize from the orientation of the suitcase in its initial and final positions (**Fig. 7.19**) that the object was rotated about a vertical axis $\mathbf{n}$ by an angle φ. From these parameters and from the location of the center of the suitcase in its initial and final positions ($\mathbf{r}_S$, $\mathbf{r}'_S$), the location of a point A on the helical axis can be constructed. $\mathbf{r}_S$ and $\mathbf{r}'_S$ are the locations of the center of the suitcase (used here to represent the geometric centers of the reference points on the suitcase), and M designates the midpoint of the line SS'. The relevant radius vector is $(\mathbf{r}_S + \mathbf{r}'_S)/2$, and $\mathbf{e}$ is the unit vector in the direction of the difference vector $(\mathbf{r}'_S - \mathbf{r}_S)$. The line SS' and $\mathbf{n}$ are skew lines in space. M and A are those points where the distance between the two lines assumes a minimum value. The line connecting M and A is perpendicular to $\mathbf{n}$ as well as to SS'. The vector $\mathbf{f}$ is a unit vector in the direction of MA. R is the radius of the cylindrical surface on which the suitcase moves. From the lines projected onto the base plane of the cylinder we deduce $|\mathbf{r}_A - \mathbf{r}_M| = R \cdot \cos(\varphi/2)$ and $|\mathbf{r}'_S - \mathbf{r}_S| \cdot \cos(\varepsilon) = 2R \cdot \sin(\varphi/2)$. As A is the point of minimum distance between the lines, the unit vector $\mathbf{f}$ is oriented perpendicular to $\mathbf{n}$ and $\mathbf{e}$. Hence, $\mathbf{f}$ can be represented by the vector product $\mathbf{f} = (\mathbf{n} \times \mathbf{e})/\cos(\varepsilon)$. After some simple intermediate calculations, the result of Eq. 7.52 is reached.

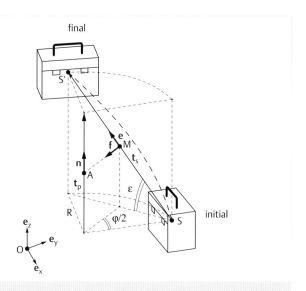

Fig. 7.19 Motion of a rigid body: interpretation of the general motion as helical motion (Chasles' theorem). The required number of reference points (not shown in the diagram) is fixed on a rigid body (suitcase). From the spatial location of the reference points in the initial and final state, the locations of the geometric centers S ($\mathbf{r}_S$) and S' ($\mathbf{r}'_S$) as well as the rotation matrix $\mathbf{D}$ are determined. The change in location of the geometric centers is described by $\mathbf{t}_S = \mathbf{r}'_S - \mathbf{r}_S$. The axis of rotation $\mathbf{n}$ and the angle of rotation φ are determined from the rotation matrix. The translation $\mathbf{t}_p$ in the direction of the helical axis is obtained by projection from $\mathbf{n}$ and $\mathbf{t}_S$. The location of the axis of rotation relative to the initial and final position of the suitcase is set by points A and M. M is the midpoint of the line SS'. The vector $\mathbf{f}$ directed from M to A is perpendicular to $\mathbf{n}$ and $\mathbf{t}_S$. The radius R and the radius vector $\mathbf{r}_A$ can be calculated by means of the unit vectors $\mathbf{e}$, $\mathbf{n}$, and $\mathbf{f}$.

Step 4: Different Interpretations of a Rotation Matrix D

Irrespective of how we wish to interpret the rotation matrix $\mathbf{D}$, as rotation by one single angle about one single axis (Eq. 7.31), as an Euler rotation sequence about three axes (Eq. 7.26), or as a Bryan–Cardan rotation sequence about three axes (Eq. 7.27), the matrix elements D_{ik} of the matrix $\mathbf{D}$ are numerically identical. These numbers are merely interpreted differently. From time to time one is confronted with the problem of switching from one interpretation to another. For example, the task may be to determine the helical axis and the angle of rotation when the three Euler angles are known, or to determine the set of Cardan angles when the helical axis and the related angle of rotation are known. All of these tasks boil down to the problem of extracting the parameters of a three-dimensional rotation from the (known) elements of a rotation matrix $\mathbf{D}$. This is possible, but in some cases there will prove to be no unequivocal solution to this problem.

Calculation of the Euler Angles from the Elements of a Rotation Matrix D

In the process of solving this, two cases have to be distinguished. Main case A (Eq. 7.54): For any given $\cos\theta$ there exist two sine values which differ in their sign. Consequently two sets of angles are obtained. For each of the three angles of each set the quadrant can be unequivocally determined from the sine and cosine functions by means of the atan2 function.

(7.54)

$$\cos\theta = D_{33}$$
$$\sin\theta = \pm\sqrt{1-(\cos\theta)^2}$$
$$\cos\psi = D_{32}/\sin\theta$$
$$\sin\psi = D_{31}/\sin\theta$$
$$\cos\phi = -D_{23}/\sin\theta$$
$$\sin\phi = D_{13}/\sin\theta$$

Special case B: If $\sin\theta = 0$, $\cos\theta$ can assume the values ± 1. Subcase 1 (Eq. 7.55): For $\cos\theta = +1$, θ has the value $0°$ or $\pm 360°$. In this case it is only the sum of the angles ϕ and ψ that can be obtained from

(7.55)

$$\cos(\phi + \psi) = D_{22}$$
$$\sin(\phi + \psi) = D_{21}$$

Subcase 2 (Eq. 7.56): For $\cos\theta = -1$, θ can assume the values $\pm 180°$. In this case it is merely the difference between angles ϕ and ψ that can be obtained.

(7.56)

$$\cos(\phi - \psi) = D_{11}$$
$$\sin(\phi - \psi) = D_{12}$$

Calculation of the Bryan–Cardan Angles from the Elements of a Rotation Matrix D

In the solving process, various cases have again to be distinguished. Main case A (see Eq. 7.57): For any $\sin\phi_2 \neq \pm 1$ there exist two cosine values $(\cos\phi_2 \neq 0)$ which differ in their sign. Accordingly, two sets of angles ϕ_1, ϕ_2, ϕ_3 are obtained. For each of the three angles of each set the quadrant can be unequivocally determined from the sine and cosine functions by means of the atan2 function.

(7.57)

$$\sin\phi_2 = D_{13}$$
$$\cos\phi_2 = \pm\sqrt{1-(\sin\phi_2)^2}$$
$$\cos\phi_1 = D_{33}/\cos\phi_2$$
$$\sin\phi_1 = -D_{23}/\cos\phi_2$$
$$\cos\phi_3 = D_{11}/\cos\phi_2$$
$$\sin\phi_3 = -D_{12}/\cos\phi_2$$

Special case B: $\cos\phi_2 = 0$. The relevant sine can assume the values ± 1. Subcase 1 (Eq. 7.58): $\cos\phi_2 = 0$, $\sin\phi_2 = +1$, corresponding to the angles $\phi_2 = -270°, +90°$. In this case it is only the sum of the other two angles ϕ_1 and ϕ_3 that can be determined.

(7.58)

$$\cos(\phi_1 + \phi_3) = D_{22}$$
$$\sin(\phi_1 + \phi_3) = D_{32}$$

Subcase 2 (Eq. 7.59): $\cos\phi_2 = 0$, $\sin\phi_2 = -1$, corresponding to the angles $\phi_2 = -90°$, $+270°$. In this case it is only the difference between the other two angles ϕ_1 and ϕ_3 that can be determined.

(7.59)
$$\cos(\phi_1 - \phi_3) = D_{22}$$
$$\sin(\phi_1 - \phi_3) = D_{32}$$

Determination of the Components of a Unit Vector u,v,w in the Direction of the Axis of Rotation n and of the Angle of Rotation φ About This Axis from the Elements of a Rotation Matrix D

As in the two problems discussed above, we need to distinguish between different cases. In the main case A we assume $\cos\varphi \neq 1$. The parameters searched for are calculated from

(7.60)
$$u^2 = \frac{D_{11} - C}{1 - C}$$
$$v^2 = \frac{D_{22} - C}{1 - C}$$
$$w^2 = \frac{D_{33} - C}{1 - C}$$

(7.61)
$$C = \cos\varphi = \frac{D_{11} + D_{22} + D_{33} - 1}{2}$$

Square roots have to be extracted from the squares; the signs of u,v,w are determined by insertion in the eigenvalue equation, Eq. 7.32. Once a valid combination of u,v,w-values and a φ-value has been established, the final choice is made by considering one of the valid relations between rotation matrices $\mathbf{D}_n(\varphi)$, that is, $\mathbf{D}(\mathbf{n}, -360° + \varphi) = \mathbf{D}(\mathbf{n}, \varphi)$ or $\mathbf{D}(-\mathbf{n}, -\varphi) = \mathbf{D}(\mathbf{n}, \varphi)$. The first relation indicates that, with the direction of the axis of rotation unchanged, the rotation can also be explained by using an angle of rotation equal to $-360° + \varphi$. The second relation indicates that a change in the direction of the axis of rotation requires the sense of the rotation to be changed as well. Depending on the problem being worked on, the investigator may be able to make a rough estimate of the axis and the angle of rotation; this will then permit a final choice to be made from the different mathematical solutions available.

Special case B: $\cos\varphi = 1$, corresponding to the angles of rotation $\varphi = 0°$, $\pm 360°$. The rotation matrix then equals the unit matrix; that is, the rotated points coincide with their images. Any direction can be chosen for the axis of rotation.

7.5.2 Parameters Describing the Relative Motion of Two Bodies

In many cases of practical interest, the problem is not in describing the motion of a body in a laboratory coordinate system but in describing the relative motion of two bodies. One example of such relative motion is the motion of the tibia relative to the motion of the femur. If one succeeds in fixing a "measurement coordinate system" on one of the bodies, for example on the femur, the problem can be reduced to that discussed in the previous section. The motion of the lower leg would then be observed in the coordinate system of the thigh and interpreted according to one of the above conventions (Euler angles, etc.). One measuring device employed in biomechanical research and defining its own coordinate system is a commercially available electromagnetic tracking device. Its transmitter is fixed on one body and its receiver on the other. The output data are the Euler angles of the transmitter with respect to the receiver and the distance coordinates between the two devices.

If, however, the locations of reference points fixed to the femur and to the tibia have been recorded simultaneously in a laboratory coordinate system (**Fig. 7.20**), several calculation steps have to be performed before the relative motion between tibia and femur can be analyzed:

1. From the geometric centers of the reference points on the femur, the translation of the femur is calculated and reversed. The identical transformation is applied to the reference points on the tibia.

2. An iterative procedure is used to determine the rotation matrix which images the already translated reference points of the femur in the final state onto its reference points in the initial state. This rotation matrix is then applied to the already translated reference points of the tibia. The effect of these

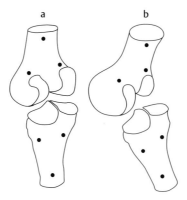

a   b

Fig. 7.20a, b Study of the relative motion of the femur and tibia (motion of the knee joint). The initial (**a**) and final (**b**) states are shown. The femur and the tibia each bear three reference points. To obtain the parameters describing the relative motion, we assume the knee joint to be rigid in both the initial and the final state. By rotating and translating the rigid configuration of the final state, we succeed in superimposing the reference points of the femur in the final state (**b**) onto those in the initial state (**a**). The reference points on the two femora are now congruent; those of the tibia, however, are not. The difference in their position and orientation allows the parameters of the relative motion between the femur and the tibia to be determined.

transformations is that the reference points of the femur in the initial and final states now coincide. The motion of the femur in the laboratory system is thus compensated for.

3. The remaining differences in the locations of the reference points on the tibia in the initial and the final states now characterize the relative motion of the tibia with respect to the femur. This motion can be analyzed as described above, like the motion of a single body in a laboratory coordinate system. The direction and location of the helical axis and the related angle of rotation or, alternatively, the translation vector and the sets of angles (Euler or Bryan–Cardan) can be determined.

Alternatively, a body-fixed coordinate system could be constructed from the radius vectors of the reference points fixed on the femur. In three-dimensional space, three reference points are required for the definition of a coordinate system. These three reference points must not lie on a line but rather on the corners of a triangle. The radius vectors of the three reference points P_1, P_2, P_3 in the laboratory coordinate system are designated $\mathbf{r}_1$, $\mathbf{r}_2$, $\mathbf{r}_3$. To construct a body-fixed coordinate system, the first unit vector $\mathbf{f}_1$ is obtained from the difference vector $\mathbf{a} = \mathbf{r}_2 - \mathbf{r}_1$ by dividing it by its magnitude:

(7.62)
$$\mathbf{f}_1 = \mathbf{a}/|\mathbf{a}|$$

Starting from the difference vector $\mathbf{b} = \mathbf{r}_3 - \mathbf{r}_1$, the vector $\mathbf{v} = \mathbf{b} - \mathbf{f}_1 \cdot (\mathbf{f}_1 \cdot \mathbf{b})$, which is perpendicular to $\mathbf{f}_1$, is constructed. Division by its magnitude yields the second unit vector.

(7.63)
$$\mathbf{f}_2 = \mathbf{v}/|\mathbf{v}|$$

The third unit vector $\mathbf{f}_3$ is defined by the vector product

(7.64)
$$\mathbf{f}_3 = \mathbf{f}_1 \times \mathbf{f}_2$$

The geometric center $\mathbf{r}_s$ of the reference points P_1, P_2, P_3 at the femur is chosen according to Eq. 7.49 as the origin of the coordinate system. The location of the reference points on the tibia (with radius vectors $\mathbf{r}_j$ in the laboratory system) is now to be expressed in the femur system. For this purpose the difference vectors $\mathbf{r}_j - \mathbf{r}_s$ given in the laboratory system are projected onto the unit vectors $\mathbf{f}_1$, $\mathbf{f}_2$, $\mathbf{f}_3$. This provides the coordinates of the tibia reference points in the system of the femur. Any change in these coordinates directly reflects the relative motion between tibia and femur.

The description of the relative motion, for example as helical motion, is still unsatisfactory, because the location and orientation of the axis are given in the laboratory or, in the example discussed above, in the femur-fixed coordinate system. If the motion of a joint is to be investigated, interest is usually focused on knowing the location and orientation of the axis in a coordinate system which is properly aligned with respect to the structures of the skeleton, and not with respect to a coordinate system that is dependent on the more or less randomly selected laboratory system or reference points on the moving object. A femur coordinate system sensibly adapted to visual interpretation of the results would be a system aligned to the "preferred directions" of the femur, that is, with one axis pointing in a longitudinal direction and another in a mediolateral direction crossing the two condyles. The relative position and orientation of the anatomical and measurement coordinate system are deduced from radiographs and/or from measurements of external anatomical landmarks. If the translation and rotation are determined (again by iteration), the data measured in the laboratory coordinate system can be imaged into the anatomical coordinate system.

In practice additional problems arise because the locations of reference points cannot be measured without measurement errors. It follows that, when fitting the rotation matrices, no exact solution exists, only a best fit. In addition, reference points on biological objects are often not absolutely fixed but may move in relation to each other or to the object. The motion of markers fixed not to bones but to the skin is just one example of this.

7.6 Describing Motions of the Joints of the Human Body

7.6.1 Visual Representation of Motions in a Plane

To describe three-dimensional movements of the body segments in orthopedics and physiotherapy, motions are usually referred to in three mutually perpendicular planes: the sagittal, coronal, and transverse planes (**Fig. 7.21**). Forward bending of the trunk is thus a motion *in the sagittal plane*, lateral bending of the trunk a motion *in the coronal plane*, and rotation of the trunk about the long axis of the body a motion *in the transverse plane*. The description of *motion in a plane* is employed not only for the whole body but also for its parts. **Fig. 7.22** shows a detail from **Fig. 7.21**. If we are interested only in the motion

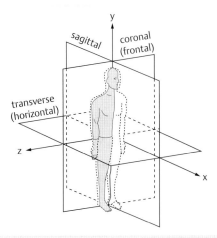

Fig. 7.21 Definition of the planes of motion and the body-fixed xyz-coordinate system.

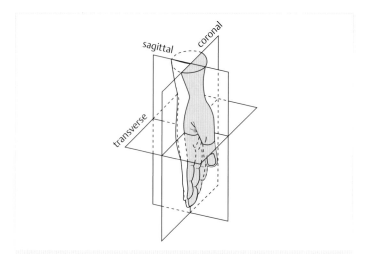

Fig. 7.22 To describe motions of the hand, the planes of motion are imagined as fixed to the lower arm, irrespective of the position of the arm.

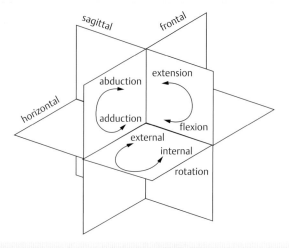

Fig. 7.23 Names of the rotations in the sagittal, frontal, and horizontal planes of motion.

of the hand, we imagine the three planes to be fixed to the lower arm, independent of the position of the arm—whether it is at the side or in front of the body or above the head.

The directions of rotation in these planes have specific names (**Fig. 7.23**). *Extension* and *flexion* designate rotations in the sagittal plane, *abduction* and *adduction* rotations in the coronal plane, and *internal* and *external rotation* rotations in the transverse plane. Specific names are also used for the motion of hands and feet. *Pronation* and *supination* designate rotations of the hand in the transverse plane and the forefoot in the coronal plane. In relation to the abduction/adduction rotations and internal/external rotations, it must be remembered that the terms shown in **Fig. 7.22** have different meanings for the right and left extremities: for example, the direction of internal rotation of the right leg is the opposite direction to internal rotation of the left leg.

In a mathematical description of rotations, reference is usually not made to rotations *in a plane* but to spatial rotations *about an axis of rotation*. An axis of rotation is perpendicular to the plane of interest. For the mathematical description of motions a body-fixed, right-handed, Cartesian xyz-coordinate system is introduced (**Fig. 7.21**). Flexions/extensions are thus rotations *about the z-axis* (or about an axis parallel to the z-axis), and similarly for abduction/adduction and pronation/supination. For the majority of practical applications in orthopedics and physiotherapy, description of motion in the planes shown in **Figs. 7.21** and **7.22** is adequate and appropriate. However, if motions occur outside the three planes shown, it is no longer so. In such cases, one is dealing with spatial rotations which can be represented in different ways.

7.6.2 Describing the Motion of Joints in Space

Many joints permit motions about more than one axis of rotation. The tibia, for example can be moved relative to the femur in flexion/extension and in abduction/adduction; in addition, rotation of the tibia about its own long axis is possible. Combined rotations may be described in different ways: by stating the helical axis and angle, or by giving sets of Euler or Bryan–Cardan angles. It is, however, a great advantage to choose a way that allows the angles of rotation obtained to be interpreted clearly and that (if possible) agrees with the traditional, orthopedic definitions.

The following section explains how joint motion is described with the aid of *joint coordinate systems*, using the example of the knee joint.[4]

To describe the motion of the lower leg relative to the thigh we imagine a Cartesian coordinate system to be fixed to the proximal articulating bone and another to the distal articulating bone: in this case, the tibia and femur (**Fig. 7.24**). In the initial state the axes of both systems are assumed to be aligned parallel to each other. The sequence of the rotations is chosen as follows: The first rotation occurs about the z_p-axis through the angle γ (extension/flexion). The second rotation occurs about the x_d-axis through the angle α (adduction/abduction). The third rotation occurs about the y_d-axis through the angle β (internal /external rotation).

The individual rotations are described by the rotation matrices

$$(7.65) \qquad \mathbf{R}_\gamma = \begin{bmatrix} \cos\gamma & -\sin\gamma & 0 \\ \sin\gamma & \cos\gamma & 0 \\ 0 & 0 & 1 \end{bmatrix}$$

$$(7.66) \qquad \mathbf{R}_\alpha = \begin{bmatrix} 1 & 0 & 0 \\ 0 & \cos\alpha & -\sin\alpha \\ 0 & \sin\alpha & \cos\alpha \end{bmatrix}$$

(7.67)
$$\mathbf{R}_\beta = \begin{bmatrix} \cos\beta & 0 & \sin\beta \\ 0 & 1 & 0 \\ -\sin\beta & 0 & \cos\beta \end{bmatrix}$$

For the combined rotation it has to be kept in mind that the first rotation occurs about an axis of the proximal segment whereas the two subsequent rotations occur about body-fixed axes of the distal segment.[4] The resulting rotation matrix **D** is the product

(7.68)
$$\mathbf{D} = \mathbf{R}_\gamma \cdot \mathbf{R}_\alpha \cdot \mathbf{R}_\beta$$

The matrix elements of **D** are

(7.69)
$$\begin{bmatrix} D_{11} & D_{12} & D_{13} \\ D_{21} & D_{22} & D_{23} \\ D_{31} & D_{32} & D_{33} \end{bmatrix} = \begin{bmatrix} \cos\gamma \cdot \cos\beta - \sin\gamma \cdot \sin\alpha \cdot \sin\beta & -\sin\gamma \cdot \cos\alpha & \cos\gamma \cdot \sin\beta + \sin\gamma \cdot \sin\alpha \cdot \cos\beta \\ \sin\gamma \cdot \cos\beta + \cos\gamma \cdot \sin\alpha \cdot \sin\beta & \cos\gamma \cdot \cos\alpha & \sin\gamma \cdot \sin\beta - \cos\gamma \cdot \sin\alpha \cdot \cos\beta \\ -\cos\alpha \cdot \sin\beta & \sin\alpha & \cos\alpha \cdot \cos\beta \end{bmatrix}$$

From the matrix elements of **D** the angles of rotation can be calculated

(7.70)
$$\alpha = \sin^{-1} D_{32}$$
$$\beta = \sin^{-1}\left(\frac{-D_{31}}{\cos\alpha}\right)$$
$$\gamma = \sin^{-1}\left(\frac{-D_{12}}{\cos\alpha}\right)$$

It should be pointed out that the distal segment does not really have to be rotated about the angles α, β, γ; for a given sequence of rotations, the set of angles merely describes the final state relative to the initial state. If a different sequence were chosen, a different set of angles would be obtained for the identical final state. The paper of Cappozzo et al[4] cited above contains an example.

The same approach to describing joint motions can also be formulated in a different way. Grood and Suntay[5] proposed directing the x-axes of the coordinate systems anteriorly, the z-axes laterally, and the y-axes longitudinally along the bones. The first rotation would occur about the z_p-axis; the second rotation about an axis perpendicular to z_p and y_d, designated a *floating axis* by Grood and Suntay; and the third rotation about the y_d-axis. It can be seen, however, from **Fig. 7.24** that after the first rotation z_d is still parallel to z_p. The axis x_d is perpendicular to z_p and y_d and is thus identical to the *floating axis*. In other words, the definition of a *floating axis* is not stringently required. An alternative formulation would be: Since the axes z_p and z_d coincide in the initial state, the first rotation can also be imagined to occur about z_d instead about z_p, while the second and third rotations occur about x_d and y_d. This is Cardan's rotation about three body-fixed axes.

For the angles α, β, γ calculated from the observation of a motion to agree with the "orthopedic" definitions, the joint coordinate systems have to be suitably defined. The coordinate system of the femur, for example (**Fig. 7.24**), is positioned so that the z_p-axis coincides with the axis for flexion/extension and the y_p-axis connects the midpoint of the condyles with the center of the femoral head. The direction of

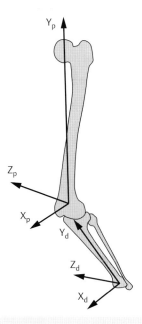

Fig. 7.24 Joint coordinate system, illustrated with the example of the knee joint. The axes of rotation of the proximal articulating bone are designated by the index p, while the axes of the distal articulating bone are designated by the index d. (Adapted, with permission, from Cappozzo et al.[4])

the x_p-axis (perpendicular to x_p and z_p) is thus specified. In vivo, the joint coordinate systems can only be defined by means of palpable or measurable anatomical landmarks on the articulating bones. Translational motion of the articulating bones (in addition to rotational motion) can be defined as translation of the origins of the coordinate systems. To do this, it is necessary to locate these origins in the same way, by using anatomical landmarks. Translational motions that are observable in vivo are, however, usually very small. Recommendations for the definition of the directions of the coordinate systems and their origins are given in the papers by Grood and Suntay[5] and Wu et al.[6,7]

If the motion of the distal segment of a joint is to be described by a sequence of Cardan angles, in exceptional cases joint positions exist where the angles of rotation cannot be unambiguously assigned. As can be noted from Eq. 7.70, β and γ are indeterminate when α equals 90° and subsequently $\cos\alpha$ equals zero. This case is termed *gimbal lock*. At the knee joint this does not occur, because maximum abduction/adduction is well below 90°. Due to its large range of motion, however, the shoulder joint can adopt a position in *gimbal lock* (**Fig. 7.25**). With the upper arm flexed forwards, the assignment of flexion/extension and internal/external rotation is unequivocal. At 90° abduction these two rotation axes coincide and the assignment of the rotations is indeterminate. In other words, one is now free to decide to describe a rotation about the common axis as flexion/extension or as internal/external rotation.

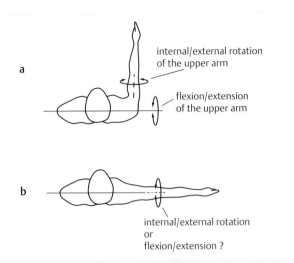

internal/external rotation
of the upper arm

a

flexion/extension
of the upper arm

b

internal/external rotation
or
flexion/extension ?

Fig. 7.25a, b Gimbal lock in the motion of the upper arm.
a Upper arm in anteflexion.
b Upper arm in 90° abduction.

References

1. Debrunner HU, Jacob HAC. Biomechanik des Fußes. 2nd ed. Stuttgart: Enke; 1998

2. Drerup B. Principles of measurement of vertebral rotation from frontal projections of the pedicles. J Biomech 1984;17(12):923–935

3. Skalli W, Lavaste F, Descrimes JL. Quantification of three-dimensional vertebral rotations in scoliosis: what are the true values? Spine 1995;20(5):546–553

4. Cappozzo A, Della Croce U, Leardini A, Chiari L. Human movement analysis using stereophotogrammetry. Part 1: theoretical background. Gait Posture 2005;21(2):186–196

5. Grood ES, Suntay WJ. A joint coordinate system for the clinical description of three-dimensional motions: application to the knee. J Biomech Eng 1983;105(2):136–144

6. Wu G, Siegler S, Allard P, et al; Standardization and Terminology Committee of the International Society of Biomechanics; International Society of Biomechanics. ISB recommendation on definitions of joint coordinate system of various joints for the reporting of human joint motion—part I: ankle, hip, and spine. J Biomech 2002;35(4):543–548

7. Wu G, van der Helm FC, Veeger HE, et al; International Society of Biomechanics. ISB recommendation on definitions of joint coordinate systems of various joints for the reporting of human joint motion—Part II: shoulder, elbow, wrist and hand. J Biomech 2005;38(5):981–992

Part III

Mechanical Aspects of the Human Locomotor System

8 Mechanical Properties of Bone and Cartilage

An organism composed only of soft tissues could survive without great problems in the ocean. When living on the land or in the air, rigid and fracture-resistant structural elements are indispensable for maintenance of the body shape and for locomotion. The strength of our bones is high enough to sustain normal, everyday loading. In addition, our bones are rigid; that is, their deformation under load is small (**Fig. 8.1**). While possessing these qualities, however, the bones must not become too massive and heavy. If overload damage occurs, bones must be able to repair themselves. In addition, bones protect vital organs such as the brain, spinal cord, heart, and lungs. Structural properties such as strength and rigidity are of importance here too.

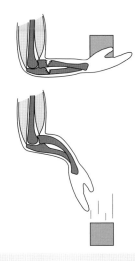

Fig. 8.1 Mechanical demands on bones. Excessively fragile or flexible bones are unable to stabilize postures or to control movements. (Adapted from Currey.[1] ©1984 Princeton University Press. Reprinted by permission of Princeton University Press.)

Apart from their duties in the mechanical field, bones play an important role in calcium metabolism and provide space for the blood-generating cells. For this reason the mechanical properties and architecture of the bones are inextricably linked with metabolic processes. One example of this interrelation is the change in bone density observed with physical activity or in the course of aging.

In joints of the human body, the shapes of the articulating bones are usually incongruent: their shapes do not fit together. Contact between incongruent bodies can occur only at points or along lines. If such points are loaded, we expect very high contact pressures. To restrict peak pressures in incongruent joints to physiologically tolerable values, therefore, the articulating surfaces are covered with articular cartilage.

Cartilage, which in relation to bone is soft, deforms under pressure, with the result that the area of the pressure-transmitting surface does not fall below a certain minimum value; this places an upper limit on the pressure. The friction properties of cartilage are also of eminent importance for the proper functioning of the joints—the friction between cartilage surfaces is so small that joints can be regarded virtually as frictionless. This is of great practical importance, since otherwise it would be difficult to move loaded joints.

8.1 Architecture of Bone Tissue

The material properties and architecture of bones can be discussed at different levels, under ultramicroscopic or microscopic magnification as well as macroscopically (as seen with the naked eye). This section does not aim to give a comprehensive description of the composition and properties of bones but is confined to those items that explain the unique mechanical properties of bones and which highlight the difficulties encountered in an exact description of these properties. For comprehensive information the reader is referred to the writings of Martin et al,[2] Currey,[3] and Tillmann and Töndury.[4]

8.1.1 Ultramicroscopic Findings

Bone is composed of cells embedded in a fibrous, organic ground substance (extracellular matrix). The extracellular matrix of mature bone consists of about 20% water. The dry material consists of 30% to 40% organic and 60% to 70% inorganic components. The organic component consists of 90% collagen, with the remaining 10% being composed essentially of glycosaminoglycans and glycoproteins.

The collagen of the bones is exactly the same as the material employed in other tissues of the body subjected to tensile stress, such as ligaments or connective tissue. In primary woven bone, the collagen fibrils are not aligned in any preferred direction. In mature lamellar bone, by contrast, the collagen fibrils can form a meshed or spiral arrangement, aligned preferentially in the longitudinal direction of the long bones.

The rigidity and strength characteristic of bone material are effected by the deposition of mineral substances in the organic ground substance (matrix). These inorganic salts comprise about 85% calcium phosphate, 6% to 10% calcium carbonate, and small admixtures of other alkaline salts. After generation of the organic matrix, these salts are first deposited in an amorphous phase; subsequently crystals bearing a close resemblance to hydroxyapatite $Ca_{10}(PO_4)_6(OH)_2$ are formed. These crystals are between 20 and 100 nm long and between 1.5 and 3.0 nm in diameter (1 nm = 10^{-9} m). They are aligned in their long axis to the collagen fibrils and are attached to the fibrils in several layers.

8.1.2 Microscopic Findings

The bone cells comprise the bone-building cells (osteoblasts), the bone-resorbing cells (osteoclasts), and the mature cells enclosed in the extracellular matrix (osteocytes). Osteoblasts produce an early stage of bone tissue, the osteoid. In the course of this phase the osteoblasts remain enclosed in the matrix and become osteocytes. Within a few days the osteoid is mineralized to about 70%; mineralization is completed within a few months. Osteoclasts resorb the collagen component of the bone tissue by an enzymatic process. The mineral component is dissolved by creation of an acidic environment.

During the growth phase, as well as during the entire lifetime, bone tissue is continuously remodeled as osteoclasts resorb bone and osteoblasts rebuild new bone, often in a different architecture. A distinction is made between primary bone (created for the first time) and secondary bone (created by reconstruction). Almost all bone present at birth, and the callus produced for the purpose of stabilization around fractures, consists of so-called *woven bone*. The collagen fibers of the woven bone have diameters in the region of 0.1 μm (1 μm = 10^{-6} m) and exhibit no preferred direction. Unordered trabeculae, the so-called *primary spongy bone*, develop from woven bone. Under the influence of mechanical loading, the primary spongy bone is transformed into spatially ordered, secondary trabecular (spongy) bone. The lamellar bone material of cortical bone also originates from woven bone. In lamellar bone, mineral and collagen are deposited in layers of about 5 μm thickness. The collagen fibers of lamellar bone have diameters in the region of 2 to 3 μm and definitely preferred orientations. The architecture of lamellar bone bears some similarity to that of technical fiber composite materials.[3,4] Lamellar, cortical bone is interspersed with osteons. Osteons are created when bone is resorbed by osteoclasts, in the form of a thin channel, which is subsequently filled with new bone deposited in layers by osteoblasts.

8.1.3 Macroscopic Findings

The small difference in the density of woven bone and lamellar bone material is due to minor differences in their organic and inorganic composition. Major differences in the density of bone tissue samples are due to the porosity of the tissue. In the cross section of long bones, an outer layer of compact bone, known as cortical bone, is visible. The internal volume of long bones is usually filled with a structure composed of thin rods (trabeculae) and plates. Bone displaying this architecture is termed *trabecular* (*spongy*) bone. The architecture of trabecular bone is not unlike that of technical foams with open pores. There is no abrupt transition from cortical to trabecular bone. The outermost bony layer of the long bones beneath the articular cartilage, for example, is called cortical bone, despite the fact that its thickness at this location is virtually the same as that typical of trabeculae.

As a rough categorization, the apparent density of cortical bone is above 1.5 g/cm³, and the apparent density of trabecular bone between 0.1 and 1.0 g/cm³. The qualifier *apparent* points to the fact that this density measurement allows for porosity; it does not describe the true density of the compact material (that is, as measured without voids). The apparent density is obtained by dividing the mass of a bone sample, cleaned of marrow and body fluids, by its volume. The apparent density should be distinguished from the density measured in the material in its compressed state (that is, without pores). With regard to this latter density, cortical and trabecular bone would exhibit only minor differences because both bone types are constructed essentially from lamellar bone. Deformation and strength of bones depend strongly on the apparent density.

8.2 Growth of Bones and Adaptation of Their Shape

As bone material is virtually undeformable, longitudinal growth of bones and adaptation of their shape can only be brought about by apposition or ablation of material on their internal or external surfaces. Longitudinal growth of the bones occurs in nonmineralized zones close to their ends. The so-called growth plate is located between the end piece (epiphysis) and the adjoining middle portion (metaphysis) of a bone. Cartilage-generating cells develop in the growth plate, forming columns in a multistage process and producing the surrounding ground substance or matrix. Where these columns join with the metaphysis, the cells change their function, grow in size, and prepare for ossification. Again in a multistage process, the mineralized cartilage is transformed into bone. By this means the metaphysis increases in length while the growth plate retains its position relative to the ends of the bone.

The fact that longitudinal growth of bone does not occur at its very ends, at the joint surface, but under the "protective shield" of the epiphysis has the advantage of avoiding mechanically induced disturbance of the growth process. Due to its high water content, cartilage is not very susceptible to pressure, so the bones can grow longitudinally while they are under compressive load from the joints in the course of daily life. Due to its architecture, however, the shear strength of the growth plate is low. In newborns the growth plate is almost plane, while with age the growth plate takes on an irregular, curved shape. The effect of this shape change is to increase shear strength. The shear strength of the growth plate is particularly low during phases of rapid growth. Shear forces are considered responsible for juvenile loosening of the femoral epiphysis (epiphysiolysis), while a ball hitting the juvenile wrist laterally can injure the growth plate of the radius.

Growth in the width of the growth plates is achieved by cell proliferation at the periphery. The concurrent modeling of the entire bone shape, with diminution of the diameter below the growth plate and adaptation of the diameter in the central portion of the long bones (diaphysis), takes place by targeted removal and deposition of bone material at the surface of the bone. Concurrent removal and deposition makes it possible to "shift" sections of the metaphysis and diaphysis relative to the long axis of the bone, thereby creating the curvature of the long bones (**Fig. 8.2**). Once skeletal maturity has been reached, the bones do not remain unaltered. Throughout life, remodeling takes place through removal and apposition of bone material, occasionally with different architecture. It is hypothesized that this continuous remodeling serves to repair microdamage as well as to adapt the mechanical properties of the bone to the in vivo loading conditions.

In the course of maturation, the growth plates close, in a particular temporal sequence, by ossification. Between about 15 and 18 years of age, all bones have attained their adult length and all growth plates

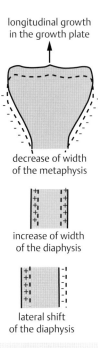

longitudinal growth
in the growth plate

decrease of width
of the metaphysis

increase of width
of the diaphysis

lateral shift
of the diaphysis

Fig. 8.2 Adaptation of bone shape by apposition (+) or resorption (−) at external or internal surfaces. (Adapted from Martin et al.[2] With kind permission of Springer Science + Business Media.)

are closed. In many cases their characteristic architecture can be spotted in radiographic images, even in old age. The course of the closure of the growth plates over time allows the definition of *skeletal age*. On average, skeletal age runs parallel to chronological age, but people whose growth plates close earlier than normal have a skeletal age that runs ahead of their chronological age, whereas those whose growth plates remain open longer than normal have a skeletal age that is lower than their chronological age. To determine skeletal age, radiographs of the hand are compared with the norm of healthy juvenile individuals. If a person's skeletal age, chronological age, and height are known (and possibly also the father's and mother's heights), it is possible to predict precisely how tall that person will be on reaching skeletal maturity.[5]

8.3 Fracture Healing

After bone fracture, inflammation together with hematoma, swelling, and pain are observed at the fracture site. Swelling and pain enforce immobilization; a splint or a cast has the same effect. Due to the surrounding soft tissues, however, absolutely rigid immobilization is unattainable: some interfragmentary motion remains. The healing of the fracture is brought about by cells originating from the periosteum and the medullary cavity (endosteum). The gap at the fracture site is first filled by fibrocartilage (**Fig. 8.3**). Cells

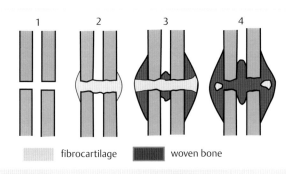

fibrocartilage   woven bone

Fig. 8.3 Stages 1 to 4 of bone healing with formation of fibrocartilage and woven bone (callus). (Adapted, with permission, from Debrunner.[6])

originating from the periosteum generate woven bone (callus), which bridges the fracture on the outer surface. Cells originating from the endosteum bridge the fracture in the medullary cavity. Callus consists of spatially disordered collagen fibers; within a relatively short time bone mineral is embedded between these fibers. The stiffness and strength of callus are lower than those of cortical bone, but the diameter of the callus formation is larger than the original diameter of the long bone. This has the effect that approximately 1 month after fracture, because of the increase of the second moment of area, the stiffness and bending strength can be equal to or even larger than those of the intact bone. From this time onwards, the callus transforms into normal bone, so that after 1 to 2 years the original shape of the bone is restored.

Healing of a fracture by formation of callus is called *secondary* healing. This in contrast to *primary* healing, in which the bone fragments unite directly by bone remodeling (that is, without callus formation). Primary healing occurs when there is direct contact between the fracture surfaces and only very small relative motion between them. The relative motion must be so small that newly formed vessels bridging the fracture gap are not sheared off. Primary healing can be observed when the fragments are screwed together with a stiff metallic plate, usually in conjunction with a longitudinally directed compressive force to further minimize the remaining relative mobility. The issue of whether secondary or primary fracture healing leads to better clinical results in the end remains at present unresolved, despite the many in vitro and animal experiments as well as clinical studies conducted in the past 40 years.

8.4   Mechanical Properties of Bone Material

8.4.1 Stress and Strain of Inhomogeneous, Anisotropic Materials

A material that is of uniform composition throughout its whole volume is termed *homogeneous*. Bone material is *inhomogeneous* because it is composed of a crystallized mineral and a fibrous organic component. A material whose mechanical properties do not depend on the direction of load or deformation is

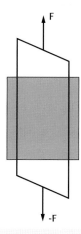

Fig. 8.4 Example of the deformation mode of an anisotropic material. Under the action of a force, the material exhibits not only a change in length in the direction of the force but in also an angular deformation.

termed *isotropic*. Due to the spatial alignment of the organic fibers in lamellar bone, the architecture of the layered lamellae in cortical bone, and the spatial configuration of the trabeculae in trabecular bone, the mechanical properties of bone (moduli of elasticity and shear, etc.) depend on the orientation in which they have been measured. Thus, bone material is *anisotropic*.

Unlike in isotropic materials, the strain occurring in anisotropic materials is not necessarily in the same direction as the applied stress. Under tensile stress a beam made of an anisotropic material may, for example, not only lengthen but also exhibit an angular deformation (**Fig. 8.4**). The deformation of inhomogeneous, anisotropic materials under the influence of external forces cannot be characterized by the three material constants (modulus of elasticity E, shear modulus G, and Poisson's ratio µ), as in the case of homogeneous, isotropic materials. To describe the relation between stress and strain, Hooke's law and the law describing shear deformation

(8.1)

$$\sigma = E \cdot \varepsilon$$
$$\tau = G \cdot \alpha$$

have to be generalized. In this generalized law the modulus of elasticity E and the shear modulus G are replaced by a term c, known as the *stiffness matrix*. In the general case, this term depends on 21 material constants. (We are dealing here with a symmetric 6 · 6 tensor with 21 independent elements.) The stress σ is replaced by a mathematical expression (a vector with six components) which depends on the three normal and the three shear stresses. The strain ε is replaced by a mathematical expression (vector with six components) which depends on the linear strains in the three spatial directions and on three angular deformations. In this formulation, the generalized Hooke's law is written as

(8.2)
$$\sigma_i = \sum_{j=1}^{6} c_{ij} \cdot \varepsilon_j$$

The index i assumes values from 1 to 6. The mathematical sum sign Σ indicates that, to calculate the i-th component σ_i of the stress vector, all products $c_{ij} \cdot \varepsilon_j$ have to be added together. The index j runs from j = 1 to j = 6. Thus, in contrast to the case of isotropic materials, the stress in a certain spatial direction will depend on the strain and the angular deformation in all three spatial directions. Conversely, a normal stress effects not only a deformation in the direction of the stress but also an angular deformation. This was the very case in the example shown in **Fig. 8.4**.

In the technical domain the generalized Hooke's law forms the basis for a description of the mechanical properties of fiber-reinforced materials. But even in such applications it proves difficult to determine the complete set of 21 material constants experimentally. When dealing with bone material, additional difficulties arise. Due to changes in bone density and architecture, the mechanical properties of bone change from one volume element to the next. In addition, bone is nonlinearly elastic: that is, the material properties depend on the magnitude of the applied strain and on the deformation velocity. In technical materials there is no equivalent to the in vivo repair and adaptation processes encountered in bone.

These comments are aimed at making it clear that, other than for those situations where a crude, approximate description of the mechanical behavior of bone will suffice, a detailed description has to be based on intricate theory and on experimental determination of a large set of material constants. For this reason, lines of reasoning are often complex and hard to follow. Nevertheless, a detailed description is indispensable if, for example, the relation between mechanical stimuli and bone adaptation is to be investigated. To this end, the state of stress and deformation under the application of external forces and moments must be known as accurately as possible. Estimates based on the properties of a homogeneous, isotropic material are inadequate.

8.4.2 Material Properties of Cortical Bone

When, in the following, the mechanical properties of bone are characterized by only a few material constants, it must be kept in mind that this constitutes a crude approximation to reality. **Table 8.1** gives an overview of the properties of human cortical bone. The numbers quoted are only approximate. The ranges of variation are due, in part, to the biological variation of the individual bones investigated and, in some cases, to varying examination methods. The stress σ_u, which effects the destruction of the sample, is called the *ultimate* (or *maximum*) stress.

The anisotropy of bone material becomes apparent when samples cut in different directions from the cortical layer of a long bone are compared. As an illustration, **Table 8.2** quotes measured results for the modulus of elasticity and the ultimate stress for samples cut longitudinally and transversely with respect to the long axis of a bone.

Material property	Approximate value
Modulus of elasticity (Young's modulus) E	$6-25 \cdot 10^9$ N/m²
Poisson's ratio μ	0.08–0.45
Shear modulus G	$0.31 \cdot 10^9$ N/m²
Ultimate stress in a tensile test	$87-151 \cdot 10^6$ N/m²
Ultimate stress in a compression test	$106-193 \cdot 10^6$ N/m²
Ultimate stress under shear loading	$53-82 \cdot 10^6$ N/m²

Table 8.1 Material properties of human cortical bone

Source: Data from Reilly and Burstein.[7]

Material property	Approximate value
Modulus of elasticity, sample oriented in longitudinal direction	$17.0 \cdot 10^9$ N/m²
Modulus of elasticity, sample oriented in transverse direction	$11.5 \cdot 10^9$ N/m²
Ultimate tensile stress, sample oriented in longitudinal direction	$133 \cdot 10^6$ N/m²
Ultimate tensile stress, sample oriented in transverse direction	$51 \cdot 10^6$ N/m²
Ultimate compressive stress, sample oriented in longitudinal direction	$193 \cdot 10^6$ N/m²
Ultimate compressive stress, sample oriented in transverse direction	$133 \cdot 10^6$ N/m²

Table 8.2 Orientation dependence of the material properties of human cortical bone

Source: Data from Reilly and Burstein.[8]

Bone material is viscoelastic; the values of the material constants depend on the deformation velocity (that is, whether deformation occurs over a short or long time interval). As an example, **Fig. 8.5** shows the dependence of the modulus of elasticity E and of the ultimate stress σ_u on the deformation velocity. The observed increase of E and σ_u indicates that with increasing deformation velocity the material is becoming *harder* and *stronger*.

Like many other materials, cortical bone exhibits mechanical fatigue under repeated loading. The stress at which fracture of a sample is observed decreases with increasing numbers of load cycles. Carter et al[10–12] reported that material fatigue depended predominantly on the magnitude of the strain, with bone density or ash content having little influence on fatigue strength. According to these authors, the ultimate stress after 10^7 load cycles is in the region of $7 \cdot 10^6$ N/m². This is considerably lower than the ultimate stress under a single load cycle as quoted in **Table 8.1**.

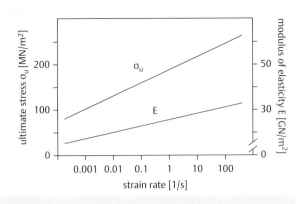

Fig. 8.5 Modulus of elasticity E and ultimate stress σ_u of cortical bone related to strain rate. (Adapted from Wright and Hayes.[9])

Fig. 8.6 shows the number of cycles to fracture in dependence on the magnitude of the strain as measured by Carter et al.[10] To check how high the risk of a fatigue fracture is when walking, running, or performing strenuous athletic exercise, estimated regions of the strain in the lower extremity are also shown in this diagram. It is concluded that fatigue fractures are not to be expected when walking. When running over long distances, occurrence of fatigue fractures is possible, especially if an individual running style with high repetitive loading coincides with low individual bone strength. Indeed, fractures of the lower

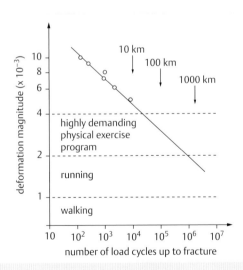

Fig. 8.6 Fatigue properties of human cortical bone in relation to the magnitude of the strain. In addition, regions of strain of the bones of the lower extremity expected to occur during strenuous exercises, running, or walking are indicated. (Adapted from Carter et al.[10])

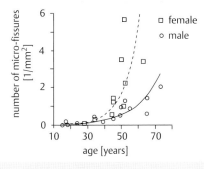

Fig. 8.7 Prevalence of microfissures in cortical bone in relation to age. (Adapted, with permission, from Schaffler et al.[17])

extremity occasionally observed in young soldiers after running long distances or marching with heavy packs are interpreted as fatigue fractures (sometimes termed *stress fractures*).[13]

The mechanical properties of cortical bone change with age.[14] These changes are assumed to be caused by structural changes in the organic and inorganic bone components. According to Burstein et al[15] and Duchemin et al,[16] the modulus of elasticity, ultimate stress, and ultimate strain decrease with age. In other words, bone becomes softer and more brittle with increasing age. In the material investigated by Burstein et al,[15] no gender-related difference in the mechanical properties was noted. The observation that microfissures in cortical bone are not rare findings agrees with the results of Burstein and coworkers. The prevalence of such fissures increases with age (**Fig. 8.7**).[17]

8.4.3 Architecture and Material Properties of Trabecular Bone

Trabecular bone is composed of a three-dimensional mesh of interconnected bone rods and plates, arranged similarly to that of open-pore technical foam materials. Except in woven bone, the rods and plates are oriented in preferred directions that are readily discernible to the naked eye on bone sections. Below the cartilaginous layer of joints, for example, the trabeculae are preferentially oriented perpendicular to the joint surface. There appears to be a second preferred direction oriented at about 90° to the first, where the rods and plates are interconnected, thus reinforcing the mesh. It is understandable from these observations that the elastic properties and the strength of trabecular bone are determined by the density, the distance, and the relative orientation and interconnection of the rods and plates. It follows furthermore that measured material properties of trabecular bone depend on the direction of testing. Trabecular bone is an anisotropic material.[18]

With increasing age the compressive strength of trabecular bone decreases.[19] At the same time the ratio of rods to plates changes (**Fig. 8.8**)[20]: the number of plates decreases while the number of rods remains

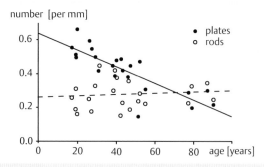

Fig. 8.8 Plates and rods of the trabecular bone of the second lumbar vertebra in relation to age. (Adapted from Delling et al.[20] With kind permission of Springer Science + Business Media.)

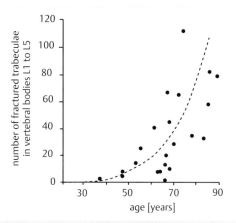

Fig. 8.9 Number of fractured trabeculae observed in specimens of the lumbar spine (first to fifth lumbar vertebra) in relation to age. (Adapted from Vernon-Roberts and Pirie.[21])

virtually constant. In specimens of trabecular bone originating from the acetabulum of the hip joint or from the central volume of vertebral bodies, fractured trabeculae in different stages of the healing process are a common finding.[20-22] The prevalence of such fractures increases with age (**Fig. 8.9**).[21] It is hypothesized that these fractures are caused by mechanical overloading; alternatively, they may result from a normal remodeling process.

Porosity is defined as that volume fraction of a bone sample not filled by bone material. The porosity of a sample of cortical bone with no voids would be zero; the porosity of trabecular bone can approach (though not reach) the value 1. If the material properties of cortical bone and those of the rods and plates of trabecular bone are assumed to be approximately equal, the material properties of samples of cortical

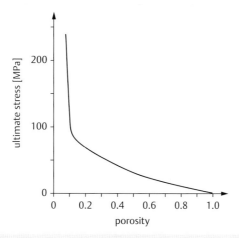

Fig. 8.10 Ultimate compressive stress of human bone in relation to porosity. (Adapted from Martin et al.[2] With kind permission of Springer Science + Business Media.)

and trabecular bone (save for anisotropic effects) can be expected to depend continuously on the degree of porosity. The modulus of elasticity of trabecular bone with porosity p can be approximated by[23]

$$(8.3) \qquad\qquad E = 15 \cdot (1-p)^3 \ [GPa]$$

This formula tells us that, with increasing porosity p (with increasing void space in the sample), the modulus of elasticity E exhibits a marked decrease. Quantitatively, the modulus of elasticity of trabecular bone ranges between 1.4 MPa and 9800 MPa.[24]

Fig. 8.10 shows the ultimate stress of samples of trabecular bone in dependence on porosity. The ultimate stress is seen to decrease with increasing porosity. With increasing porosity (or decreasing apparent density) trabecular bone becomes *softer* and *weaker*. The ultimate stress observed in samples of trabecular bone covers the entire stress range depicted in **Fig. 8.10**. Depending on the type of bone and the source of the samples, published data range between 0.2 MPa and 378 MPa.[24] Samples of trabecular bone are usually not irreparably damaged by one single overload episode, but subsequently still exhibit some strength, though at a reduced level (see, for example, Keaveny et al[25]). The residual strength of mechanically damaged bones (fractured osteoporotic vertebrae, for example) constitutes a vital safety factor for the functioning of the locomotor system. The ultimate strain of trabecular bone is about 4%,[26,27] and is independent of porosity and apparent density.

When a sample of trabecular bone is viewed with the naked eye, the alignment of the trabeculae in preferred directions is obvious beyond any doubt. In the past, describing the intuitively observed anisotropy in

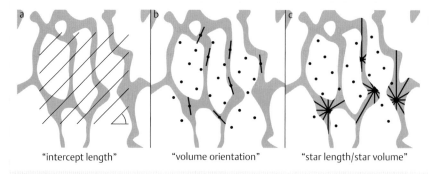

"intercept length"   "volume orientation"   "star length/star volume"

Fig. 8.11a–c Illustration of the parameters "mean intercept length" (**a**), "volume orientation" (**b**), and "star length/star volume" (**c**) used to describe the anisotropy of trabecular bone. (Adapted, with permission, from Odgaard et al.[29])

quantitative, mathematical terms posed considerable difficulties. The remarkable progress made in recent years, however, allows the spatial anisotropy of the mesh to be described in numerical terms and these data to be linked with the anisotropy of the mechanical properties. Parameters describing the local anisotropy ("fabric") of the spatial mesh can be defined. In parallel, the deformation of such meshes under the influence of external forces can be computed using the finite element method or, alternatively, it can be measured directly. The comparison of calculated and measured results reveals how well a specific anisotropy parameter actually describes the mechanical properties of a sample of trabecular bone.[28-30]

Fig. 8.11 illustrates three proposals for a quantitative description of the local anisotropy of trabecular bone.[29] The figure uses a two-dimensional model, but the concepts are applied in three dimensions. The sample of trabecular bone shown appears intuitively to be preferentially oriented in the vertical direction. An attempt can be made to describe the preferred direction by superimposing a line grid in different orientations (**Fig. 8.11a**) and observing the lengths of the grid lines (*intercept length*) intersecting the trabeculae. In the example shown, we expect long intercept lengths when the grid is oriented vertically and short lengths when the grid is oriented horizontally.

Alternatively (**Fig. 8.11b**), points can be selected at random within the bone volume and the direction in which straight lines through these points exhibit the longest intercept with the bone volume (*volume orientation*) is observed. In the example shown, these directions would preferentially point to the vertical; a second preferred direction would point approximately to the horizontal. As a further alternative (**Fig. 8.11c**), the orientation of local bone volume elements can be quantified if points are again selected at random within the bone volume and the distance of the bone surface as seen from these points in different directions is recorded (described as *star length* and *star volume*). In addition to orientation, these parameters also quantify the interconnection of the rods and plates in the trabecular bone.

Due to recent improvements in the spatial resolution of computed tomography, it is now possible to reconstruct the lattice of trabecular bone not only from in vitro bone samples, but also in vivo from tibia and radius (see, for example, Boutroy et al[31]). If further progress allows in vivo imaging of trabecular architecture in other regions of the skeleton as well, we can expect important new insights into bone growth and remodeling.

8.5   Determination of Bone Density

The spatial density of bone (grams per cubic centimeter) cannot be determined directly in vivo. Measurement of the absorption of γ- or X-rays allows determination only of an area density (grams per square centimeter). However, if a body is irradiated from a variety of directions, the distribution of the spatial density can be calculated from the set of area densities measured.

When passing through matter, the intensity of γ- or X-radiation decreases (is attenuated). For radiation of a given energy it holds that

(8.4) $$I = I_0 \cdot \exp(-\mu \cdot x)$$

In this formula, exp is the exponential function; I_0 and I denote the intensity of the incoming and outgoing beam; x is the thickness of the layer; μ is the coefficient of absorption of the material. μ depends on the atomic number (ordinal number in the periodic system of elements) of the irradiated element (or the atomic numbers of all elements contained in a mixed sample), on the density of the matter, and on the energy of the radiation. Eq. 8.4 holds for a homogeneous material layer of thickness x. If an inhomogeneous layer is irradiated, for example a layer containing (nonabsorbing) voids, Eq. 8.4 remains valid if we accept x as the summed effective thickness of the material in the path of the beam.

If the absorption coefficient μ of bone is known from a calibration experiment, it is possible to determine the effective thickness of bone material in vivo from the measured I_0 and I. If the density ρ [g/cm³] of bone material is known from an additional in vitro calibration experiment, the area density at the location of the irradiation is given by

(8.5) $$d = x \cdot \rho \ \ [g/cm^2]$$

If, in addition to bone mineral, soft tissue is located in the path of the radiation, an error occurs when the above formula is used, because the soft tissue also contributes to the absorption of the radiation, though to a much lesser extent than the mineral component. To correct for this error, one can irradiate the body twice, but with rays of different energy. With two materials in the path of the beam, for example bone and water (as a substitute for soft tissue), the absorption law reads

(8.6) $$I = I_0 \cdot \exp(-\mu_1 \cdot x_1 - \mu_2 \cdot x_2)$$

with μ_1 and μ_2 as absorption coefficients and x_1 and x_2 as thicknesses of the layers of the two materials. The fact that the absorption coefficients are energy-dependent is made use of to determine the thickness of the two layers if the absorption is measured at two different radiation energies. Performing measurements at radiation energies A and B provides two equations

(8.7)
$$I_A = I_{0A} \cdot \exp(-\mu_{1A} \cdot x_1 - \mu_{2A} \cdot x_2)$$

(8.8)
$$I_B = I_{0B} \cdot \exp(-\mu_{1B} \cdot x_1 - \mu_{2B} \cdot x_2)$$

from which, so long as the (energy-dependent) absorption coefficients μ_{1A}, μ_{2A}, μ_{1B}, and μ_{2B} are known, the thicknesses x_1 and x_2 of the layers can be determined. The source of radiation utilized comprises either two radioactive elements or X-ray tubes powered by two different voltages. If X-ray tubes are employed, it must be noted that these do not emit radiation of a fixed energy, but an energy spectrum with a fixed maximum energy, the value of which is determined by the input voltage. The determination of the thickness of the two layers then relies on formulae similar to those given above.

Conventional radiographs (**Fig. 8.12**) image bones because bones absorb more of the X-radiation than do the surrounding tissues. However, such radiographs are ill suited to a quantitative appraisal of the area density of the bones. This is because the relationship between the blackness of the film and the radiation dose received is not linear, and is further influenced by the film development. Digital radiographs avoid these errors, but there is no avoiding the problem that every area element of the film not only receives radiation directly from the direction of the X-ray tube—it also receives scattered radiation from every volume element in the irradiated body.

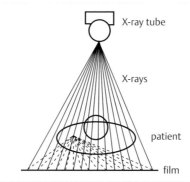

Fig. 8.12 Ray path in conventional radiography. Dashed lines represent scattered X-rays originating from one volume element of the irradiated body.

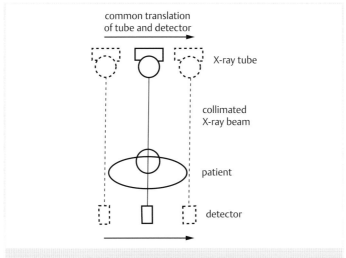

Fig. 8.13 Ray path in dual energy X-ray absorptiometry (DXA). The X-ray tube and the detector are moved across the body together.

The procedures of dual photon absorptiometry (DPA) and dual energy X-ray absorptiometry (DXA) employ collimated γ- or X-radiation (**Fig. 8.13**) to reduce the perturbing influence of scattered radiation. A collimator is a device (for example, a lead block with a small drilled hole) that produces a beam with a small cross section that flares only slightly. The beam hits a detector mounted behind a second collimator, which serves to suppress scattered radiation. The radiation source and the detector are moved together. All materials and structures in the path of the beam contribute to its attenuation. Measurements are performed with two energies to determine the layer thickness of bone separately from that of water, fat, and soft tissue.

The bone density measured by DPA or DXA is designated *bone mineral density* and is stated in units of grams per square centimeter [g/cm²]; for lumbar spine measurements, the result is sometimes given in units of grams per centimeter [g/cm]. For this purpose, the area density is multiplied by the width of the vertebrae; the result quantifies the amount of bone material in the lumbar spine per centimeter in a craniocaudal direction. The *bone mineral content* is the amount of bone mineral (in grams) of a whole organ. To obtain this, the area density of the organ (for example, a vertebra) is multiplied by its width and height. If volume of the organ [cm³] and its bone mineral content [g] are known, the *mean volumetric bone density* of the organ [g/cm³] can be obtained as the quotient of these two parameters. (Unfortunately, the terms *bone mineral density* for area or volume density and *bone mineral content* for total mineral content are not always used consistently in the scientific literature.)

Computed tomography (CT) uses the absorption data of an object irradiated by X-rays in many different directions (**Fig. 8.14**) to calculate a three-dimensional model of the density distribution of the object under

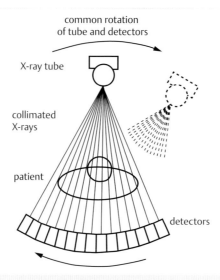

Fig. 8.14 Ray path in computed tomography (CT, quantitative CT). The X-ray tube and the array of detectors are moved concurrently in such a way that every volume element of the body is irradiated many times from different directions.

investigation. Since CT applications in the human body involve volume elements that differ greatly in their absorption of X-rays (bone, soft tissue, void spaces, surrounding air, and so on), the density calculated in each volume element is quoted, not in absolute units, but in Hounsfield units:

$$(8.9) \qquad\qquad H = 1000 \cdot ((\rho / \rho_w) - 1.0)$$

where H is the density in Hounsfield units, ρ designates the computed density of the material and ρ_w the density of water. According to this formula, a volume filled with water has zero density in Hounsfield units. A volume filled with fat has negative values in Hounsfield units, because the density ρ of fat is lower than that of water. A volume filled with bone has positive values in Hounsfield units, because the density ρ of bone is higher than that of water.

To convert density values given in Hounsfield units into density values of bone mineral, calibration objects are measured together with the bones or body segments under investigation. Following a proposal by Genant et al,[32] differently concentrated solutions of K_2HPO_4 in water are used for this purpose. The absorption of X-rays by K_2HPO_4 is very similar to the absorption by the mineral component of bone. The measured Hounsfield units of a calibration object are employed to convert the density of the object into an equivalent density of K_2HPO_4 in units of milligrams per cubic centimeter [mg/cm³]. This protocol is called *quantitative computed tomography* (QCT). Whereas density values in Hounsfield units measured on different X-ray units are not directly comparable due to inadvertent or uncontrolled shifts in machine calibration or changes in tube voltage, density data given in units of mg/cm^3 K_2HPO_4 are independent of the apparatus and thus permit direct comparisons. As QCT determines real density data and not only area or line densities, it is possible—unlike with DPA or DXA—to obtain data separately for partial volumes filled with cortical or trabecular bone.

If the tomograph employs one fixed tube voltage, the density of only one material can be determined in each volume element. If more than one material is present, for example bone and fat, a systematic error occurs. Repetition of the measurement with a different X-ray energy (double energy quantitative computed tomography, DQCT) would allow two materials to be discriminated, as with DPA and DXA. This procedure has, however, not been adopted for routine clinical application due to the increased radiation exposure and the comparatively small diagnostic benefit. For a comparison of the precision and reproducibility of QCT, DPA, and DXA when determining bone density and bone mineral density, the reader is referred to Mazess.[33]

8.6 Clinical Applications of a Bone Density Measurement

The clinical applications of bone density measurements include the monitoring of fracture healing, follow-up of diseases such as bone metabolism disorders or osteoporosis, treatment monitoring (effects of medication or exercise on density increase), and in vivo prediction of fracture risk. Conventional radiographs are normally sufficient to monitor fracture healing. Repeated measurements of bone density (by whatever method) for treatment or disease monitoring make sense if the natural course of a disease is to be documented, or if the measurement results would have implications for further treatment. On the other hand, bone density measurements are of limited use in cases where no therapy is currently available for the bone disease concerned.

Laboratory (in vitro) studies of bone specimens can investigate the relationships between the strength of a bone and its dimensions (diameter, cross-sectional area, wall thickness) and its trabecular and cortical bone density. If these geometrical parameters and bone densities are then measured in vivo in patients, individualized predictions of bone strength are possible. For example, Lotz and Hayes[34] and Hayes et al[35] used QCT to investigate the relationship between trabecular bone density at the junction of the femoral neck with the femur and the strength of the femur. The experimental setup was designed to simulate a fall onto the side, as the authors considered this type of fall to be the primary cause of fractures of the proximal femur occurring in the elderly. **Fig. 8.15** shows the relationship between bone density and the strength of the specimens investigated, together with the regression line describing the mean, statistical relation between these parameters. As seen in the figure, femoral strength increases approximately linearly with bone density. The strength is very low at bone densities below 100 mg/mL K_2HPO_4. There is also a close correlation between the bone mineral content of the proximal femur and strength when the femur

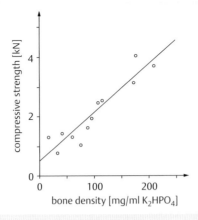

Fig. 8.15 Strength of the proximal femur in relation to bone density. (Adapted from Hayes et al.[35])

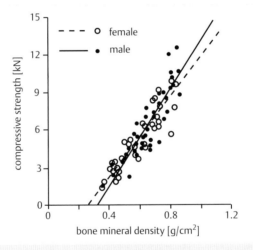

Fig. 8.16 Compressive strength of the central layer of lumbar vertebrae in relation to bone mineral density. (Adapted, with permission, from Ebbesen et al.[37])

is subjected to a loading mode that simulates the load in erect stance.[36] Another example is a study by Ebbesen et al[37] which investigated the relationship between compressive strength and bone mineral density in specimens of lumbar vertebrae (central part, endplates removed). The results show (**Fig. 8.16**) that strength increased approximately linearly with bone mineral density. There was virtually no difference between specimens from male and female subjects.

In both fractures of the femoral neck and compression fractures of lumbar vertebrae, the scatter of the measured data with respect to the regression lines indicates that strength depends on parameters in addition to bone density and size, though to a lesser extent. The material properties of bone might have interindividual differences which cannot be detected by a density measurement. Differences in the individual architecture of cortical and trabecular bone will also influence bone strength.

8.7 Adaptation of Bones to Mechanical Demands

The overall shape of bones is genetically determined. This enables the anthropologist to determine provenance from fragments of human or animal bones. However, it has long been conjectured, on the basis of striking individual differences in cortical and trabecular bone architecture, that bones are not unalterable structures but can adapt, within certain limits, to the mechanical demands made on them. Wolff[38] postulated the architecture of cortical and trabecular bone to follow a mathematical law. Wolff was inspired in his hypothesis by the similarity between the alignment of the trabecular rods in the proximal femur and the course of the principal stress trajectories constructed by a contemporary engineer in objects made of homogeneous material and of identical shape. Roux[39] held the view that the adaptation of bones was based on a self-regulating mechanism. In the period that followed, both hypotheses became blended in the oft-cited *Wolff's law*.[40]

Wolff's law is not a law as, for example, Kepler's laws are laws: no concrete consequences can be deduced from it. When Wolff's law is cited in the scientific literature, it represents the hypothesis that changes in the mechanical demands bring about changes in the bone structure, or—to put it the other way around—that a change in bone structure allows conclusions to be drawn about a change in the mode of mechanical loading. In the following, some examples are discussed which may be interpreted as evidence of the adaptation of bones to mechanical demands. Incidentally, bone is not exceptional in being able to adapt to mechanical demands: muscles, tendons, and skin also exhibit adaptation of this kind.

8.7.1 Adaptation of Shape and Architecture

Bone material has high compressive strength, but low tensile strength. To prevent fractures, therefore, bending of bones should be avoided. **Fig. 8.17** illustrates the load **H** on the hip joint and the force **F** of the abductors during the stance phase of slow gait. The direction of **H** almost coincides with the direction of the femoral neck. Distal to the trochanter, the sum of forces **H** and **F** act on the femoral diaphysis; this force is directed approximately along the long axis of the bone. We may conclude from this that the shape of the femur is modeled so that the femoral neck and diaphysis are loaded essentially in compression, not in bending.

The walls of a bone of rectangular, longitudinal cross section (**Fig. 8.18**), under load by a compressive force **F**, would tend to bulge outwards due to expansion of the trabecular bone and the bone marrow. This would lead to tensile stress in the outer layers of the convex cortical wall. If, however, the wall

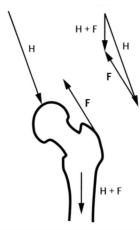

Fig. 8.17 Compressive loading of the femoral neck by the load **H** acting on the hip joint. The compressive loading exerted on the femoral shaft is equal to the sum of **H** and the force of the abductor muscles **F**.

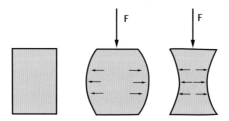

Fig. 8.18 Explanatory model for the waisted shape of long bones. In a bone with inwardly curving walls, the bending moment due to the load **F** and the bending moment due to the internal pressure counteract each other. (Adapted from Frost.[41])

curved inwards to begin with, the bending moment caused by the force **F** (tending to bend the wall further inwards) could be compensated by the outward-directed bending moment caused by the internal pressure (tending to bend the wall outwards). In this way, the deformation of the wall remains small. This argument[41] explains very well the "waisted" shape of our bones (phalanges of the hand, vertebral bodies, femur).

In bone sections, preferred orientations of the trabeculae near joint surfaces can be discerned with the naked eye. The trabeculae are preferentially oriented perpendicular to the thin layer of cortical bone below the cartilage. In a second preferred orientation, at 90° to the first, there are trabeculae connecting the rods among themselves. The mechanical interpretation of this is that the trabeculae oriented perpendicular to the joint surface are subjected to compression and not to bending. The sideways bracing has the effect

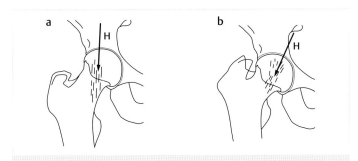

Fig. 8.19a, b Orientation of the trabeculae in the femoral neck before (**a**) and 10 years after (**b**) variation osteotomy. (Adapted from Pauwels.[42])

of reducing the length of the rods, thus increasing their ability to resist bending. Pauwels[42] observed the orientation of the trabecular bone of the femoral head before and after a variation osteotomy (**Fig. 8.19**). The osteotomy changed the direction of force **H** on the hip joint, and the orientation of the trabeculae followed this change.

8.7.2 Effects of Decreased or Increased Physical Activity

The mass of the bones (total mineral content of the body) and the mass of the muscles (mass of the soft tissues net of body fat) are correlated throughout life.[43] Rauch et al[44] showed that during adolescence the increase in bone mass parallels the increase in muscle mass. These observations comply with the hypothesis that the mineral content of bones and thus their strength are regulated by the mechanical loading. It is, however, also possible that the two processes—the increase of both bone and muscle mass—are determined genetically and are not causally related.

It has long been known that long-term bedridden subjects experience a loss of bone density. **Fig. 8.20** shows the result of bone mineral density measurements in the os calcis of three healthy young men over the course of 30 to 36 weeks' confinement to bed and the following recovery period. Since the start of manned space flight, the loss of bone mineral in astronauts owing to weightlessness has been documented. **Fig. 8.21** shows data from 18 astronauts who spent between 126 and 438 days in space (LeBlanc et al[46] cited by Cavanagh et al[47]). They performed physical exercises on board, but this still did not allow bone mineral loss to be completely avoided. For comparison, **Fig. 8.21** shows the loss of bone density in a bedridden cohort.

Conversely, an increase in physical activity brings about an increase in bone mineral, as is shown in examples in sport. Nilsson and Westlin[48] investigated bone mineral density in the distal femur of four cohorts: top-ranking athletes, competitive athletes, and physically active and physically inactive controls (**Table 8.3**). The disciplines comprised weight lifting, hammer throwing, soccer, and swimming.

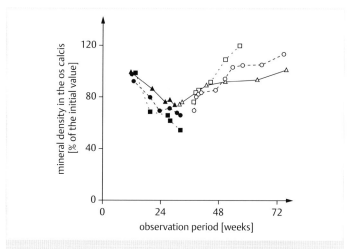

Fig. 8.20 Bone mineral density of the os calcis during (closed symbols) and after (open symbols) 30 to 36 weeks of bed rest. (Adapted from Donaldson et al.[45])

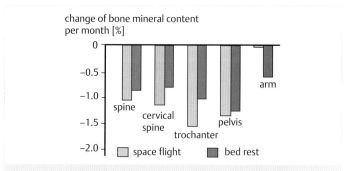

Fig. 8.21 Decrease of bone mineral density during space flight in comparison to bed rest. (Adapted, with permission, from Cavanagh et al.[47])

Jones et al[49] documented the cortical thickness of the humerus of the dominant and the nondominant arm of professional tennis players (**Table 8.4**). The layer thickness in the dominant arm was noticeably increased compared to the nondominant arm. In addition, the external diameter of the humerus of the dominant arm, as measured both anteroposteriorly and mediolaterally, was about 10% larger than in the nondominant arm.

Granhed et al[50] investigated the bone mineral density of the L3 vertebral body of weight lifters in relation to training intensity (**Fig. 8.22**). Density increased markedly with increasing intensity of the training, that is, with the mass lifted annually for training purposes. For comparison: the bone mineral density of an age-matched control group who did not engage in this athletic discipline ranged between 2 and 5 g/cm.[51]

Study cohort	n	Bone mineral density [g/cm³]
Top-ranking athletes	9	0.252 (0.049)
Competitive athletes	55	0.236 (0.049)
Controls, active	24	0.213 (0.031)
Controls, inactive	15	0.168 (0.037)

Table 8.3 Bone mineral density in the distal femur

Source: Data from Nilsson and Westlin.[48]

Note: Mean age of study participants was 22.5 years. Numbers in parentheses represent one standard deviation.

Location	n	Gender	Dominant arm [cm]	Control arm [cm]
Anterior	44	M	0.76 (0.09)	0.55 (0.06)
	23	F	0.61 (0.07)	0.49 (0.07)
Posterior	43	M	0.71 (0.10)	0.51 (0.07)
	22	F	0.58 (0.08)	0.46 (0.06)

Table 8.4 Thickness of the cortical bone of tennis players, measured 11 cm proximal to the elbow joint

Source: Data from Jones et al.[49]

Note: Numbers in parentheses represent one standard deviation.

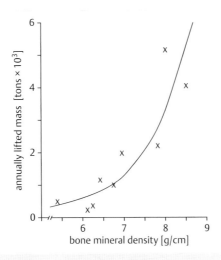

Fig. 8.22 Bone mineral density in the lumbar spine of weight lifters in relation to training intensity. (Adapted from Granhed et al.[50])

Jämsä et al[52] observed an increase in bone mineral density of the proximal femur dependent on mechanical loading. The magnitude of the loading was estimated from the data of an acceleration sensor attached to the body. All in all, it can be concluded that physical activities that involve high and/or impact loading bring

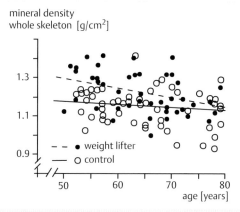

Fig. 8.23 Bone mineral density in the skeleton of former weight lifters and controls in relation to age. (Adapted, with permission, from Karlsson et al.[55])

about an increase of bone density.[53,54] Disciplines such as cycling, swimming, running, or walking lead to only small increases or, sometimes, even a decrease.

If the sport is discontinued, a decrease of bone density can be observed. Karlsson et al[55] documented the bone mineral density of the entire body in former weight lifters and controls in the age range between 50 and 80 years (**Fig. 8.23**). Although at the age of 50 bone density was still higher among the former weight lifters than in the controls, above the age of 65 there was no difference between the two cohorts. Granhed et al[56] investigated the bone mineral density of the L3 vertebral body in wrestlers and weight lifters (**Fig. 8.24**). In young athletes (12–20 years of age) bone density increased strongly with age, and it remained approximately constant during the high-performance period (20–40 years of age). If the sport was given up at over the age of 40, there was then virtually no difference between the former athletes and controls.

As an alternative to sport, a current discussion relates to whether increased bone density could be brought about by whole body vibration. This is an attractive proposal, because standing on a vibration platform requires no personal effort, and because at vibration frequencies between 10 Hz and 30 Hz a large number of loading cycles can be applied in a short time. However, there are some risks related to whole body vibration, one of which is that resonances may be induced in the body. If a resonance is induced, the amplitude of the vibration becomes substantially larger than the amplitude of the vibration platform. The resonance frequency of the lumbar spine is around 10 Hz. It remains to be shown that should a resonance be induced, no injury to bones or soft tissues will follow.

If the platform vibrates with a sinusoidal oscillation of amplitude A and frequency υ

(8.10)
$$x(t) = A \cdot \sin(2\pi\upsilon t)$$

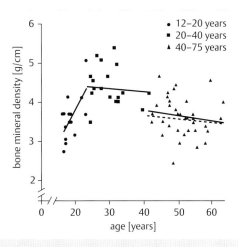

Fig. 8.24 Age dependence of bone mineral density in L3 vertebra of weight lifters and wrestlers in the starting phase of high-intensity training (solid circles), in the high-performance phase aged between 20 and 40 years (solid squares), and after cessation of the high-performance phase (solid triangles). Also shown are the regression lines for the three cohorts. The dashed line characterizes the average bone mineral density of subjects who never engaged in athletic training. (Adapted from Granhed et al.[56])

the acceleration a(t) of the platform (mathematically, the second derivative with respect to time) is given by

(8.11)
$$a(t) = -4\pi^2 \upsilon^2 \cdot A \cdot \sin(2\pi \upsilon t)$$

Problems with exposure to whole body vibration may arise if the acceleration of the platform exceeds the gravitational acceleration g. On moving downwards, the platform loses contact with the body (it moves downwards faster than the body falls). During its subsequent upward movement, the platform "collides" with the falling body, and very high peak loads may result.

Whether whole body vibration can bring about a lasting increase in bone density remains to be shown. Drerup et al[57] observed in vivo the bone density in the central volume of the L3 vertebral bodies of 14 subjects who had been exposed on average for 19.9 years to whole body vibration as drivers of earth-moving machinery in an open coal pit. Their spines had been exposed to vibration in the frequency range between 1 and 15 Hz in addition to irregular shock loads. **Fig. 8.25** depicts the measured density values in the study group in relation to age. For comparison, the age-dependent normal values of bone density[58] are also shown in **Fig. 8.25**. There was no discernable difference between the bone density in the exposed study cohort and that in nonexposed persons.

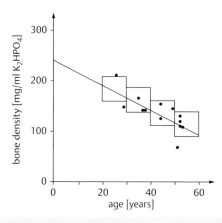

Fig. 8.25 Trabecular bone density of L3 vertebra (n = 14) after long-term exposure to whole body vibration in comparison to normal, age-appropriate values (squares). Mean duration of exposure, 19.9 years. (Adapted, with permission, from Drerup et al.[57])

8.7.3 Mechanical Control Signals for Bone Remodeling

The only way for remodeling of bones to take place is by the addition (apposition) or removal (ablation) of bone material on the surface of the bone. This is carried out by the osteoblast and osteoclast cell populations. What is not known is the signaling that controls these cells to ensure that the remodeling occurs, as it does, in a biomechanically advantageous fashion. However, some conjectures put forward in the past can now be regarded as disproved.

Compressive, tensile, or shear stress alone can be rejected, because the description of the state of stress in a volume element depends on the orientation of the coordinate system. For each volume element there exists an orientation such that only compressive or tensile stress exists on the surfaces of the element. The so-called principal stress trajectories describe this orientation within the volume of the structure under mechanical stress. For each volume element, however, there also exists a second orientation of the coordinate system, in which only shear stresses occur on the surfaces of the element. Which of the coordinate system orientations to employ in describing the state of stress, however, is an arbitrary matter of choice. So bone remodeling cannot be dependent on a single type of stress.

Neither are the paths of the principal stress trajectories, which inspired Wolff, candidates for a signaling system. Unlike in a structure filled with continuous material, principal stress trajectories have no actual existence in a discontinuous structure like bone. The agreement between the alignment of the trabeculae in bone as observed by Wolff and the pathways of the principal stress trajectories in a structure that geometrically resembles that bone must be regarded as accidental.[59]

Entities that are potential candidates for the regulation of bone remodeling include the local deformation (strain), the change of the deformation in space (strain gradient) and over time (strain rate), the local strain energy (strain energy density), and the movement of fluid (fluid flow) in the channels connecting the osteocytes.[60] If deformation is the relevant control signal, observations in humans and in animal experiments suggest that a deformation threshold exists below which there is no activity of the bone cells. On the other hand, it does appear that very small mechanical signals can also trigger bone remodeling.[61,62] In animal experiments an important issue seems to be whether the imposed load causes a normal, physiologic deformation pattern or whether the pattern is "unusual" for the bone in question.[63] Another topic of discussion is the relevance of microfractures of the trabecular bone; a high prevalence of such fractures in trabecular bone in the region of the hip joint and in vertebral bodies has been documented by several investigators. Such fractures can be regarded as pathologic as they indicate inadequate bone strength in relation to the loading regime. On the other hand, it is possible that these fractures form part of a physiological process in the course of which old, brittle bone is replaced by new bone better adapted to the mechanical requirements. Straightening a bone with a suboptimally healed fracture requires ablation of bone material at the convex surfaces and apposition at the concave surfaces. How the locally active bone-resorbing and bone-building cells detect the overall convex or concave shape of the bone and make use of this information to guide their activity is, however, still unclear. Apart from direct stimulation of the bone by mechanical signals, it is also possible that external loads stimulate the muscles first, and that they in turn stimulate the bone remodeling. The intermediate processes between a mechanical stimulus (whether direct or indirect) and the activity of osteoclasts and osteoblasts that eventually results are at present unknown.

8.8   Structure and Mechanical Properties of Cartilage

Cartilage is composed of cells, chondroblasts and chondrocytes, which produce the extracellular matrix. The extracellular matrix is composed of collagen fibers, proteoglycans, further organic compounds, and water. Anatomically, three types of cartilage are distinguished: hyaline cartilage, fibrocartilage, and elastic cartilage.[4] Hyaline cartilage covers the joint surfaces, and fibrocartilage forms the intervertebral discs and joint menisci, while the outer ear and the epiglottis are made up of elastic cartilage. The different types of cartilage are differentiated by the density of their cells, the alignment of their collagen fibers, and, in the case of elastic cartilage, by an additional content of elastic material.

Fig. 8.26 illustrates the structure of the hyaline cartilage covering the joint surfaces. The collagen fibers are anchored deeply in a zone adjacent to the subchondral trabecular bone; in the central cartilage layer they are oriented perpendicular to the joint surface. Close to the surface the orientation changes and the fibers now run predominantly tangential to the surface. This tangential orientation allows the fibers to absorb shear forces arising through friction of the joint surfaces. Hyaline cartilage consists of about 30%

joint surface

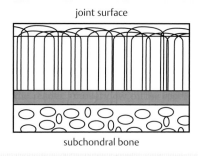

subchondral bone

Fig. 8.26 Course (schematic) of collagen fibers in hyaline cartilage. (Adapted from Martin et al.[2] With kind permission of Springer Science + Business Media.)

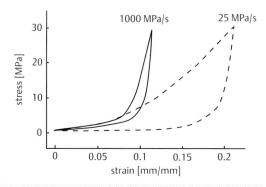

Fig. 8.27 Stress–strain diagram of cartilage samples observed at two different strain rates. (Adapted, with permission, from Milentijevic and Torzilli.[64])

collagen and proteoglycans and 70% water. The water is not free but bound by electrochemical forces to the hydrophilic proteoglycans. Hyaline cartilage contains no blood vessels or nerve fibers. Compressive load acting briefly on a cartilaginous surface is transmitted to the underlying bone as hydrostatic pressure. Compressive loading of longer duration stimulates fluid transport and deformation increases markedly. **Fig. 8.27** illustrates the viscoelastic properties of hyaline cartilage using stress–strain diagrams of explanted samples for different rise times of the applied load. There is a certain similarity between the mechanical properties of cartilage and the properties of a fiber-reinforced plastic material or gel. In such materials, fibers of high tensile strength are embedded in a virtually incompressible ground substance. Shear forces between the fibers and the ground substance resist deformation of the material.

The deformation of the hyaline cartilage ensures that a contact area comes into being between primarily incongruent joint surfaces under load. As an example, **Fig. 8.28** shows the region of the patellar surface

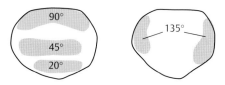

Fig. 8.28 Contact areas between patella and femur as a function of the bending angle of the knee. (Adapted from Seedholm et al.[65])

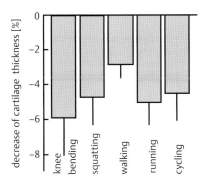

Fig. 8.29 Decrease in retropatellar cartilage thickness after 30 deep knee bends, 20 seconds of squatting, 5 minutes of walking, 200 m running, walking up and down stairs (54 steps), and 10 minutes of cycling. (Adapted, with permission, from Eckstein et al.[68])

subjected to compressive stress in relation to the bending angle of the knee. Even if the load on the joint is several times the body weight, only a fraction of the joint surface is ever under pressure—a fraction that shifts with the knee's angle of bend. Thus, during motion the cartilage is subjected to brief phases of loading and unloading. In a joint under compressive stress, fluid flow directed to the periphery of the loaded zone is initiated in the hyaline cartilage, as the subchondral bone is virtually impermeable.[66] The cartilage layer bulges at the periphery of the loaded zone and water can escape there. This fluid contributes to the preservation of the low friction between the joint surfaces. Conversely, unloading of the joint leads to fluid inflow and reconstitution of the original thickness of the cartilage layer.

Recent technical improvements in magnetic resonance imaging allow in vivo measurement of cartilage thickness and volume with a precision in the order of 5% to 10%.[67] After dynamic loading (walking, running, squatting), a 3% to 5% reduction in the thickness of the retropatellar cartilage was observed (**Fig. 8.29**).[68] There was no difference between trained athletes and controls. After 50 squats, Eckstein et al[67] observed a 6% decrease in the thickness of the patellar cartilage. If the same persons carried out 100 squats, the cartilage thickness was not further reduced. After 90 minutes recovery time the cartilage was restored to its original thickness. Taken as a whole, the thickness of the cartilage layer of the hip or knee shows only minor changes under short-duration compressive loading (walking, running). For this reason, and because it is only around 1.5 to 2.5 mm thick, cartilage cannot contribute noticeably to the damping of peak values of joint loads.

8.9   Frictional Properties of Cartilage

The friction in healthy joints is extraordinarily small; joints make almost no resistance to passive movements. The resistance "felt" during passive movements is entirely due to stretching of the soft tissues around the joints. Resistance to passive movements can, however, become perceptible if severe arthritis has roughened the joint surfaces or they have become irregularly shaped after fracture. From the mechanical point of view, the axis of rotation of a stiff joint is effectively shifted to the periphery of the joint's surface, resulting in a tendency to "lever" the articulating bone out of the joint.

In engineering a distinction is made between different types of friction. *Solid-state friction* exists when there is direct contact between imperfections in the flatness of the two materials. *Boundary friction* exists when the surfaces are wetted by a lubricant, so that in the absence of motion the contact occurs partly via the flatness imperfections and partly via the lubricant trapped between the flatness imperfections. During relative motion between the surfaces, the lubricant can form a film effectively separating the two surfaces (*fluid film lubrication*). If the articulating bones are incongruent, the adhesion of the lubricant on the surfaces effects that during motion the lubricant is pressed into the intraarticular space. This mechanism is designated *hydrodynamic friction*. All effects mentioned above contribute to the friction properties of human joints. The thickness of the fluid film on the cartilaginous joint surfaces is in the order of 0.5 µm. The viscosity of the synovial fluid facilitates the formation of hydrodynamic lubrication. In healthy joints the coefficient of dynamic friction between cartilage and cartilage amounts to less than 0.02.

8.10   Adaptation and Mechanically Induced Impairment of Cartilage

In contrast to bone, knowledge on the adaptation of hyaline cartilage to the mechanical demands is fragmentary. Eckstein et al[69] observed no difference of the cartilage thickness of the knee joint between triathletes with a high training workload and controls not engaged in sport activities. A comparison between the morphology of the cartilage of the knee joint of competitive sportsmen (weight lifters and sprinters) and controls who never engaged in weight training exhibited no difference with respect to cartilage thickness and joint surfaces.[67] According to the authors the results lead to the conclusion that different cartilage thicknesses are not indicators of the individual loading history. The authors hypothesize that a load-dependent increase of the cartilage thickness does not occur because this would not effect any mechanical advantage. Other potential training effects as changes in the fiber architecture or in the biochemical composition are at present not accessible by noninvasive means.

With increasing age the thickness of the hyaline cartilage layer decreases due to the advancement of the subchondral bone. In addition the cartilage surface may be subject to mechanical wear and tear. Risk factors held responsible for the destruction of the hyaline cartilage are previous injury of the cartilage, fractures of the underlying bone, overweight and age.[70] Episodes of short-duration overloading can injure the cartilage surface or lead to fissures of the tissue. For example, subjects exposed to physically demanding work, especially knee bending, are at a higher risk for an arthrosis of the knee joint. Here it is possible that the damage to the cartilage is due to the on average higher loading. On the other hand it is also possible that irregular peak loads, which cannot be evaded in physically demanding work, are responsible for the damage and the resulting arthrosis. Athletes with a history of a lesion of a joint have a higher risk to develop an arthrosis than unimpaired athletes.[71] Individual differences in the "normal" physical activity do not lead to differences of the risk to develop an arthrosis.[72]

Partial loading of a joint over a period of few weeks can effect a measurable decrease of the cartilage thickness. Hinterwimmer et al[73] documented by means of magnetic resonance imaging the thickness decrease of the cartilage of the knee joint during 7 weeks of partial loading induced by a fracture of the ankle joint (**Fig. 8.30**). Whether such changes are reversible and whether after longer phases of partial loading or complete unloading cartilage is subject to a higher injury risk, is presently unresolved.

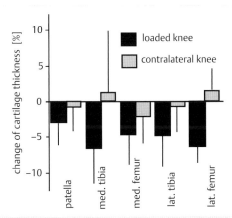

Fig. 8.30 Change in the thickness of the cartilage layer in the knee joint after 7 weeks' partial loading, in comparison with the contralateral knee. med., medial; lat., lateral. (Adapted, with permission, from Hinterwimmer at al.[73])

References

1. Currey JD. The Mechanical Adaptations of Bones. Princeton: Princeton University Press; 1984

2. Martin RB, Burr DB, Sharkey NA. Skeletal Tissue Mechanics. New York: Springer; 1998

3. Currey JD. Bones: Structure and Mechanics. Princeton: Princeton University Press; 2002

4. Tillmann B, Töndury G, eds. Bewegungsapparat. 3rd ed. Stuttgart: Thieme; 2003. Leonhardt H, Tillmann B, Töndury G, Zilles K, eds. Rauber/Kopsch, Anatomie des Menschen; Band 1

5. Tanner JM, Whitehouse RH, Marshall WA, Healy MJR, Goldstein H. Assessment of Skeletal Maturity and Prediction of Adult Height (TW2 Method). London: Academic Press; 1983

6. Debrunner AM. Orthopädie. Orthopädische Chirurgie. Bern: Huber; 2002

7. Reilly DT, Burstein AH. Review article. The mechanical properties of cortical bone. J Bone Joint Surg Am 1974;56(5):1001–1022

8. Reilly DT, Burstein AH. The elastic and ultimate properties of compact bone tissue. J Biomech 1975;8(6):393–405

9. Wright TM, Hayes WC. Tensile testing of bone over a wide range of strain rates: effects of strain rate, microstructure and density. Med Biol Eng 1976;14(6):671–680

10. Carter DR, Caler WE, Spengler DM, Frankel VH. Fatigue behavior of adult cortical bone: the influence of mean strain and strain range. Acta Orthop Scand 1981;52(5):481–490

11. Carter DR, Caler WE, Spengler DM, Frankel VH. Uniaxial fatigue of human cortical bone. The influence of tissue physical characteristics. J Biomech 1981;14(7):461–470

12. Carter DR, Caler WE. Cycle-dependent and time-dependent bone fracture with repeated loading. J Biomech Eng 1983;105(2):166–170

13. Milgrom C, Giladi M, Stein M, et al. Stress fractures in military recruits. A prospective study showing an unusually high incidence. J Bone Joint Surg Br 1985;67(5):732–735

14. Kiebzak GM. Age-related bone changes. Exp Gerontol 1991;26(2-3):171–187

15. Burstein AH, Reilly DT, Martens M. Aging of bone tissue: mechanical properties. J Bone Joint Surg Am 1976;58(1):82–86

16. Duchemin L, Bousson V, Raossanaly C, et al. Prediction of mechanical properties of cortical bone by quantitative computed tomography. Med Eng Phys 2008;30(3):321–328

17. Schaffler MB, Choi K, Milgrom C. Aging and matrix microdamage accumulation in human compact bone. Bone 1995;17(6):521–525

18. Keaveny TM, Hayes WC. A 20-year perspective on the mechanical properties of trabecular bone. J Biomech Eng 1993;115(4B):534–542

19. McCalden RW, McGeough JA, Court-Brown CM. Age-related changes in the compressive strength of cancellous bone. The relative importance of changes in density and trabecular architecture. J Bone Joint Surg Am 1997;79(3):421–427

20. Delling G, Vogel M, Hahn M. Neue Vorstellungen zu Bau und Funktion der menschlichen Spongiosa — Ist die Theorie von der Imbalance zwischen Osteoklasten und Osteoblasten noch haltbar? In: Schneider E, ed. Biomechanik des menschlichen Bewegungsapparates. Hefte zur Zeitschrift Der Unfallchirurg, Heft 261. Berlin: Springer; 1997:173–184

21. Vernon-Roberts B, Pirie CJ. Healing trabecular microfractures in the bodies of lumbar vertebrae. Ann Rheum Dis 1973;32(5):406–412

22. Ohtani T, Azuma H. Trabecular microfractures in the acetabulum. Histologic studies in cadavers. Acta Orthop Scand 1984;55(4):419–422

23. Martin RB. Determinants of the mechanical properties of bones. J Biomech 1991;24(Suppl 1):79–88

24. Goldstein SA. The mechanical properties of trabecular bone: dependence on anatomic location and function. J Biomech 1987;20(11-12):1055–1061

25. Keaveny TM, Wachtel EF, Kopperdahl DL. Mechanical behavior of human trabecular bone after overloading. J Orthop Res 1999;17(3):346–353

26. Goldstein SA, Goulet R, McCubbrey D. Measurement and significance of three-dimensional architecture to the mechanical integrity of trabecular bone. Calcif Tissue Int 1993;53(Suppl 1):S127–S132, discussion S132–S133

27. Ford CM, Keaveny TM. The dependence of shear failure properties of trabecular bone on apparent density and trabecular orientation. J Biomech 1996;29(10):1309–1317

28. Odgaard A. Three-dimensional methods for quantification of cancellous bone architecture. Bone 1997;20(4):315–328

29. Odgaard A, Kabel J, van Rietbergen B, Dalstra M, Huiskes R. Fabric and elastic principal directions of cancellous bone are closely related. J Biomech 1997;30(5):487–495

30. Cowin SC. Remarks on the paper entitled 'Fabric and elastic principal directions of cancellous bone are closely related'. J Biomech 1997;30(11-12):1191–1193

31. Boutroy S, Bouxsein ML, Munoz F, Delmas PD. In vivo assessment of trabecular bone microarchitecture by high-resolution peripheral quantitative computed tomography. J Clin Endocrinol Metab 2005;90(12):6508–6515

32. Genant HK, Ettinger B, Cann CE, Reiser U, Gordan GS, Kolb FO. Osteoporosis: assessment by quantitative computed tomography. Orthop Clin North Am 1985;16(3):557–568

33. Mazess RB. Bone densitometry of the axial skeleton. Orthop Clin North Am 1990;21(1):51–63

34. Lotz JC, Hayes WC. The use of quantitative computed tomography to estimate risk of fracture of the hip from falls. J Bone Joint Surg Am 1990;72(5):689–700

35. Hayes WC, Piazza SJ, Zysset PK. Biomechanics of fracture risk prediction of the hip and spine by quantitative computed tomography. Radiol Clin North Am 1991;29(1):1–18

36. Lochmüller EM, Miller P, Bürklein D, Wehr U, Rambeck W, Eckstein F. In situ femoral dual-energy X-ray absorptiometry related to ash weight, bone size and density, and its relationship with mechanical failure loads of the proximal femur. Osteoporos Int 2000;11(4):361–367

37. Ebbesen EN, Thomsen JS, Beck-Nielsen H, Nepper-Rasmussen HJ, Mosekilde L. Lumbar vertebral body compressive strength evaluated by dual-energy X-ray absorptiometry, quantitative computed tomography, and ashing. Bone 1999;25(6):713–724

38. Wolff J. Das Gesetz der Transformation der Knochen. Berlin: Hirschwald; 1892

39. Roux W. Der züchtende Kampf der Teile oder die "Teilauslese" im Organismus (Theorie der funktionellen Anpassung). Leipzig: Engelmann; 1881

40. Roesler H. The history of some fundamental concepts in bone biomechanics. J Biomech 1987;20(11-12):1025–1034

41. Frost HM. Orthopaedic Biomechanics. Springfield: Thomas; 1973

42. Pauwels F. Atlas zur Biomechanik der gesunden und kranken Hüfte. Berlin: Springer; 1973

43. Ferretti JL, Capozza RF, Cointry GR, et al. Gender-related differences in the relationship between densitometric values of whole-body bone mineral content and lean body mass in humans between 2 and 87 years of age. Bone 1998;22(6):683–690

44. Rauch F, Bailey DA, Baxter-Jones A, Mirwald R, Faulkner R. The 'muscle-bone unit' during the pubertal growth spurt. Bone 2004;34(5):771–775

45. Donaldson CL, Hulley SB, Vogel JM, Hattner RS, Bayers JH, McMillan DE. Effect of prolonged bed rest on bone mineral. Metabolism 1970;19(12):1071–1084

46. LeBlanc A, Schneider V, Shackelford L, et al. Bone mineral and lean tissue loss after long duration space flight. J Musculoskelet Neuronal Interact 2000;1(2):157–160

47. Cavanagh PR, Licata AA, Rice AJ. Exercise and pharmacological countermeasures for bone loss during long-duration space flight. Gravit Space Biol Bull 2005;18(2):39–58

48. Nilsson BE, Westlin NE. Bone density in athletes. Clin Orthop Relat Res 1971;77:179–182

49. Jones HH, Priest JD, Hayes WC, Tichenor CC, Nagel DA. Humeral hypertrophy in response to exercise. J Bone Joint Surg Am 1977;59(2):204–208

50. Granhed H, Jonson R, Hansson T. The loads on the lumbar spine during extreme weight lifting. Spine 1987;12(2):146–149

51. Hansson T, Roos B, Nachemson A. The bone mineral content and ultimate compressive strength of lumbar vertebrae. Spine 1980;5(1):46–55

52. Jämsä T, Vainionpää A, Korpelainen R, Vihriälä E, Leppäluoto J. Effect of daily physical activity on proximal femur. Clin Biomech (Bristol, Avon) 2006;21(1):1–7

53. Suominen H. Bone mineral density and long term exercise. An overview of cross-sectional athlete studies. Sports Med 1993;16(5):316–330

54. Guadalupe-Grau A, Fuentes T, Guerra B, Calbet JA. Exercise and bone mass in adults. Sports Med 2009;39(6):439–468

55. Karlsson MK, Johnell O, Obrant KJ. Is bone mineral density advantage maintained long-term in previous weight lifters? Calcif Tissue Int 1995;57(5):325–328

56. Granhed H, Jonson R, Keller T, Hansson T. Short and Long Term Effects of Vigorous Physical Activity on Bone Mineral in the Human Lumbar Spine [thesis]. Göteborg: University of Göteborg; 1988

57. Drerup B, Granitzka M, Assheuer J, Zerlett G. Assessment of disc injury in subjects exposed to long-term whole-body vibration. Eur Spine J 1999;8(6):458–467

58. Felsenberg D, Kalender WA, Banzer D, et al. Quantitative computertomographische Knochenmineralgehaltsbestimmung. Fortschr Röntgenstr 1988;148(4):431–436

59. Huiskes R. If bone is the answer, then what is the question? J Anat 2000;197(Pt 2):145–156

60. Cowin SC. Bone stress adaptation models. J Biomech Eng 1993;115(4B):528–533

61. Rubin C, Turner AS, Bain S, Mallinckrodt C, McLeod K. Anabolism. Low mechanical signals strengthen long bones. Nature 2001;412(6847):603–604

62. Judex S, Rubin CT. Is bone formation induced by high-frequency mechanical signals modulated by muscle activity? J Musculoskelet Neuronal Interact 2010;10(1):3–11

63. Lanyon LE. Functional strain in bone tissue as an objective, and controlling stimulus for adaptive bone remodelling. J Biomech 1987;20(11-12):1083–1093

64. Milentijevic D, Torzilli PA. Influence of stress rate on water loss, matrix deformation and chondrocyte viability in impacted articular cartilage. J Biomech 2005;38(3):493–502

65. Seedholm BB, Takeda T, Tsubuku M, Wright V. Mechanical factors and patellofemoral osteoarthrosis. Ann Rheum Dis 1979;38(4):307–316

66. Wong M, Carter DR. Articular cartilage functional histomorphology and mechanobiology: a research perspective. Bone 2003;33(1):1–13

67. Eckstein F, Hudelmaier M, Putz R. The effects of exercise on human articular cartilage. J Anat 2006;208(4):491–512

68. Eckstein F, Lemberger B, Gratzke C, et al. In vivo cartilage deformation after different types of activity and its dependence on physical training status. Ann Rheum Dis 2005;64(2):291–295

69. Eckstein F, Faber S, Mühlbauer R, et al. Functional adaptation of human joints to mechanical stimuli. Osteoarthritis Cartilage 2002;10(1):44–50

70. Scott CC, Athanasiou KA. Mechanical impact and articular cartilage. Crit Rev Biomed Eng 2006;34(5):347–378

71. Kern D, Zlatkin MB, Dalinka MK. Occupational and post-traumatic arthritis. Radiol Clin North Am 1988;26(6):1349–1358

72. Hannan MT, Felson DT, Anderson JJ, Naimark A. Habitual physical activity is not associated with knee osteoarthritis: the Framingham Study. J Rheumatol 1993;20(4):704–709

73. Hinterwimmer S, Krammer M, Krötz M, et al. Cartilage atrophy in the knees of patients after seven weeks of partial load bearing. Arthritis Rheum 2004;50(8):2516–2520

9 Structure and Function of Skeletal Muscle

Muscles are biological machines that convert chemical energy, derived from the reaction between food substrate and oxygen, into mechanical work and heat. Muscle strength can be defined as the ability of skeletal muscles to develop force to initiate, decelerate, or prevent movement. Force alone, however, is not enough for the performance and control of movements, stabilization of posture, and prevention of injury to the musculoskeletal system. For optimum control and performance of the musculoskeletal system, therefore, muscular endurance and muscle coordination are also required. Muscular endurance can be defined as the ability to maintain a specified force for a given period of time. However, this definition is not universally applicable, as endurance varies with the type of mechanical work performed.

9.1 Skeletal Muscle Morphology

Skeletal muscle is the largest organ in the body. It accounts for approximately 40% of total body weight and is organized into hundreds of separate entities, or body muscles, each of which has been assigned a specific task to enable the great variety of movements that are essential to normal life. Each muscle is composed of muscle fibers and connective tissue. The muscle fibers are the active elements, while connective tissues are the passive elements and serve as the connection between the muscle fibers and the skeleton. The muscle fibers are arranged in parallel and normally extend from one tendon to another (**Fig. 9.1**). A thin layer of connective tissue, the endomysium, surrounds each individual muscle fiber. The individual fibers together with their endomysium are arranged in bundles (fascicles) and each bundle is surrounded by another layer of connective tissue, the perimysium. Muscle fiber bundles have a diameter of approximately 1 to 3 mm. The whole muscle is enclosed by the epimysium. The epimysium is continuous with the fascia, which allows the muscle to slide with respect to surrounding tissues. The connective tissue of the muscle also contains blood vessels and nerves (**Fig. 9.1a**).

Muscle fibers, or muscle cells, are cable-like structures composed of tightly packed subunits, myofibrils, that fill up most of the volume of the fibers (**Fig. 9.1b**). Satellite cells are located between the basal membrane and the cell membrane of the muscle fiber. These cells are the muscle fiber stem cells, also called myogenic progenitor cells. Given that fully differentiated muscle fibers are postmitotic, the only cells that can divide to serve in different repair and regeneration processes are the satellite cells. The satellite cells are not innervated but are influenced by the microenvironment and chemical signal substances produced in the muscle fibers.

In humans, the length of the muscle fibers may vary between a few millimeters and many centimeters. It is generally assumed that the length of a muscle fiber can be about 60% of the total muscle length. The

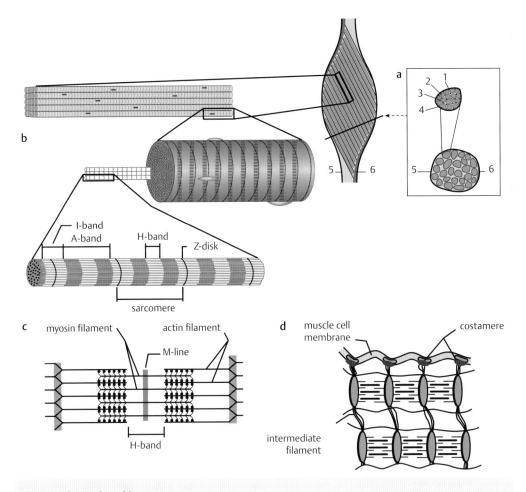

Fig. 9.1a–d Muscle architecture.

a Relationship between muscle fibers and connective tissue in a pennate skeletal muscle: 1, capillary within the endomysium; 2, muscle fiber; 3, endomysium; 4, perimysium; 5, epimysium; 6, fascia of the muscle.

b Muscle fascicle with muscle fibers and myofibrils.

c Single sarcomere, showing Z-disks and myosin and actin filaments.

d Two myofibrils connected with intermediate filaments and costameres responsible for the perpendicular transmission of force to the extracellular matrix.

mean diameter of a muscle cell is approximately 50 µm, especially in untrained individuals. The relationship between the muscle cell diameter and muscle fiber length is called the *aspect ratio*; a muscle cell with a diameter of 50 µm and a length of 15 cm is 3000 times longer than it is thick; that is, it has an aspect ratio of 3000.

The myofibrils are made up of filaments, called myofilaments. The myofilaments are arranged in sarcomeres, which are the contractile units of the muscle fibers. Sarcomeres are arranged in series and in

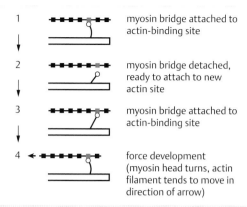

1   myosin bridge attached to actin-binding site

2   myosin bridge detached, ready to attach to new actin site

3   myosin bridge attached to actin-binding site

4   force development (myosin head turns, actin filament tends to move in direction of arrow)

Fig. 9.2 Sequence of events in cross-bridge construction and force generation. Starting from the initial state (1), the cycle begins with the detachment of the myosin head from the actin molecule (2). The head now moves to a new site (3), force is developed due to deformation of the molecule, and the filaments shift relative to each other (4).

parallel and are responsible for force generation and shortening of the muscle fiber. The sarcomere is defined as the part of the myofibril enclosed between the so-called Z-disks or Z-lines (**Fig. 9.1b**). From the Z-disk, (thin) actin myofilaments project towards the middle of each sarcomere and in the central region of each sarcomere they interdigitate with (thick) myosin filaments. Each (thick) myosin filament is surrounded by a hexagonal array of (thin) actin filaments. When a muscle is in a relaxed state there is some overlap between the myosin and the actin filaments.

Force is generated in the sarcomere through interaction between the actin and myosin filaments (**Fig. 9.1c**).[1-4] Structures called cross-bridges form part of the (thick) myosin filaments. They attach to the backbone of these filaments in such a way as to enable them to attach to sites on the (thin) actin filaments that are close by. The cross-bridges are functionally identical and act independently. The probability of a cross-bridge attaching to an actin filament is influenced by local biochemical conditions such as the calcium ion concentration. At any given time during activity of a muscle, some cross-bridges are attached to the actin filaments but others are detached or moving towards new attachment sites (**Fig. 9.2**).

When attachment occurs, the cross-bridges undergo structural deformation. Force is generated and the thin filament (actin) is pulled along the thick filament (myosin). The myofilaments slide in relation to each other and the overlap between the filaments increases; at the same time, the sarcomere shortens (**Fig. 9.3**). According to the theory of contraction, the length of the myosin filaments is assumed to be constant and not to contribute to the shortening of the sarcomere. Therefore, the shortening of a sarcomere is assumed to occur only via the sliding of the filaments relative to each other. The total shortening of the myofibril is the sum of the length changes occurring in the sarcomeres arranged in series in that myofibril. Supposing

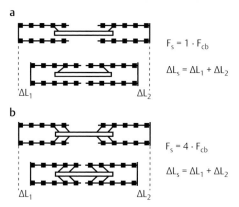

Fig. 9.3a, b Effects of parallel versus serial arrangement of cross-bridges in a sarcomere. **a** Two bridges in series, **b** four bridges in parallel. F_{cb}, force in a cross-bridge; F_s, force of a sarcomere; ΔL_1, ΔL_2, changes in length of the halves of the sarcomere; ΔL_s, change in length of the sarcomere. The force in **b** is four times the force in **a**; the maximum change in length is the same in both.

we have two myofibrils, one consisting of ten sarcomeres and the other of five sarcomeres arranged in series. The amount of shortening of the former will be twice that of the latter.

It is assumed that active muscle force originates exclusively from cross-bridges. As a consequence, active force generated at any given time is dependent on the number of parallel cross-bridges attached to the thin (actin) filaments. Because of the sarcomeres within a myofibril are arranged in series, the force generated by one unit has to be maintained and transmitted to the next unit, and thus the force of the whole structure is equal to the force of a single unit, that is, the force of one sarcomere. The force being transmitted from one half of the sarcomere, that is, from the Z-disk to the myosin filament via the actin filament, must be equal to the force transmitted to the actin filament via the myosin filament in the other half of the sarcomere (**Fig. 9.4**).[5] It follows that an equal number of active cross-bridges should be attached in both parts of the sarcomere. If the number of active cross-bridges is small, the force developed is low. If the number of active cross-bridges increases, the force developed will also increase.

In general it is believed that forces developed in the sarcomeres are propagated to the tendon through musculotendinous junctions. This model is true for muscle fibers ending close to the tendon or fascia of the muscle. Some muscle fibers, however, end within the muscle belly. In these cases it is generally believed that the force generated in the sarcomere is transmitted via shear forces to the endomysium of the muscle cell. It follows that forces developed in a muscle fiber are transmitted not only in the longitudinal direction but also perpendicularly. Forces can therefore be transmitted perpendicularly between sarcomeres and

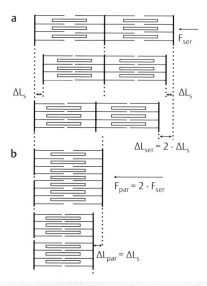

Fig. 9.4a, b Effect of serial (**a**) versus parallel (**b**) arrangement of sarcomeres. F_{ser} and F_{par} designate the maximum forces generated in the serial or parallel arrangement. ΔL_s is the change in length in a sarcomere; ΔL_{ser} and ΔL_{par} are the maximum attainable length changes in the serial or parallel arrangement. The maximum force in **a** is half of the maximum force in **b**; the maximum change in length in **a** is twice the maximum change in length in **b**.

neighboring myofibrils and between myofibrils and the muscle cell membrane. The transmitted forces perpendicular to the direction of the muscle fiber occur through the interaction of intermediate filaments, for example desmin filaments, and through the muscle fiber's connections to costameres located in the muscle cell membrane (see **Fig. 9.1d**). In addition, muscle fibers also contain dystrophin and dystrophin-associated proteins. This protein complex connects the cytoskeleton of the muscle fiber to the extracellular matrix. The main functions of this complex are to transmit forces generated in the sarcomeres to the extracellular matrix and to stabilize the cell membrane during muscular contractions (**Fig. 9.5**).

Titin is an important molecule within the sarcomere and creates a continuous filament system throughout the length of the myofibril. It is suggested that titin serves as a stretch sensor at the cellular level and may act in protein up- and down-regulation as well as influencing various gene activities.

9.2   The Force–Length Relationship

Sarcomeres arranged in series are called myofibrils. Muscle fibers are a collection of myofibrils arranged in parallel. Thus, muscle fibers are a collection of sarcomeres arranged both in series and in parallel. The maximum force developed in a muscle fiber will increase in proportion to the quantity of myofibrils

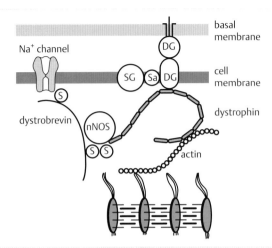

Fig. 9.5 Dystrophin and dystrophin-associated proteins (also called dystrophin–glycoprotein complex) play a central role in the lateral force transmission from the Z-disks to the extracellular matrix. DG, dystroglycan complex; nNOS, neuronal nitrogen oxide synthase; S, syntrophin; Sa, sarcospan; SG, sarcoglycan complex.

arranged in parallel; in other words, the force is proportional to the cross-sectional area of the muscle fiber (**Fig. 9.4**). Experiments have shown that the amount of force developed in a muscle fiber depends on the length of the muscle fibers at the time of activation and the contraction velocity. These dependencies are understood to be determined by the filament system and by the parallel and serial arrangement of sarcomeres within the muscle fibers.[6–10]

Since the late nineteenth century, it has been known that the force developed by a muscle of constant length (that is, during isometric contraction) varies with its length at the start of the contraction. The muscle generates less force when it is in a very much shortened or lengthened state than it does at a mid-range length. The isometric force–length relationship can be measured directly when a muscle is maximally stimulated at a variety of discrete lengths and the resulting force is recorded. When the maximum force at each length is plotted against the length, a relationship like that shown in **Fig. 9.6** is obtained. The force–length curve represents the results of many experiments plotted on the same graph, which is an artificial connection of individual data points from isometric experiments. Therefore, the force–length relationship is strictly valid only for isometric contractions. The structural basis for the force–length relationship was elucidated in the early 1960s. Basically, the force–length relationship in skeletal muscle is understood as a direct function of the overlap between actin and myosin filaments.[1,9]

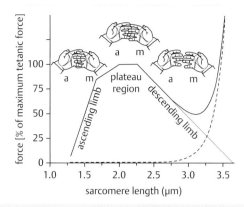

Fig. 9.6 Maximum tetanic force in relation to sarcomere length. The dashed curve describes the elastic tensile force generated when a muscle is stretched beyond its optimal length. The solid curve describes the sum of active force and passive tensile force. At three sarcomere lengths the overlap of the myosin and actin filaments is visualized using the example of the fingers of the two hands sliding with respect to each other. In this example, the fingers of one hand represent the myosin (m) and the fingers of the other hand the actin (a) filaments.

9.2.1 Descending Limb of the Force–Length Curve

The region of the force–length curve in which the force decreases as the sarcomere length increases is known as the *descending limb*. Beyond a certain muscle fiber length, force development is no longer possible. The length of a myosin filament is 1.65 μm and that of an actin filament 2.0 μm. At a sarcomere length of 3.65 μm—equal to the sum of the filament lengths—there is no overlap between the actin and the myosin filaments. Thus, in this situation, although biochemical processes might permit actin–myosin interaction by removing the inhibition on the actin filament, no myosin cross-bridges are located close to the actin active sites, and therefore no force generation can occur.

9.2.2 Plateau Region of the Force–Length Curve

Force increases with decreasing muscle length up to a sarcomere length of 2.2 μm. For sarcomere lengths in the range between 2.0 and 2.2 μm, muscle force remains constant. While shortening of the sarcomere length over the 2.2 to 2.0 μm range results in greater filament overlap, it does not result in increased force generation because no additional cross-bridge connections are made. The reason for this is the bare region (not containing cross-bridges) of the myosin molecule, which is 0.2 μm long. The region of the force–length curve over which length change results in no change in force generation is called the *plateau region*. The maximum tetanic force of the muscle in this region is termed F_0. The length at which F_0 is attained is known as optimal length, termed L_0.

9.2.3 Ascending Limb of the Force–Length Curve

The region of the force–length curve where force increases as length increases is called the *ascending limb*. When sarcomeres shorten to below 2.0 μm, actin filaments from one side of the sarcomere double-overlap with the actin filaments on the opposite side. In other words, at these lengths, actin filaments overlap both with themselves and with the myosin filaments. Under these double-overlap conditions, the actin filament from one side of the sarcomere interferes with cross-bridge formation on the other side, resulting in decreased muscle force output. The region where shortening between 2.0 and 1.87 μm occurs is known as the *shallow* ascending limb of the force–length curve. This region is distinguished from the next portion of the force–length curve, which is known as the *steep* ascending limb. At these very short lengths, the myosin filament actually begins to interfere with shortening as it abuts the sarcomere Z-disk, leading to a rapid reduction of force.

9.2.4 Passive Force–Length Curve

The dashed line in **Fig. 9.6** represents the force generated if a muscle is passively stretched to various lengths. Near the optimal length L_0, passive tension is almost zero. However, as the muscle is stretched to longer lengths, passive force increases dramatically. The increase in passive force that occurs when the muscle is stretched may play an important role in re-establishing myofilament overlap in the absence of muscle activation. These relatively long lengths can be attained physiologically. In such situations, large passive forces directed at re-establishing muscle length will be encountered.

The structures responsible for the increase in passive resistive force are located both outside and inside the myofibrils. According to Cavagna[11] and Heerkens et al[12] the parallel elastic elements of muscle (intramuscular connective tissue) are responsible for the force exerted by a passive muscle when it is stretched beyond its optimum length. As collagen is the major protein in muscle, the tensile properties of passive muscles are primarily dependent on the amount and type of collagen present.[13] Although intramuscular connective tissue enables forces (actively developed by the muscle or passively imposed on the muscle) to be transmitted safely and effectively by the entire tissue, information on the connective tissue component of skeletal muscle is relatively sparse.

Recent studies have shown the origin of passive muscle tension also to be located within the myofibrils themselves. A new structural protein, *titin*, sometimes referred to as *connectin*, may be the source of this passive tension.[14,15] This large protein molecule spans each half-sarcomere and is anchored to the Z-disk, connecting the thick myosin filaments end to end. Titin is thought to play a basic role in maintaining the structural integrity of the sarcomere and to produce passive force when muscle sarcomeres are stretched. Furthermore, titin is believed to produce a high percentage of the passive force that is developed in most muscles in the plateau region and the descending limb of the force–length curve. Once a sarcomere is stretched beyond thick and thin filament overlap, cross-bridge attachment becomes impossible, and the forces required to re-establish myofilament overlap are thought to come primarily from the passive elastic forces of the highly stretched titin. In addition to passively supporting the sarcomere, titin stabilizes the myosin lattice so that high muscle forces do not disrupt the orderly hexagonal array. If titin is selectively destroyed, normal muscle contraction may cause significant myofibrillar disruption.

9.3 The Force–Velocity Relationship

Skeletal muscle has an inherent capacity to adjust its active force to precisely match the load exerted on it during shortening, or to regulate the resistive force during muscle elongation. This property distinguishes muscle from a simple elastic structure and is based on the fact that active force generation is continuously adjusted to the speed of the contractile system. The maximum force that a muscle can develop depends not just on its length but also on the velocity of the contraction. It can be observed that the active force developed by a skeletal muscle is higher when the contraction velocity is low and decreases as the contraction velocity increases. Thus, when the load is high, the active muscle force is increased to the required level by reducing the speed of contraction. Conversely, when the load is low, the active force can be made correspondingly small by increasing the speed of shortening.

Fig. 9.7 shows the relationship between force and velocity of an isolated whole sartorius muscle of the frog, published by Hill.[8] Like the force–length relationship, the force–velocity relationship is a curve that represents the results of several experiments plotted together on the same graph. A muscle is stimulated

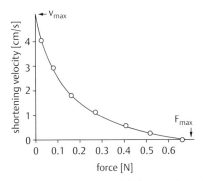

Fig. 9.7 Empirical relation between force and contraction velocity of a muscle, documented for the sartorius muscle of the frog. The relation was described by Hill[8] by means of a hyperbola.

maximally and allowed to shorten or to lengthen against a constant load. The contraction velocity during shortening or lengthening is measured and then plotted as a function of the load.

According to Hill, the relationship between the magnitude of force **F** and the contraction velocity v during a concentric (shortening) contraction may be described by the equation

(9.1) $$(F + a) \cdot v = b \cdot (F_{max} - F)$$

In this equation, a and b are experimentally derived constants. The values of a and b are estimated at approximately 0.25. F_{max} is the maximum tetanic force developed at a given muscle length. The maximum force development is achieved at a contraction velocity v equal to zero. The maximum contraction velocity v_{max} is observed at force F equal to zero (**Fig. 9.7**). The Hill equation can be used to predict the relative change in muscle force occurring as a muscle is allowed to contract.

The reason why muscle force is related to contraction velocity is because a certain amount of time is required for the cross-bridges between actin and myosin to attach and detach—the rate at which they cycle through attachment/detachment is therefore a constant.[3,7,16] At any point in time, the force generated by a muscle depends on the number of cross-bridges attached. When the contraction velocity increases, the filaments slide past one another faster and faster, fewer cross-bridges can be attached, and therefore force decreases. Conversely, as the relative filament velocity decreases, more cross-bridges have time to attach and generate force, so that force increases. This account does not aim to give a full description of the foundation of the force–velocity relationship, but only to provide some insight into how cross-bridge rate constants can affect force generation as a function of velocity.

9.4 Theoretical Modeling of Skeletal Muscle Behavior

The purpose of skeletal muscle modeling is to predict static and dynamic behavior in different situations. The model of a muscle is constructed from single elements with known mechanical properties. Elements may be combined to represent properties of the whole muscle. Hill[6] developed a muscle model consisting of two basic elements: a contractile element and an elastic element (**Fig. 9.8a**). The contractile element models the myofilaments responsible for active force development. The elastic element describes the passive elastic properties of the structure. The mechanical property of the elastic element equals the elastic property of a spring (see Chapter 2). Like a spring, the elastic elements store energy during elongation and release virtually all the energy as they return to their original length.

In its simplest form, the Hill[6] model is constructed from a contractile element connected in series with a passive elastic element. In this model, the contractile elements are considered to have force–length as well as force–velocity characteristics similar to those described for muscle fibers. As the two elements are connected in series, both are subject to the identical tensile force. The change in length of the combined

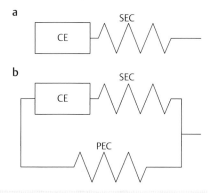

Fig. 9.8a, b Hill's muscle model. The contractile properties are represented by the contractile element CE. The elastic properties are represented by the series elastic component SEC (in series to the contractile element) and the parallel elastic component PEC (parallel to the contractile element).

a Basic model for description of the active properties of a muscle.

b Basic model for description of the active and passive properties of a muscle.

model is the sum of the length changes occurring in each element of the model. The velocity of shortening and lengthening of the model is the sum of the velocities of both elements of the model.

The combined function of the elastic and contractile elements connected in series seems to be important for producing fine, coordinated movements.[17,18] It follows from the model that, during contraction of a muscle, force will increase slowly. This is assumed to be due to the simultaneous shortening of the contractile and lengthening of the elastic elements. The length changes of the contractile and elastic elements counteract each other, allowing a smooth movement to occur without any jerking. In other words, the elastic elements dampen rapid increases in muscle force.[19]

If a muscle fiber is shorter than its optimum length, further shortening of the fiber leads to a decrease in force development accompanied by simultaneous shortening of the series elastic element (in series to the contractile element). When the contraction velocity of a muscle fiber increases, the force is reduced (because of the force–velocity relationship) and the series elastic element is again allowed to shorten. As a consequence, the overall length change in the model that combines contractile and elastic elements is greater than the length change that would be possible with an isolated contractile element.

To explain the mechanical behavior of passive muscles, a third element is introduced: the parallel elastic element (**Fig. 9.8b**). The parallel elastic element is arranged in parallel to the contractile element. As the stiffness and the tensile strength of the contractile element are assumed to be negligibly small, the parallel elastic element is the source of the force preventing rupture of contractile elements during passive elongation of a muscle. On the other hand, the force of the parallel elastic element is negligibly small compared with the maximum force of the contractile element, so when maximum active force is generated, the parallel elastic element will resist only a small fraction of the external force and will consequently shorten.

9.5 Mechanical Properties of Tendons

Tendinous tissue behaves like a nonlinear elastic structure. **Fig. 9.9** shows an example of a force–length characteristic of tendon, based on data published by Woo et al.[20] A specimen consisting of a tendon and its insertion into bone (tendon–bone complex) was investigated. Starting from its resting length, the tendon–bone complex was elongated up to rupture or failure at the site of insertion, and the opposing (resistive) force was measured. The stiffness of the complex at each point of the curve is defined as the ratio of force increase and length increase, that is, $\Delta F/\Delta L$ [N/m]. The figure shows that the stiffness of the tendon is a function of elongation. With minor elongation of the tendon, stiffness is low, so, for example, small changes in force have relatively large effects on tendon length. As elongation increases, stiffness increases as well. In the linear portion of the curve, stiffness is virtually constant. The stress σ_{max} (force divided by cross-sectional area) of a tendon at the point of rupture amounts to approximately 100 MPa; the strain ε_{max} at rupture is in the region of 10% of the starting length.

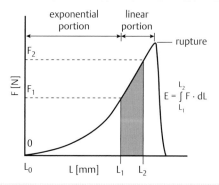

Fig. 9.9 Force–length characteristic of a tendon, using the example of the flexor digitalis tendon of the pig.[20] The graph shows the force of the tendon in relation to its length, starting from its length L_0 in the unloaded state. Force as a function of length shows first an approximately exponential behavior pattern followed by an approximately linear portion. Upon further increase of the force, rupture occurs at the tendon–bone interface. The shaded area below the curve is a measure of the energy E stored when the force changes from F_1 to F_2 and the tendon length changes from L_1 to L_2.

The series elastic elements located in tendinous tissue are important for optimum function of active muscles. When a muscle develops force, the length of the tendon increases and the muscle is allowed to shorten. Because of the change in tendon length, a muscle–tendon unit will have an increased operating range relative to the range of muscle fibers alone. If the muscle–tendon unit is strained by small forces during a movement, the length change in the unit will occur at the tendon because of its lower stiffness. The result is that a fraction of the length change that would have to be accommodated by muscle fibers is actually taken up by tendons. Thus, by attaching muscles to bones via compliant (elastically elongating) tendons, the length changes of the muscle fibers are reduced. Length changes of muscles and their tendons may also have opposite signs. When the force of a muscle–tendon unit with constant length is reduced, the tendon is allowed to shorten, while muscle length will increase. Length changes of tendons also dampen sharp increases in muscle force, so the time elapsing until the muscle force reaches its maximum value is, in fact, increased.[18]

Plastic deformation of tendons is negligible; after release, a stretched tendon will return to its original length. The energy expended on stretching the tendon is stored as potential energy and released almost completely as the force exerted on the tendon decreases to zero. The loss of energy is less than 10%. The force–length characteristics of tendons are dependent only to a minor extent upon the velocity of stretching. Therefore, the deformation energy stored in a tendon during stretching is given by the area below the force–length curve.[20–22]

(9.2)
$$E = \int F \cdot dL \ [Nm]$$

In this formula E denotes the energy, F the magnitude of the resistive force, and dL the change in length. The integral extends from the resting length of the tendon (with zero force F) up to the length reached under the force applied. The amount of stored energy increases as stretching increases (see Chapter 3). At higher forces the tendon is rather stiff and the change in length relative to the change in force will be small. Therefore, in this situation the increase in stored energy will be small as well. A greater amount of energy could be stored if the length change in the tendon were increased. In real life these increased ranges of elongation are obtained during stretch–shortening cycles occurring in a variety of movements. During a stretch–shortening cycle the initial stretching of the muscle–tendon unit is followed by active shortening of the complex. During the stretching phase energy is stored in the unit.

The potential energy stored in a muscle–tendon unit is released by decreasing the force exerted on the structure. If this is done slowly, the energy will become available slowly; if it is done at a rapid rate, the energy will be released rapidly as well. The amount of energy released per unit of time, the power P, is given by

(9.3)
$$P = F \cdot v$$

where F is the force and v the shortening velocity of the muscle–tendon unit.

It is of practical importance that tendons can store energy during a stretch–shortening cycle at a relatively low rate. Upon lengthening, the tendon then acts as an energy reservoir that can be emptied at a high rate to effect movements with high speed and power.[5] This situation may be compared with shooting an arrow with a bow. The potential energy of the bow is increased when the active muscles pull on the string, thereby deforming the bow. When the string is suddenly released, the deformation energy is set free and the arrow will be launched with high power, resulting in a high velocity.

9.6 Force Regulation in Skeletal Muscles

An excitatory impulse generated naturally in the central nervous system or artificially by an electrical signal generator creates a so-called *action potential* (specific electrical field) at the relevant muscle fibers. The tensile force developed by a single fiber in response to a single action potential invading the axon terminals is called a twitch. As the frequency of the stimulating impulses increases, twitches begin to overlap. At frequencies above a certain limit, single twitches can no longer be discriminated and tetanic contraction develops. The frequency limit, where tetanic contraction or tetanic force generation occurs, varies among different fibers and individual motor units. This limit is normally observed in the range between 10 and 100 Hz (**Fig. 9.10**). The higher the frequency of stimulation of the muscle fibers, the greater is the force produced in the muscle as a whole.

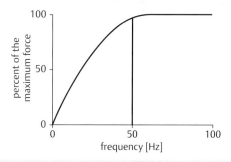

Fig. 9.10 Dependence of the force of a muscle fiber on the stimulation frequency, the force–frequency curve. At stimulation frequencies higher than about 10 Hz, single twitches merge to form a constant output force. In the lower region of the force–frequency curve, small changes in stimulation frequency effect large variations in force output. In contrast, at high frequencies a change in frequency effects only a small change in force, if any. Changing the frequency from 50 Hz to 100 Hz effects, for example, only a negligibly small change in force. Stimulation frequency of motor units is usually in the order of 10 to 60 Hz. In this region, force depends strongly on frequency.

Skeletal muscle fibers possess a wide spectrum of morphologic, contractile, and metabolic properties. Muscle fibers are classified as fast or slow, oxidative or nonoxidative, and glycolytic or nonglycolytic.[23,24] Often, only three different types are described; for details see **Table 9.1**. The three types differ characteristically with respect to speed of shortening, force generation, and endurance. Fast-contracting fiber types (type IIb) shorten approximately two to three times faster than slow-contracting fibers (type I). The specific tensile stress (force divided by cross-sectional area) of fast muscle fiber types is higher than that of slow muscle fibers. In general, slow muscle fibers (type I) have the greatest endurance, followed by type IIa and type IIb fibers.

Designation of motor unit	Muscle fiber type
Fast fatigable unit (FF)	Type IIb, fast glycolytic fiber
Fast fatigue-resistant unit (FR)	Type IIa, fast oxidative glycolytic fibers
Slow unit	Type I, slow oxidative fiber

Table 9.1 Relation between motor units and muscle fiber types

The functional unit of force generation in a muscle is the sarcomere (in fact, the half-sarcomere, due to sarcomere symmetry). The functional unit of force generation of the muscle is the motor unit. A motor unit comprises an α-motoneuron and the muscle fibers innervated by it. This unit is the smallest part of the muscle that can be made to contract independently. Motoneurons have their cell bodies in the ventral root of the spinal cord. The axons of the neurons terminate at the motor endplate of the fibers. When stimulated, all the fibers of a motor unit respond simultaneously. The fibers of a motor unit are said to show an "all-or-nothing response" to stimulation: they contract either maximally or not at all.

Motor units are usually classified according to the physiological properties of their muscle fibers.[24] These properties are the motor unit twitch tension, the tetanic tension recorded at an intermediate stimulation frequency, and the fatigability of the unit in response to a specific stimulation protocol (**Fig. 9.11**). In general, motor units belong to three different groups. Those that have a fast contraction time and a low fatigue index are known as fast fatigable (FF) units. Those that have a fast contraction time and a high fatigue index are designated fast fatigue-resistant (FR) units. Those that have slow contraction times, and which are most resistant to fatigue, are classified as slow (S) units.

A whole muscle is subdivided into many motor units, each of which comprises a single motoneuron and its related muscle fibers. The muscle fibers belonging to one motoneuron have the same physiological, biochemical, and ultrastructural properties. The number of muscle fibers belonging to a motor unit, and the number of motor units within a whole muscle, vary widely. This is closely related to the degree of control required of the muscle. The muscle fibers within a motor unit are interspersed among fibers of other motor units. The functional consequence of this dispersion is that the forces generated by a unit will spread over a larger tissue area. This may minimize mechanical stress in focal regions within the muscle.

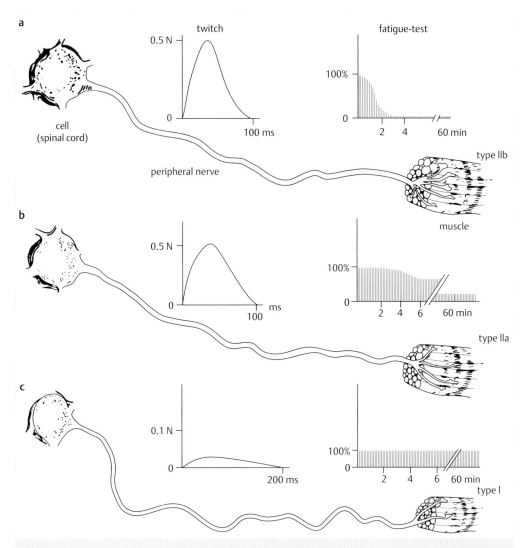

Fig. 9.11a–c Anatomical and physiologic properties of three different types of motor units. (Adapted from Edington and Edgerton.[25])

a Type IIb has large axons innervating a large number of muscle fibers. Such units produce large forces but are subject to rapid fatigue.

b Type IIa has medium size axons innervating a large number of muscle fibers. Such units produce lower forces than Type IIb but are less subject to fatigue.

c Type I has small axons innervating only few fibers. Such a unit develops only a low force but is able to maintain this force over a longer period of time.

The nervous system can vary muscle force output by two mechanisms. By varying the stimulation frequency, the force will be changed: when the frequency of stimulation is increased, the force output will increase as well. Thus, the force output is positively related to the discharge rate of a motor unit. This

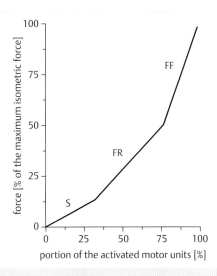

Fig. 9.12 Recruitment of motor units in relation to the active, isometric muscle force. At low-force levels, type S (slow) units are recruited first; with increasing force, type FR (fatigue-resistant) units and then type FF (fast fatigable) units are recruited. (Adapted from Edgerton et al.[30])

phenomenon is termed *temporal summation*. Alternatively, muscle force can be varied by changing the number of motor units that are active at a given time. For relatively low-force contractions, few motor units are activated, while for higher force generation, more units are activated.[26] The process by which motor units are added as muscle force increases is termed *recruitment*.

In their classical study, Henneman et al[27] showed that, at very low forces, low-amplitude voltage signals of short duration ("spikes") were observed at the nerve. As muscle force increased, the size of the spikes also increased in a very orderly fashion: as force continued to increase, the units recruited exhibited larger and larger spikes. The entire process was reversed as force decreased. From these observations it was concluded that, at low muscle force levels, motor units with the smallest axons and the lowest threshold and depolarization frequency were recruited first. As force increased, larger and larger axons with higher activation thresholds and higher excitation amplitudes were recruited. This is known as the "size principle" and provides an anatomical basis for the orderly recruitment of motor units to produce a smooth contraction. In later studies (for example, that by Binder and Mendell[28]) it was determined that, in general, small motor axons innervate slow motor units (type I) and larger motor axons innervate fast motor units (types IIa and IIb). These findings were confirmed in studies on human motor units.[29,30]

Based on the above findings, the following scheme was proposed for the voluntary recruitment of motor units (**Fig. 9.12**). At very low excitation levels, the smallest axons with the lowest threshold to activation are activated first. As voluntary effort increases, most of the next-largest axons are recruited, activating

195

the type IIa fibers. During maximal effort, the largest axons innervating type IIb fibers are activated. This activation pattern seems reasonable, since the most frequently activated S units are those with the greatest endurance. The FF units, which are rarely activated, have the lowest endurance. In addition, the S units (type I), which are activated first, develop the lowest tension, so that low tension is generated as contraction begins. This provides a mechanism for smoothly increasing tension as first S units, then FR units, and finally FF units are recruited.

9.7   Relationship between Force and Electromyography (EMG)

Electromyography gives a method for recording and processing the electrical signals of an activated muscle. The twitch of a muscle fiber is initiated by electrochemical processes at the muscle fiber membrane. These electrical impulses propagate throughout the muscle fiber. The resulting electrical potentials are measured by fine intramuscular needle electrodes or electrodes attached on the skin. The electrical potential of a motor unit, representing the sum of the individual action potentials generated in the muscle fibers of the motor unit, has an amplitude in the range between 200 µV and 3 mV. The duration of the potentials is normally between 2 ms and 15 ms, depending on the muscle examined. In processing the EMG, it is usually the frequency and amplitude of the signals that are analyzed.

There is general agreement on the usefulness of the EMG as an indicator of the activation pattern of a motor pool. Electromyography is frequently used to study the activity of individual muscles in the maintenance of posture and during normal or abnormal patterns of movement. Such recordings can be combined with film or video recordings, helping to define the relationship between the position of a joint, or limb, and the EMG signal.

Some important, still unresolved problems in orthopedic biomechanics could be resolved if it were possible to predict the magnitude of the muscle force (in newtons) from the recorded electromyographic signal. In the past, several studies have been aimed at elucidating this relation. There is agreement that the EMG signal reflects the activity of a muscle. However, it is not possible at present to predict the resulting force from the recorded EMG signals. In most cases there is not even proportionality between muscle force and signal amplitude. Only in special cases—that is, under isometric contractions—may proportionality between integrated EMG (area below the curve) and force be assumed. In such experiments it is important for the electrical activity from the total area of the muscle to be measured. If the moment arm of the muscle is known, the force can be calculated from the moment developed.

The derived factor of proportionality between EMG signal and force can be used to predict muscle force from the EMG signal only. However, this method has its limitations. The factor of proportionality between EMG signal and muscle force determined for one muscle may not be valid for another muscle. Other muscles may have different moment arms, changing the relation between the EMG signal and force.

Factors determined from one individual subject cannot be transferred to another subject, and placement of surface electrodes is poorly reproducible among subjects. In addition, the EMG signal seems to depend on the velocity of the muscle length change. For example, EMG is being measured from a muscle that is shortening at 5% v_{max}. The force generated by this muscle will be approximately 75% of maximum isometric tension. If the EMG from the same muscle is measured under conditions where it is shortening at only 1% of v_{max}, much more tension will be generated due to the slower contraction velocity. The EMG signal will, however, be identical in both situations. These findings are due to the fact that all motor units are already activated when generating 75% of maximum force.[31–33] Owing to the shortening of the muscle, not all cross-bridges are able to attach. When the velocity is reduced, the activity and the EMG signal remain virtually unchanged, but the force increases because more cross-bridges have sufficient time to attach. In an attempt to overcome these difficulties, efforts are made to obtain information on the velocity dependence of the EMG signal and to apply a theoretically derived or experimentally determined correction when predicting muscle force from the EMG signal of a contracting or elongating muscle.

In conclusion, EMG measurements provide valuable information on muscle activation patterns, but an EMG record should be interpreted with caution in terms of force. In special circumstances—that is, in purely isometric situations or when dealing with slow length changes—forces might be calibrated and estimated.

9.8 Muscle Architecture

A typical muscle fiber in an adult man has a diameter in the range of 50 to 70 μm. The length varies from a few millimeters to more than 10 cm. Muscle fibers are generally attached to tendon plates or aponeuroses, which have a continuous transition into the more rounded tendons that run outside the muscle. Skeletal muscles are distinguished from one another with respect to fiber length, ratio of fiber length versus muscle length, and the orientation of the fibers relative to the long axis of the muscle.[34–38] While the diameter of muscle fibers is relatively consistent between muscles of different sizes, the geometric arrangement (spatial architecture) of these fibers can be quite different. The architecture of the muscle fibers at the microscopic level together with the distribution of fiber types is responsible for the contractile properties at the macroscopic level.

Most muscles may be seen as a collection of fibers arranged in parallel. For the sake of simplicity, the arrangement of muscle fibers (muscle architecture) is regarded as falling into two types. Muscles with fibers extending parallel to the force-generating axis are termed *parallel* muscles. Muscles with fibers oriented at an angle relative to the force-generating axis are termed *pennate* muscles (**Fig. 9.13**). For both parallel and pennate muscles, the ratio of muscle fiber length to muscle length ranges approximately between 0.2 and 0.6. In other words, even in strictly parallel muscles, the fibers extend at most over only 60% of the muscle length.

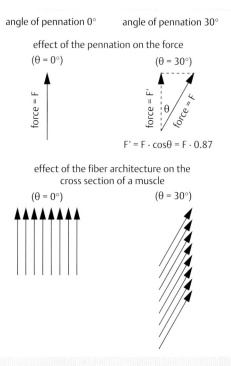

angle of pennation 0°   angle of pennation 30°

effect of the pennation on the force
($\theta = 0°$)   ($\theta = 30°$)

force = F

force = F' θ force = F

$F' = F \cdot \cos\theta = F \cdot 0.87$

effect of the fiber architecture on the
cross section of a muscle
($\theta = 0°$)   ($\theta = 30°$)

Fig. 9.13 Effect of pennation. Muscle fibers arranged in the longitudinal direction of the muscle transmit their entire force on the tendon. Muscle fibers directed at an angle with respect to the tendon transmit only part of their force in the longitudinal direction of the tendon. In the example shown, the longitudinal tendon force at an angle of pennation of 30° amounts to 87% of the muscle fiber force.

The mechanical properties of muscles arranged in parallel are governed by the same principles of series and parallel arrangement as discussed above for sarcomeres. Based on this organization, it follows that the total change in length of a muscle equals the length change in the muscle fibers. The force–length and force–velocity relationship of a parallel muscle are similar to those of a single muscle fiber. The muscle force is equal to the sum of forces generated by the individual fibers. The mechanics of pennate muscle, however, are more complicated. The geometric arrangement of the individual muscle fibers in relation to the longitudinal axis of the muscle affects the relationship between muscle fiber and muscle length change. A number of architectural studies performed in human upper and lower limb muscles have demonstrated that pennation angles range from 0° to 30°.[38] If muscle fibers are arranged at an angle ϕ in relation to the longitudinal axis of the tendon, the magnitude of the force component **F′** of the force **F** developed in the muscle fibers and transmitted to the tendon (**Fig. 9.13**) will be

(9.4) $|\mathbf{F'}| = |\mathbf{F}| \cdot \cos\phi$

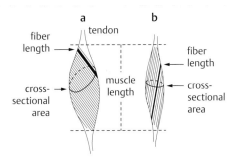

Fig. 9.14a, b Muscles with differing architecture.
a Muscle with short fibers and large physiologic cross section.
b Muscle with long fibers and small physiologic cross section.

At an angle of pennation greater than zero, cos ϕ will always be less than 1 and only a fraction of the muscle fiber force will be transmitted in the direction of the axis of the tendon. Therefore, in pennate muscles, the force actually transmitted to the tendon will be less than the sum of forces developed in the individual muscle fibers. When a pennate muscle contracts, the angle of pennation increases.

What is the rationale behind a design inducing part of the force generated not to be transmitted to the tendon? In several locations in the body it would be difficult to accommodate muscles with pennation angles equal to zero, because large numbers of longitudinally arranged fibers lead to large cross sections of the muscles. Thus it may be hypothesized that pennation is a space-saving strategy as it reduces the anatomical cross-sectional area at the expense of reducing the longitudinal force transmission to the tendon. On the other hand, pennation permits more muscle fibers to be attached along a tendon, thus compensating for the reduced force.

Different models are proposed to explain the effect of pennation on the force-producing capacities of skeletal muscle.[5,35,36,39] These models, in general, are based on muscle geometry, volume constraints, pennation angles between muscle fibers and tendon, homogeneity of sarcomere length, and numbers of sarcomeres in series, as well as on the relationship between the force–length characteristics of muscle fibers and tendon elasticity. The issue is, however, still under discussion.

The anatomical cross-sectional area of a muscle is in general not proportional to its maximum force because of differences in muscle architecture. To correlate the maximum force capacity with the cross-sectional area of a muscle, the physiological cross-sectional area (PCSA) is to be calculated. The PCSA represents the sum of cross-sectional areas of the muscle fibers, measured perpendicular to their longitudinal direction (**Fig. 9.14**). The physiological cross-sectional area is proportional to the maximum force capacity of a muscle. This area is hardly ever identical to the cross-sectional area of a muscle in the traditional anatomical planes, as seen, for example, in magnetic resonance imaging. The physiological cross-sectional area is calculated as follows:

(9.5) $$PCSA = m / (\rho \cdot l)$$

where m represents muscle mass (g), ρ muscle density (1.056 g/cm^3 for mammalian muscle), and l the mean length of the muscle fibers within the muscle.

The content of this formula may be visualized as follows. Muscle mass divided by density equals muscle volume. If the muscle were cylindrical in shape, dividing volume by length (fiber length) would represent the cross-sectional area of the cylinder. Since fiber length is not equal to cylinder length, however, the area calculated according to the above formula is only a theoretical parameter characterizing a cylinder with a length equal to that of the fibers. In general, PCSA and maximum force development are not strictly proportional to muscle mass. Knowing the mass of the muscle or any change in this mass does not, therefore, permit any prediction about the magnitude of the muscle force or any change to this force.

Strictly speaking, every muscle is unique in terms of its architecture. However, by ignoring the finer differences and taking them in functional groups, some generalizations can be made (**Table 9.2**). Muscles with greater angles of pennation generally contain more fibers and thus can exert greater total force. By contrast, a muscle containing fibers with a small angle of pennation generally benefits from more effective transmission of force to the tendon. In addition, muscles with long fibers appear to be designed for a large working range because excursion range is proportional to the length of the muscle fibers. This occurs primarily because there are more functional units (sarcomeres) arranged in series in the direction of movement. The gross architecture of a muscle may also influence its shortening properties. In general, the longer a given muscle and the more parallel the alignment of its fibers, the greater its capacity for length changes and its shortening velocity. Consequently, a muscle's architectural features need to be taken into account when evaluating its functional role in various activities.

Orientation to tendon	Functional advantage	Types of muscles
Parallel arrangement (angle of pennation < 10°)	More effective transmission of force on tendon Greater extent and speed of shortening Greater economy of maintaining tension	Predominantly type I fibers
Pennate arrangement (angle of pennation > 10°)	Greater physiological cross-sectional area to enhance force and power generation	Predominantly type II fibers

Table 9.2 Effect of fiber architecture on mechanical properties of skeletal muscle

Fig. 9.15a compares the force–length and force–velocity curves of two muscles with equal muscle fiber lengths and pennation angles. The muscle mass of the second muscle is assumed to be twice the mass of the first. Both muscles have the same basic shape of the force–length curve; however, the force curve from the muscle with the greater mass is shifted to larger force values. The same holds for the force–velocity curves. The muscle with the greater mass exhibits a larger maximum force F_{max}, but both curves exhibit the same basic shape. If both curves were plotted on relative scales, the two muscles would appear to have identical properties. Stress—that is, force divided by cross-sectional area—is equal between the two muscles.

Fig. 9.15b shows two muscles with identical physiological cross section and pennation angles but with different fiber lengths. As shown in the figure, the peak force of the force–length curve is identical but the muscle with the longer fibers exhibits a greater range of length changes and an increased maximum contraction velocity v_{max} compared with the muscle with the shorter fibers. These two examples show that muscle architecture has a profound influence on functional properties. The contractile units (the sarcomeres) are identical in both examples.

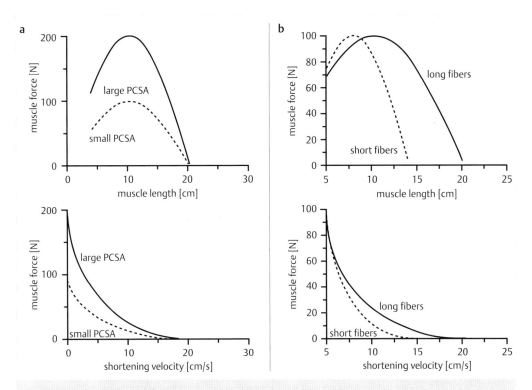

Fig. 9.15a, b Force–length and force–velocity relation of muscles with differing architecture.

a Force–length and force–velocity relation of two muscles with equal fiber lengths but different physiological cross-sectional areas (PCSA).

b Force–length and force–velocity relation of two muscles with different fiber lengths but equal physiological cross-sectional areas.

As a joint rotates, the change in length of a muscle is dependent on the distance between the insertion of the muscle and the center of rotation. **Fig. 9.16** compares two muscles with different distances between their insertion and the center of rotation. When movement occurs with a given interval of rotation, the change in length of the muscle with the shorter distance will, for purely geometric reasons, be less than that of the muscle with the longer distance. In general, a muscle with a long distance between insertion and center of rotation will have longer muscle fibers. This is interpreted as adaptation to the mechanical requirements. However, the range of length changes made possible by the architectural design is not always fully exploited in real life. The architectural design of a muscle is also assumed to be adapted to parameters such as velocity and acceleration of joint movements.[40] However, knowledge in this field is still fragmentary.

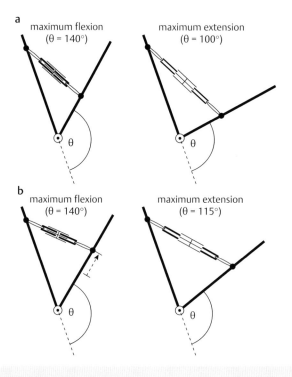

Fig. 9.16a, b Change in the range of motion of a joint due to a change in the distance between the insertion of a muscle and the center of rotation. The joint in **a** has a range of motion (difference between maximum extension and flexion) of 40°. When the distance between the insertion and the center of rotation is increased (**b**), the range of motion decreases to 25°. This decrease is due to the fact that, because of the increase in the distance between insertion and center of rotation, the length change in the sarcomeres per degree of rotation increases.

9.9 Skeletal Muscle Mechanics

Skeletal muscles are designed to initiate movements, to decelerate movements, to resist external loads so that movement does not occur, and to provide the body with a substantial part of its necessary heat. Muscle activity may be static or dynamic. Static muscle work is defined as contraction with constant muscle length. Dynamic muscle activity is defined as contraction during which muscle length changes. Contractions may be classified into three types: isometric, concentric, and eccentric.

9.9.1 Isometric Contraction

When a muscle develops force but no movement occurs as muscle length remains constant, static equilibrium exists. This contraction is called *isometric*. Often, a situation in which force increases with no observable change in length of the muscle–tendon unit is also called isometric contraction. In reality, there is a shortening of the muscle fibers and simultaneous elongation of the tendon in this case.

9.9.2 Concentric Contraction

When a muscle is able to shorten against a given load, movement occurs. This type of contraction is termed *concentric*. The force developed under concentric muscular action is always less than the maximum isometric force F_{max} developed at optimum muscle length. The shortening velocity of contraction is increased when muscles work against small loads. When the load against which the muscle contracts is reduced to almost zero, the maximum velocity of contraction v_{max} is achieved. The velocity of contraction v_{max} is characteristic of each muscle and depends on muscle fiber distribution and architectural characteristics. During concentric muscular activity, mechanical work E is performed:

(9.6)
$$E = F \cdot (-\Delta L)$$

In this equation F and ΔL designate the force and the length change in the muscle. When muscles shorten, the change in length is counted negative and thus mechanical work is positive. The mechanical power P of a muscle is defined as the work performed per unit of time.

(9.7)
$$P = F \cdot (-v)$$

In this equation v is the contraction velocity of the muscle. The velocity is counted negative when a muscle shortens and the power is thus positive. Because of the relationship between force and contraction velocity (see Section 9.3), maximum power occurs at a contraction velocity of approximately one-third of v_{max}.

9.9.3 Eccentric Contraction

If a muscle is activated in such a fashion that its length under a given external load is observed to increase, the contraction is called *eccentric*. According to the above equations, the work and power delivered during eccentric contractions are negative. This means that the muscle absorbs energy. During eccentric contractions, the muscle force may exceed by far the maximum isometric force F_{max}. The increase in force is due to summing of active and passive resistive force. This passive force is directed at restoring muscle length when muscles are stretched during an activity (see **Fig. 9.6**). This property is fundamental to many everyday movement patterns. There is currently considerable scientific interest in studying the behavior of muscles during eccentric contractions. Eccentric contractions are physiologically common. In addition, muscle pain and some muscle injuries seem to be associated with eccentric muscular activity.

Note: Muscle contractions are sometimes classified as isometric, concentric, or eccentric depending on whether "the external force equals the muscle force, or is smaller or larger than the muscle force." Mechanically, this statement is incorrect as, according to Newton's third law, the muscle force is invariably opposite and equal to the external force exerted on the muscle. This holds for all three types of muscle contraction. The difference between the different contractions is defined by the length change in the muscle and the resulting movement under application of the force.

Muscle activity during movements of the body seldom involves pure forms of isometric, concentric, or eccentric contractions. This is due to body segments being periodically subjected to impact forces, as in walking or running, or to gravity lengthening the muscles. A sequence of an eccentric followed by a concentric contraction is referred as a *stretch–shortening cycle*. The purpose of stretching is to make the final concentric contraction more powerful than one resulting from a pure concentric contraction alone. The observed increase in force is due to the fact that in the range between maximum stretch and when optimum muscle length is reached, the force developed is equal to the sum of the active force (effected by innervation) and the passive force (effected by the stretching).

If the force output of the muscle is enhanced during a stretch–shortening cycle, it is to be expected that the work efficiency will be increased as well. Mechanical efficiency is defined as the ratio of external work performed to the extra energy production:

(9.8) $$\text{Mechanical efficiency} (\%) = E_{ext} \cdot 100 / (E_{tot} - e)$$

In this equation E_{ext} is the external work, E_{tot} the energy expended, and e the resting metabolic rate.[41,42] The increase in mechanical efficiency is assumed to be related to the enhancement of resistive forces when elastic structures in the muscle or at the muscle–tendon unit are lengthened.[11,19,43–47]

Muscles generate force and transmit this force via tendons to the bones. With respect to the axis of rotation of a joint, a muscle force **F** produces a moment (or torque) **M**. The moment is defined as the cross product of the vectors **L** and the muscle force **F**:

(9.9) $$\mathbf{M} = \mathbf{L} \times \mathbf{F}$$

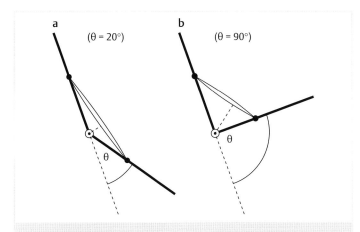

Fig. 9.17a, b Change in the moment arm of a muscle in relation to the state of flexion of a joint. The dashed line designates the moment arm, which is the perpendicular distance of the line of action of the muscle force from the center of rotation. At a small flexion angle ($\theta = 20°$) the moment arm is relatively small (**a**). With increasing flexion of the joint (for example $\theta = 90°$) the moment arm increases (**b**). The moment arm reaches its maximum value at $\theta = 180°$. The moment arm is only one of the two factors determining the moment, which also depends on the muscle force.

Vector **L** points from the axis of rotation to the point of force application at the bone. The moment developed thus depends on the amount of force developed, the magnitude of **L**, and the angle between the line of force and the direction of **L**. Therefore, the moment may be changed by changing the force or the point of force application and thus the angle.

The moment arm of a muscle is defined as the perpendicular distance between the line of application of the muscle force and the center of rotation of a joint. For purely geometric reasons the moment arm of a muscle will change as a function of joint position in the range between maximum extension and maximum flexion. **Fig. 9.17** illustrates this with the case of a simple hinge joint crossed by a muscle. It is observed that, close to maximum extension of the joint, the moment arm is small. As joint flexion increases, the moment arm of the muscle also increases. The moment arm would assume its maximum value at a flexion angle of 180° (not attainable in vivo). If the distances of the points of insertion of a muscle from the axis of rotation are equal to both sides of the axis, the moment arm will change in proportion to the sine of half the flexion angle. Thus, close to maximum extension, a given force will effect a low moment; as the flexion angle increases, the moment will increase as well.

As described above (see Chapter 1 and Chapter 4), the moment is given by the vector product of moment arm and force. During actual activities in vivo, the moment varies within broad limits. This variation is due

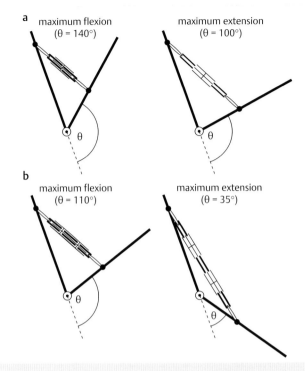

Fig. 9.18a, b Change in the range of motion of a joint due to a change in muscle length. With short muscle fibers (**a**) the joint may be mobile between 140° and 100°. Longer muscle fibers (**b**) influence the minimum and maximum length of the muscle. Thus the limits of flexion and extension change to 110° and 35°, so that the range of motion changes to 75°.

to the fact that muscle force varies in dependence on muscle length, contraction velocity, and the number of motor units recruited. The relationship between muscle length, state of rotation of a joint, and moment is illustrated in **Fig. 9.18**. Supposing a muscle–joint system is configured in such a way that, when extending from 140° to 100°, the muscle changes from its minimum to its maximum length. What would happen if the muscle length were significantly increased? Since more sarcomeres are added in series to take up the length change, the range of length change will increase. As shown in the illustration, the muscle could now extend to 35° (instead of 100°). The minimum length at which the longer muscle is not able to develop force will also increase. Therefore, the lower limit of range of motion will be changed as well, from 140° to 110°. When the joint angle changes, the relative change in sarcomere length will depend on muscle fiber length. In muscles with long fiber lengths, the relative change in sarcomere length per degree of rotation will be small. Therefore, according to the force–length relationship, the change in force as the joint rotates will be minor. If, however, muscle fiber length is short, the change in length of the sarcomeres will be increased and the force developed will change during movement of the joint.

For skeletal muscle, a close relationship can be assumed to exist between muscle architecture, geometric relation to bones and joints, and mechanical muscle properties like force generation, length change, and velocity. This indicates that the architectural specialization observed in numerous muscles has profound functional consequences. Muscles might be able to perform a large range of tasks mainly as a result of their intrinsic design rather than by being triggered by a specific set of command signals from the central nervous system. This design probably allows the central nervous system to act as a coordinator of different actions rather than as a definer of a particular activity.

9.10 Muscular Strength Training

Maximum muscular strength is defined as the maximum load a person can move once. Typically, it is determined in terms of the *one repetition maximum* (1RM) measured during a single performance of a single standardized movement. Strength training is muscular activity that aims to increase the 1RM. Muscular strength is inversely and independently associated with mortality from all causes in humans, even after adjusting for cardiovascular/cardiorespiratory fitness and other potential confounders.[48] Muscular strength determines a major part of physical working capacity. Improved muscular strength has a profound effect on everyday activity level and energy expenditure. An average 20-year-old can lift an external load of the magnitude of their own body weight in a half squat position (90° flexion of the knee joints). From this age onwards, strength reduces by an average of 10% per decade. The major part of the strength reduction seems to relate to behavioral changes; only a minor part is explained by aging processes. However, despite reductions in muscle strength, the training response seems to be similar in young and old persons when expressed as a percentage improvement in strength.

In strength training it is important to be aware of the fact that the training load is of major importance. McDonagh and Davies[49] summarized 11 studies relating to training load and repetitions. They found that training loads below 66% of the 1RM gave no increase in muscular strength even with repetitions of up to 150 contractions per day. Training loads above 66% of the 1RM increased the maximum voluntary contraction (1RM) by 0.2% to 2% per day. Loads greater than 66% with as few as 10 repetitions per day produced a significant increase in strength. The increases in dynamic strength were greatest when the heavier loads were used.[50]

Muscular strength and power are central qualities in performance. A variety of training methods are applied in an effort to increase strength and power, mostly in activities demanding acceleration and explosive force development. Strength is defined as the integrated result of several force-producing muscles performing maximally, either isometrically or dynamically, during a single voluntary effort in a defined task. Power is the product of force times velocity, that is, it is the ability to produce as much force as possible in the shortest possible time. The classic force–velocity curve shows that the maximum force in a concentric activity is less than that in an isometric contraction. The highest power is attained when the contraction velocity is 25% to 30% of the maximum value, at which point the force is approximately 30% to 40% of the maximum isometric strength (**Fig. 9.19**).

The development of training methods has traditionally been based upon the principle of specificity, and training is supposed to be task-specific in terms of contraction type, contraction force, movements, and velocity.[51-53] There are basically two different mechanisms by which muscular strength is increased: *muscular hypertrophy* and *neural adaptation* (**Fig. 9.20**).

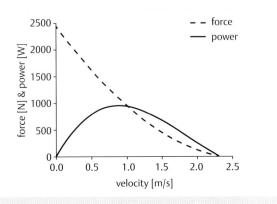

Fig. 9.19 Relationship between force (N), power (W), and contraction velocity during a concentric muscular contraction.

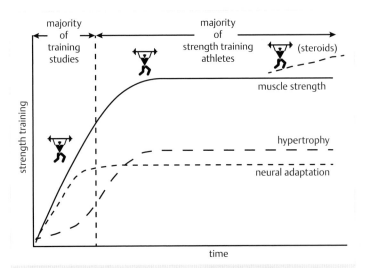

Fig. 9.20 Increase in force through muscular hypertrophy and neural adaptation. (Adapted from Sale.[54])

9.10.1 Muscular Hypertrophy

Muscular hypertrophy is an effect of strength training. There is a strong correlation between the cross-sectional area of the muscle and its ability to develop force.[53] This increase is associated with a large increase in the myofibril content of the muscle fibers. During systematic strength training over time, hypertrophy will be observed for all muscle fiber types. A muscle's ability to develop force is also dependent on many other different factors, the most common of which are the initial position, speed of lengthening, speed of shortening, eccentric initial phase, types of muscle fibers, number of motor units active at the same time, impulse frequency, and the substrate available for the muscle exercise.[52] Training for hypertrophy should emphasize eccentric/concentric actions with high loads, and with more than six repetitions.[55] Delayed onset of muscular soreness appears to trigger hypertrophy (some of the cellular events in the process of hypertrophy are shown in **Fig. 9.21**). This is the rationale behind the suggested practice in bodybuilding[55] to induce muscular hypertrophy by carrying out 5–6 sets of 8–12 repetitions (65–90% of the 1RM) until complete exhaustion. Typically, short breaks (1–2 minutes) between the sets are used to induce maximum mechanical and metabolic stress and hence maximum anabolic effects on the muscles.

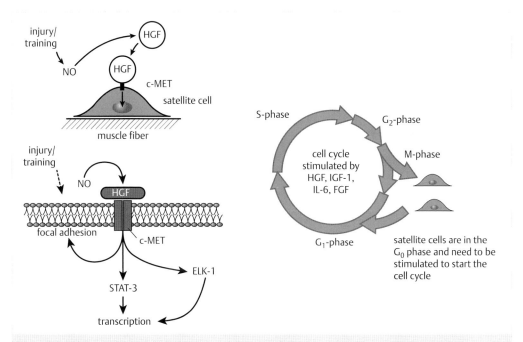

Fig. 9.21 Satellite cells are in the G_0 phase, but they can enter a new cell cycle when stimulated by hepatocyte growth factor (HGF). During muscle training or after injuries, nitrogen oxide (NO) is released, which increases the production of HGF. HGF binds to the c-MET receptor in the satellite cell membrane. Progression through the cell cycle is further stimulated by insulin growth factor (IGF), interleukin-6 (IL-6), and fibroblast growth factor (FGF) in addition to HGF. STAT-3, signal transducer and activator of transcription 3.

Increased muscle mass, however, does not necessarily increase high-velocity strength. Tesch and Larsson[55] reported an impaired ability to develop torque at high velocity in bodybuilders compared to a reference group of competitive weight lifters. Although changes in the ability to develop torque at high velocities may be a consequence of the altered architecture of hypertrophied muscle, they may also be related to velocity specificity.

In certain activities, increased body weight due to hypertrophy is not desirable because it means the individual has to transport a higher body mass. For this reason, other training modalities have been developed.

9.10.2 Neural Adaptations to Strength Training

Over the past few decades, strength training has become more focused on neural adaptation.[52] "Neural adaptation" (Behm and Sale[52]) is a descriptive term encompassing several phenomena, such as selective activation of motor units, ballistic contractions, increased frequency (rate coding), increased reflex potential, increased recruitment of motor units and increased co-contraction of antagonists,[56] and increased ability to coordinate other muscles involved in the movement.[57]

For neural adaptation, it is important to stress all motor units, but especially the high-threshold "fast-twitch" motor units. Nardone et al[58] have shown that, unlike Henneman's size principle with orderly recruitment of motor units, with eccentric training some high-threshold/fast-twitch motor units fired before the slow-twitch/low-threshold motor units. This indicates that training should include both eccentric and concentric contractions. For increases in the rate of force development, even higher forces and even lower numbers of repetitions are recommended. Adaptations resulting from this high-intensity training seem to be rapid recruitment of motor units combined with an elevated motoneuron firing rate.[59–61]

Two major principles for achieving maximum neural adaptations have been suggested. The first is to train the fastest motor units which develop the greatest force at loads between 85% and 95% of the 1RM. It is suggested that this training intensity will ensure maximum voluntary contraction.[52] The second suggested principle is to perform dynamic explosive movements with few repetitions (three to seven) and with a training resistance between 85% and 100% of the 1RM.[53] The principle of high-intensity progressive dynamic maximum strength training comprises few repetitions and high loads, for example more than 85% of the 1RM. If the goal is to increase the rate of force development and maximum strength without changes in body weight, a training regime of three to four sets of four to six repetitions using the maximum mobilization of force, or maximum intended velocity in the concentric phase, is recommended.[52,53,62–65] Training at such high intensities is documented to be effective in improving muscular strength and power, improving work economy and neural adaptations[66–68] without increasing muscle mass or body weight.

There are several indirect lines of evidence suggesting that neural adaptation to strength training exists: (1) the disproportionate increase in muscle strength at the beginning of a training program, (2) the specificity of strength training adaptations, (3) strength gains acquired after imagined strength training, and (4) "cross-education" of strength after unilateral training.

Disproportionate Increase in Muscle Strength at the Beginning of a Training Program

The "specificity of training" hypothesis set forth by Sale et al[69] suggests that greater performance enhancements are acquired when training tasks are similar to performance tasks. Several studies have reported that an increase in dynamic lifting strength is disproportionately greater than isometric strength gains after dynamic resistance training.[56,62,70] Jones and Rutherford[63] showed a gain in the 1RM of 200%, accompanied by only 5% hypertrophy. Hoff and Almåsbakk[64] showed an increase in the 1RM of 35% in well-trained individuals without changes in body weight or muscle size, indicating that neural adaptations might be present after early stages of strength training. It is unlikely that adaptations at the muscle level alone can account for such a vast increase in strength.

Specificity of Strength Training Adaptations

The suggested number of sets in rate of force development or maximum strength training is often between 3 and 5, so that one exercise in a training session typically includes 20 repetitions.[53] If the goal is to increase the rate of force development and maximum strength through neural adaptation without changes in body weight, a training regime of four to six repetitions in three or four sets using the maximum mobilization of force, or maximum intended velocity in the concentric phase, is recommended.[52,53,62–64]

Rutherford and Jones[57] showed that 12 weeks of dynamic strength training improved dynamic strength by approximately 200% while isometric strength increased by only about 15% to 20%. Almåsbakk and Hoff[62] found that bench press training with maximum intended velocity in the concentric phase with either a negligible load (0.37 kg) or a heavy load (80–85% of the 1RM) for 6 weeks similarly improved bench press velocity at submaximum loads. Conversely, submaximum bench press velocities were not improved in an alternative training group employing heavy loads but with different exercises for the same muscles. These studies indicate a high degree of training specificity, such as the coordination of agonists, synergists and antagonists, and postural stability.

Strength Gains after Imagined Strength Training

Yue and Cole[71] had one group of subjects performing repeated maximum isometric abduction contractions of their fifth digit. Another group imagined performing these contractions, while a third group served as controls. The actual training group and the imagined training group increased their maximum voluntary contractions by 30% and 20% respectively, while the control group increased by only 3.7%. Similar results have been reported for the plantar flexors.[72]

Cross-Education of Strength after Unilateral Training

One of the strongest lines of indirect evidence that neural adaptations are responsible for strength gains is the "cross-education" of strength on the contralateral side after unilateral strength training. This effect has been extensively documented; a meta-analysis has reported it to be about 8%,[73-76] and this has been corroborated by a large randomized controlled trial.[77] Many investigations however, have reported contralateral strength gains between 18% and 77%. This might be due to differences in experimental design or to differences in training programs and the muscle studied. Neural adaptations are likely to be responsible for the cross-education effect, as magnetic resonance imaging did not reveal any changes in the cross-sectional area of the untrained limb muscles.

Studies on the effect of various training paradigms on the central nervous system indicate that neural adaptations are task-specific. These neural adaptations are normally examined by means of the H-reflex and V-waves. The H-reflex is used to assess the excitability of spinal α-motoneurons, whereas V-waves measure the magnitude of motor output from α-motoneurons. The H-reflex is analogous to the mechanically induced stretch reflex. The difference between the two reflexes is that the H-reflex bypasses the muscle spindle. Both the H-reflex and the V-wave are elicited after electrical stimulation of peripheral nerves. The responses can be seen as defined waves and measured by EMG. Changes in H-reflexes are interpreted as changes in the motoneuron pool and modulation caused by descending neural drive, giving us more direct evidence of neural adaptations.[78,79] V-waves are an electrophysiological variant of H-reflexes elicited during muscle contraction with supramaximal stimulus intensities. It is assumed that the peak-to-peak amplitude of the V-wave reflects the magnitude of the efferent neural drive.[80,81]

Longitudinal studies using resistance training have demonstrated increased V-wave responses in various muscles.[81-88] Recent experiments have reinforced the concept that neural adaptations are highly specific both to the training and to the task.[85] In several studies the training interventions have focused on maximum intended velocity in the concentric phase of the exercise. Del Balso and Cafarelli[81] reported that 4 weeks of isometric plantar flexion exercise resulted in increased normalized V-wave responses (+57%). The V-wave response suggests increased efferent neural drive from spinal motoneurons to the muscles, likely caused by increased motoneuron recruitment and/or firing frequency mediated by enhanced corticospinal drive, motoneuron excitability, and/or changes in presynaptic inhibition.[74-76,79,82,86]

Adaptations at the cortical level have been difficult to prove.[87,88] However, the strength gains after imagined contractions[71] indicate adaptations at the cortical level. Lee et al[89] demonstrated enhanced cortical activation of the contralateral, untrained limb after strength training, and a recent study[90] showed an increase in left corticospinal tract structures and a significant reduction in the left putamen after 4 weeks of unilateral strength training of the right limb. This is the first study that provides evidence for strength-training-related changes in white matter and putamen in the healthy adult brain.

9.11   Endurance Training

Cardiorespiratory endurance is one of the fundamental components of physical fitness. Endurance is defined as the organism's ability to work at relatively high intensity for a long time.[91,92] $\dot{V}O_2$max (maximum oxygen consumption or maximum aerobic capacity) is the maximum rate of oxygen consumption as measured during incremental exercise. $\dot{V}O_2$max reflects the aerobic physical fitness of the individual. $\dot{V}O_2$max is expressed as an absolute rate in, for example, liters per minute, or, more commonly, as a relative rate, in milliliters of oxygen per kilogram of body mass per minute [$mL \cdot kg^{-1} \cdot min^{-1}$]. Absolute values of $\dot{V}O_2$max are typically 40% to 60% higher in men than in women. The average untrained healthy man has a $\dot{V}O_2$max of 35–40 $mL \cdot kg^{-1} \cdot min^{-1}$ and the average untrained healthy woman a $\dot{V}O_2$max of 25–35 $mL \cdot kg^{-1} \cdot min^{-1}$.

Endurance performance imposes great demands on both the cardiovascular system and the employed locomotor organs. An efficient oxygen transport system is vital. Endurance activities are demanding in terms of aerobic power, but performance is also influenced by somatic factors (for example, gender, age, and body dimensions), psychological factors (such as attitude and motivation), environment (for example, altitude and temperature), and, probably primarily, by training adaptation.[91,92] Endurance activities are favored by a predominance of slow-twitch (type 1) muscle fibers. Endurance is dependent upon the ability to supply the active cells with adequate amounts of oxygen and essential nutrients, while eliminating heat, carbon dioxide, and other waste products and sustaining homeostasis in other parts of the body. When exercising, humans must transport oxygen from ambient air, down the respiratory passage to the lungs, through the cardiovascular system, and into the muscle cells. In turn, carbon dioxide must be transported from the muscle cell to ambient air. Therefore, there are several steps at which the oxygen transport pathways may be limited.

Cardiorespiratory endurance ($\dot{V}O_2$max) has long been recognized as one of the fundamental components of physical fitness and performance in endurance events. Since accumulation of lactic acid is associated with skeletal muscle fatigue, anaerobic metabolism cannot contribute at a quantitatively significant level to the energy expended in endurance events. Therefore, during these events, maximal steady-rate $\dot{V}O_2$ functions as the primary determinant of the maximum work rate.

Endurance training stresses the factors that allow exercise at moderate to high intensity for extended periods of time. $\dot{V}O_2$max is probably the single most important factor in aerobic endurance activities.[93] The highest work rate, oxygen uptake ($\dot{V}O_2$max), or heart rate (HR) in dynamic work using large muscle groups, where production and elimination of lactate are balanced, is defined as the lactate threshold.[94] The anaerobic threshold determines the fraction of the maximum aerobic power that can be sustained for an extended period of time.[94] Work economy, or C, is defined as the ratio of work output to oxygen cost. However, gross intraindividual variations in oxygen cost during activities have been reported.[95,96] The causes of this variability are not well understood, but it seems likely that anatomical features, mechanical skill, neuromuscular skill, and storage of elastic energy are important.

The level of physical activity is important for preserving cardiovascular health. A higher level of physical activity and fitness appears to reduce all-cause mortality and cardiovascular disease mortality.[97–102] Maximum aerobic capacity or $\dot{V}O_2$max has been found to be a strong predictor of mortality in both healthy individuals and patients with cardiovascular disease, indicating that the risk increases when $\dot{V}O_2$max and stroke volume are decreased[103] in addition to an increased HR. Young endurance-trained persons have a larger stroke volume compared with moderately active persons because they have a higher diastolic filling rate and left ventricular emptying rate.

Various training intensities are used to increase $\dot{V}O_2$max and heart stroke volume—for example, low, moderate, or high intensities. Recent studies, however, have shown that high-intensity interval training has superior effects to low- and moderate-intensity training for increasing $\dot{V}O_2$max and peak stroke volume,[104] and was the single best predictor of both cardiac and all-cause deaths among patients with cardiovascular disorders.[105] These findings indicate that exercises which induce gain in $\dot{V}O_2$max should be beneficial not only in increasing functional capacity but also in survival prospects.

Trained individuals are primarily limited by the heart's ability to pump blood; that is, by their cardiac output. Cardiac output is defined as stroke volume (SV) times HR per minute. In a resting situation a normal subject will need 5 L blood per minute. If the resting HR is 50/min, it follows that the stroke volume is 100 mL. One sign of increased endurance is reduction in the resting HR. A resting HR of 40/min indicates that the stroke volume has increased to 125 ml, an increase of 25%. The stroke volume of the heart of a trained athlete can be twice that of a sedentary person. Studies indicate that stroke volume increases as a function of work load. The increased stroke volume up to the level of $\dot{V}O_2$max in trained athletes has been the rationale behind high-intensity aerobic training.

The training intensity in interval aerobic training is based upon the percentage of maximum $\dot{V}O_2$max or HR. Maximum HR can be measured during a maximum HR test; however, in general, maximum HR (HRmax) can be predicted using the equation "220 − age in years." This means that, for a person aged 30 years, the predicted HRmax would be (220 − 30) = 190. Huge variation is observed using this equation, but in most cases it is sufficient to estimate the intensity at which HRmax endurance training should be performed. Intermittent exercise at 90% to 95% of HRmax for 3–8 minutes involves a major load on the oxygen-transporting organs. With training at this intensity, the improvement in $\dot{V}O_2$ ranges from 10% to 30% within an 8- to 10-week training period.[106,107] However, individual variations related to the initial level of fitness and the duration and frequency of training are observed. When training is at lower intensities (for example, 60–80% of HRmax), only a 5% to 10% improvement in $\dot{V}O_2$max has been observed.[104,106,108–111]

During the first 1–2 minutes of interval training an oxygen deficit occurs due to the adjustment of respiration, circulation, and, especially, the stroke volume. The attainment of this state coincides with the adaptation of cardiac output (that is, SV · HR) and pulmonary ventilation.[110] It has been shown experimentally that cardiac output attains its highest values at a load that produces $\dot{V}O_2$max.[104] It should be emphasized that the maximum stroke volume is attained during and not after exercise. It is a misconception that the advantage of interval training is that frequent recovery periods per se should produce effective training of the central circulation.[104]

At present it is in general recommended that training to increase aerobic capacity should be performed in four 4-minute intervals at a training intensity of 90% to 95% of HRmax or $\dot{V}O_2$max, with a 4-minute walking period between the training intervals. However, in patients with cardiovascular disorders, different physiological tests must be performed first to identify the appropriate training prescription.[111]

References

1. Huxley AF, Peachey LD. The maximum length for contraction in vertebrate striated muscle. J Physiol 1961;156:150–165

2. Huxley AF. Muscle structure and theories of contraction. Prog Biophys Biophys Chem 1957;7:255–318

3. Huxley A. Muscular contraction. Annu Rev Physiol 1988;50:1–16

4. Huxley HE. Molecular basis of contraction in cross-striated muscle. In: Bourne G, ed. The Structure and Function of Muscle. Vol. 1. 2nd ed. New York, NY: Academic Press; 1973:301–387

5. Huijing PA. Elastic potential of muscle. In: Komi V, ed. Strength and Power in Sport. Oxford: Blackwell; 1992:151–168

6. Hill AV. First and Last Experiments in Muscle Mechanics. Cambridge: Cambridge University Press; 1970

7. Hill AV. The effect of load on the heat of shortening of muscle. Proc R Soc Lond B Biol Sci 1964;159:297–318

8. Hill AV. The heat of shortening and the dynamic constants of muscle. Proc R Soc Lond B Biol Sci 1938;126:136–195

9. Gordon AM, Huxley AF, Julian FJ. The variation in isometric tension with sarcomere length in vertebrate muscle fibres. J Physiol 1966;184(1):170–192

10. Edman KAP, Reggiani C. The sarcomere length-tension relation determined in short segments of intact muscle fibres of the frog. J Physiol 1987;385:709–732

11. Cavagna GA. Storage and utilization of elastic energy in skeletal muscle. Exerc Sport Sci Rev 1977;5:89–129

12. Heerkens YF, Woittiez RD, Kiela J, et al. Mechanical properties of passive rat muscle during sinusoidal stretching. Pflugers Arch 1987;409(4-5):438–447

13. Kovanen V, Suominen H, Heikkinen E. Mechanical properties of fast and slow skeletal muscle with special reference to collagen and endurance training. J Biomech 1984;17(10):725–735

14. Wang K, McCarter R, Wright J, Beverly J, Ramirez-Mitchell R. Viscoelasticity of the sarcomere matrix of skeletal muscles. The titin-myosin composite filament is a dual-stage molecular spring. Biophys J 1993;64(4):1161–1177

15. Labeit S, Kolmerer B. Titins: giant proteins in charge of muscle ultrastructure and elasticity. Science 1995;270(5234):293–296

16. Pollack GH. The cross-bridge theory. Physiol Rev 1983;63(3):1049–1113

17. Joyce GC, Rack PMH, Westbury DR. The mechanical properties of cat soleus muscle during controlled lengthening and shortening movements. J Physiol 1969;204(2):461–474

18. Rack PMH, Westbury DR. Elastic properties of the cat soleus tendon and their functional importance. J Physiol 1984;347:479–495

19. Bressler BH, Clinch NF. The compliance of contracting skeletal muscle. J Physiol 1974;237(3):477–493

20. Woo SLY, Gomez MA, Amiel D, Ritter MA, Gelberman RH, Akeson WH. The effects of exercise on the biomechanical and biochemical properties of swine digital flexor tendons. J Biomech Eng 1981;103(1):51–56

21. Butler DL, Grood ES, Noyes FR, Zernicke RF. Biomechanics of ligaments and tendons. Exerc Sport Sci Rev 1978;6:125–181

22. Fung YC. Biomechanics. Mechanical Properties of Living Tissues. New York: Springer; 1981

23. Brooke MH, Kaiser KK. Muscle fiber types: how many and what kind? Arch Neurol 1970;23(4):369–379

24. Bruke RE. Motor units anatomy, physiology, and functional organization. In: Brookhart JM, Mountcastle VB, Brooks VB, Geiger SR, eds. Handbook of Physiology. Bethesda, MD: American Physiological Society; 1981:345–422

25. Edington DW, Edgerton VR. Biology of Physical Activity. Boston: Houghton Mifflin; 1976

26. Bodine SC, Roy RR, Eldred E, Edgerton VR. Maximal force as a function of anatomical features of motor units in the cat tibialis anterior. J Neurophysiol 1987;57(6):1730–1745

27. Henneman E, Somjen G, Carpenter DO. Functional significance of cell size in spinal motoneurons. J Neurophysiol 1965;28:560–580

28. Binder MD, Mendell LM, eds. The Segmental Motor System. New York: Oxford University Press; 1990

29. Milner-Brown HS, Stein RB, Yemm R. The contractile properties of human motor units during voluntary isometric contractions. J Physiol 1973;228(2):285–306

30. Edgerton VR, Roy RR, Bodine SC, Sacks RD. The matching of neuronal and muscular physiology. In: Borer KT, Edington DW, White TP, eds. Frontiers of Exercise Biology. Champaign, IL: Human Kinetics; 1983

31. Bigland-Ritchie B, Johansson R, Lippold OCJ, Smith S, Woods JJ. Changes in motoneurone firing rates during sustained maximal voluntary contractions. J Physiol 1983;340:335–346

32. Bigland-Ritchie B, Johansson R, Lippold OC, Woods JJ. Contractile speed and EMG changes during fatigue of sustained maximal voluntary contractions. J Neurophysiol 1983;50(1):313–324

33. Loeb GE, Gans C. Electromyography for Experimentalists. Chicago: University of Chicago Press; 1986

34. Woittiez RD, Huijing PA, Rozendal RH. Influence of muscle architecture on the length-force diagram of mammalian muscle. Pflugers Arch 1983;399(4):275–279

35. Gans C, de Vree F. Functional bases of fiber length and angulation in muscle. J Morphol 1987;192(1):63–85

36. Otten E. Concepts and models of functional architecture in skeletal muscle. Exerc Sport Sci Rev 1988;16:89–137

37. Huijing PA, van Lookeren Campagne AA, Koper JF. Muscle architecture and fibre characteristics of rat gastrocnemius and semimembranosus muscles during isometric contractions. Acta Anat (Basel) 1989;135(1):46–52

38. Lieber RL, Fazeli BM, Botte MJ. Architecture of selected wrist flexor and extensor muscles. J Hand Surg Am 1990;15(2):244–250

39. Epstein M, Herzog W. Theoretical Models of Skeletal Muscle: Biological and Mathematical Considerations. Chichester: Wiley; 1998

40. Lieber RL, Boakes JL. Sarcomere length and joint kinematics during torque production in frog hindlimb. Am J Physiol 1988;254(6 Pt 1):C759–C768

41. Aura O, Komi PV. Effects of prestretch intensity on mechanical efficiency of positive work and on elastic behavior of skeletal muscle in stretch–shortening cycle exercise. Int J Sports Med 1986;7(3):137–143

42. Aura O, Komi PV. Mechanical efficiency of pure positive and pure negative work with special reference to the work intensity. Int J Sports Med 1986;7(1):44–49

43. Cavagna GA, Citterio G, Jacini P. Effects of speed and extent of stretching on the elastic properties of active frog muscle. J Exp Biol 1981;91:131–143

44. Cavagna GA, Dusman B, Margaria R. Positive work done by a previously stretched muscle. J Appl Physiol 1968;24(1):21–32

45. Bobbert MF, Huijing PA, van Ingen Schenau GJ. An estimation of power output and work done by the human triceps surae muscle-tendon complex in jumping. J Biomech 1986;19(11):899–906

46. Alexander R. Elastic Mechanisms in Animal Movement. Cambridge: Cambridge University Press; 1988

47. Alexander R. The spring of your step: The role of elastic mechanisms in human running. In: de Groot G, Hollander AP, Huijing PA, van Ingen Schenau GJ, eds. Biomechanics XI-A. Amsterdam: Free University Press; 1988:17–25

48. Ruiz JR, Sui X, Lobelo F, et al. Association between muscular strength and mortality in men: prospective cohort study. BMJ 2008;337:a439

49. McDonagh MJN, Davies CTM. Adaptive response of mammalian skeletal muscle to exercise with high loads. Eur J Appl Physiol Occup Physiol 1984;52(2):139–155

50. Dons B, Bollerup K, Bonde-Petersen F, Hancke S. The effect of weight-lifting exercise related to muscle fiber composition and muscle cross-sectional area in humans. Eur J Appl Physiol Occup Physiol 1979;40(2):95–106

51. Sale DG. Neural adaptations in strength training. In: Komi PV, ed. Strength and Power in Sport. Oxford: Blackwell; 1992:249–295

52. Behm DG, Sale DG. Velocity specificity of resistance training. Sports Med 1993;15(6):374–388

53. Jones DA, Rutherford OM, Parker DF. Physiological changes in skeletal muscle as a result of strength training. Q J Exp Physiol 1989;74(3):233–256

54. Sale DG. Neural adaptation to resistance training. Med Sci Sports Exerc 1988;20(5 Suppl):S135–S145

55. Tesch PA, Larsson L. Muscle hypertrophy in bodybuilders. Eur J Appl Physiol Occup Physiol 1982;49(3):301–306

56. Behm DG. Neuromuscular implications and applications of resistance training. J Strength Cond Res 1995;9(4):264–274

57. Rutherford OM, Jones DA. The role of learning and coordination in strength training. Eur J Appl Physiol Occup Physiol 1986;55(1):100–105

58. Nardone A, Romanò C, Schieppati M. Selective recruitment of high-threshold human motor units during voluntary isotonic lengthening of active muscles. J Physiol 1989;409:451–471

59. Komi PV. Training of muscle strength and power: interaction of neuromotoric, hypertrophic, and mechanical factors. Int J Sports Med 1986;7(Suppl 1):10–15

60. Schmidtbleicher D, Bührle M. Neuronal adaptation and increase of cross-sectional area studying different strength training methods. In: Johnson B, ed. Biomechanics XB. Champaign, IL: Human Kinetics; 1987:615–620

61. Häkkinen K, Alén M, Komi PV. Neuromuscular, anaerobic, and aerobic performance characteristics of elite power athletes. Eur J Appl Physiol Occup Physiol 1984;53(2):97–105

62. Almåsbakk B, Hoff J. Coordination, the determinant of velocity specificity? J Appl Physiol (1985) 1996;81(5):2046–2052

63. Jones DA, Rutherford OM. Human muscle strength training: the effects of three different regimens and the nature of the resultant changes. J Physiol 1987;391:1–11

64. Hoff J, Almåsbakk B. The effects of maximum strength training on throwing velocity and muscle strength in female team-handball players. J Strength Cond Res 1995;9:255–258

65. Hoff J, Helgerud J. Endurance and strength training for soccer players: physiological considerations. Sports Med 2004;34(3):165–180

66. Østerås H, Helgerud J, Hoff J. Maximal strength-training effects on force–velocity and force-power relationships explain increases in aerobic performance in humans. Eur J Appl Physiol 2002;88(3):255–263

67. Heggelund J, Fimland MS, Helgerud J, Hoff J. Maximal strength training improves work economy, rate of force development and maximal strength more than conventional strength training. Eur J Appl Physiol 2013;113(6):1565–1573

68. Kraemer WJ, Adams K, Cafarelli E, et al; American College of Sports Medicine. American College of Sports Medicine position stand. Progression models in resistance training for healthy adults. Med Sci Sports Exerc 2002;34(2):364–380

69. Sale DG, Upton AR, McComas AJ, MacDougall JD. Neuromuscular function in weight-trainers. Exp Neurol 1983;82(3):521–531

70. Mortiani T, de Vries HA. Neural factors versus hypertrophy in the time course of muscle strength gain. Am J Phys Med Rehabil 1979;58:115–130

71. Yue G, Cole KJ. Strength increases from the motor program: comparison of training with maximal voluntary and imagined muscle contractions. J Neurophysiol 1992;67(5):1114–1123

72. Zijdewind I, Toering ST, Bessem B, Van Der Laan O, Diercks RL. Effects of imagery motor training on torque production of ankle plantar flexor muscles. Muscle Nerve 2003;28(2):168–173

73. Munn J, Herbert RD, Gandevia SC. Contralateral effects of unilateral resistance training: a meta-analysis. J Appl Physiol (1985) 2004;96(5):1861–1866

74. Fimland MS, Helgerud J, Gruber M, Leivseth G, Hoff J. Functional maximal strength training induces neural transfer to single-joint tasks. Eur J Appl Physiol 2009;107(1):21–29

75. Fimland MS, Helgerud J, Solstad GM, Iversen VM, Leivseth G, Hoff J. Neural adaptations underlying cross-education after unilateral strength training. Eur J Appl Physiol 2009;107(6):723–730

76. Fimland MS, Helgerud J, Gruber M, Leivseth G, Hoff J. Enhanced neural drive after maximal strength training in multiple sclerosis patients. Eur J Appl Physiol 2010;110(2):435–443

77. Munn J, Herbert RD, Hancock MJ, Gandevia SC. Training with unilateral resistance exercise increases contralateral strength. J Appl Physiol (1985) 2005;99(5):1880–1884

78. Aagaard P, Simonsen EB, Andersen JL, Magnusson P, Dyhre-Poulsen P. Increased rate of force development and neural drive of human skeletal muscle following resistance training. J Appl Physiol (1985) 2002;93(4):1318–1326

79. Scaglioni G, Ferri A, Minetti AE, et al. Plantar flexor activation capacity and H reflex in older adults: adaptations to strength training. J Appl Physiol (1985) 2002;92(6):2292–2302

80. Aagaard P. Training-induced changes in neural function. Exerc Sport Sci Rev 2003;31(2):61–67

81. Del Balso C, Cafarelli E. Adaptations in the activation of human skeletal muscle induced by short-term isometric resistance training. J Appl Physiol (1985) 2007;103(1):402–411

82. Aagaard P, Simonsen EB, Andersen JL, Magnusson P, Dyhre-Poulsen P. Neural adaptation to resistance training: changes in evoked V-wave and H-reflex responses. J Appl Physiol (1985) 2002;92(6):2309–2318

83. Duchateau J, Semmler JG, Enoka RM. Training adaptations in the behavior of human motor units. J Appl Physiol (1985) 2006;101(6):1766–1775

84. Gondin J, Duclay J, Martin A. Soleus- and gastrocnemii-evoked V-wave responses increase after neuro-muscular electrical stimulation training. J Neurophysiol 2006;95(6):3328–3335

85. Schubert M, Beck S, Taube W, Amtage F, Faist M, Gruber M. Balance training and ballistic strength training are associated with task-specific corticospinal adaptations. Eur J Neurosci 2008;27(8):2007–2018

86. Folland JP, Wakamatsu T, Fimland MS. The influence of maximal isometric activity on twitch and H-reflex potentiation, and quadriceps femoris performance. Eur J Appl Physiol 2008;104(4):739–748

87. Carroll TJ, Riek S, Carson RG. The sites of neural adaptation induced by resistance training in humans. J Physiol 2002;544(Pt 2):641–652

88. Jensen JL, Marstrand PC, Nielsen JB. Motor skill training and strength training are associated with different plastic changes in the central nervous system. J Appl Physiol (1985) 2005;99(4):1558–1568

89. Lee M, Gandevia SC, Carroll TJ. Unilateral strength training increases voluntary activation of the opposite untrained limb. Clin Neurophysiol 2009;120(4):802–808

90. Palmer HS, Håberg AK, Fimland MS, et al. Structural brain changes after 4 wk of unilateral strength training of the lower limb. J Appl Physiol (1985) 2013;115(2):167–175

91. Astrand P-O, Rohdahl K. Textbook of Work Physiology. New York: McGraw-Hill; 1986

92. Maughan RJ. Marathon running. In: Reilley T, Snell P, Williams C, et al, eds. Physiology of Sports. London: Spon; 1969:121–152

93. Saltin B. Maximal oxygen uptake: limitations and malleability. In: Nazar K, Terjung RT, eds. International Perspectives in Exercise Physiology. Champaign, IL: Human Kinetics; 1990:26–40

94. Davis JA. Anaerobic threshold: review of the concept and directions for future research. Med Sci Sports Exerc 1985;17(1):6–21

95. Conley DL, Krahenbuhl GS. Running economy and distance running performance of highly trained athletes. Med Sci Sports Exerc 1980;12(5):357–360

96. Helgerud J. Maximal oxygen uptake, anaerobic threshold and running economy in women and men with similar performances level in marathons. Eur J Appl Physiol Occup Physiol 1994;68(2):155–161

97. Paffenbarger RS Jr, Hyde RT, Wing AL, Hsieh CC. Physical activity, all-cause mortality, and longevity of college alumni. N Engl J Med 1986;314(10):605–613

98. Oldridge NB, Guyatt GH, Fischer ME, Rimm AA. Cardiac rehabilitation after myocardial infarction. Combined experience of randomized clinical trials. JAMA 1988;260(7):945–950

99. Blair SN, Kohl HW III, Paffenbarger RS Jr, Clark DG, Cooper KH, Gibbons LW. Physical fitness and all-cause mortality. A prospective study of healthy men and women. JAMA 1989;262(17):2395–2401

100. Farrell SW, Kampert JB, Kohl HW III, et al. Influences of cardiorespiratory fitness levels and other predictors on cardiovascular disease mortality in men. Med Sci Sports Exerc 1998;30(6):899–905

101. O'Connor GT, Buring JE, Yusuf S, et al. An overview of randomized trials of rehabilitation with exercise after myocardial infarction. Circulation 1989;80(2):234–244

102. Jolliffe JA, Rees K, Taylor RS, Thompson D, Oldridge N, Ebrahim S. Exercise-based rehabilitation for coronary heart disease. Cochrane Database Syst Rev 2001;(1):CD001800

103. Myers J, Prakash M, Froelicher V, Do D, Partington S, Atwood JE. Exercise capacity and mortality among men referred for exercise testing. N Engl J Med 2002;346(11):793–801

104. Helgerud J, Høydal K, Wang E, et al. Aerobic high-intensity intervals improve VO_{2max} more than moderate training. Med Sci Sports Exerc 2007;39(4):665–671

105. Kavanagh T, Mertens DJ, Hamm LF, et al. Prediction of long-term prognosis in 12 169 men referred for cardiac rehabilitation. Circulation 2002;106(6):666–671

106. American College of Sports Medicine Position Stand. The recommended quantity and quality of exercise for developing and maintaining cardiorespiratory and muscular fitness, and flexibility in healthy adults. Med Sci Sports Exerc 1998;30(6):975–991

107. Rognmo Ø, Hetland E, Helgerud J, Hoff J, Slørdahl SA. High intensity aerobic interval exercise is superior to moderate intensity exercise for increasing aerobic capacity in patients with coronary artery disease. Eur J Cardiovasc Prev Rehabil 2004;11(3):216–222

108. Pollock ML. The quantification of endurance training programs. In: Wilmore JH, ed. Exercise and Sport Sciences Reviews. New York, NY: Academic Press; 1973: 155–188

109. Helgerud J, Engen LC, Wisløff U, Hoff J. Aerobic endurance training improves soccer performance. Med Sci Sports Exerc 2001;33(11):1925–1931

110. Helgerud J, Kemi OJ, Hoff J. Pre-season concurrent strength and endurance development in elite soccer players. In: Hoff J, Helgerud J, eds. Football: New Developments in Physical Training Research. Trondheim: NTNU; 2002:55–66

111. Mezzani A, Hamm LF, Jones AM, et al. Aerobic exercise intensity assessment and prescription in cardiac rehabilitation: a joint position statement of the European Association for Cardiovascular Prevention and Rehabilitation, the American Association of Cardiovascular and Pulmonary Rehabilitation and the Canadian Association of Cardiac Rehabilitation. Eur J Prev Cardiology 2013;20(3):442–467

Further Reading

Aagaard P, Simonsen EB, Andersen JL, Magnusson SP, Halkjaer-Kristensen J, Dyhre-Poulsen P. Neural inhibition during maximal eccentric and concentric quadriceps contraction: effects of resistance training. J Appl Physiol (1985) 2000;89(6):2249–2257

Adrian ED, Bronk DW. The discharge of impulses in motor nerve fibres: Part II. The frequency of discharge in reflex and voluntary contractions. J Physiol 1929;67(2):i3–i151

Basmajian JV, DeLuca CJ. Muscles Alive. Their Functions Revealed by Electromyography. 5th ed. Baltimore: Williams & Wilkins; 1985

Bergh U, Sjödin B, Forsberg A, Svedenhag J. The relationship between body mass and oxygen uptake during running in humans. Med Sci Sports Exerc 1991;23(2):205–211

Bührle M, Schmidtbleicher D. The influence of maximal strength training on movement velocity. Leistungssport 1977;7:3–10

Bunc V, Heller J. Energy cost of running in similarly trained men and women. Eur J Appl Physiol Occup Physiol 1989;59(3):178–183

Costill DL, Thomason H, Roberts E. Fractional utilization of the aerobic capacity during distance running. Med Sci Sports 1973;5(4):248–252

Ekblom B, Hermansen L. Cardiac output in athletes. J Appl Physiol 1968;25(5):619–625

Fitts RH, Widrick JJ. Muscle mechanics: adaptations with exercise-training. Exerc Sport Sci Rev 1996;24:427–473

Gledhill N, Cox D, Jamnik R. Endurance athletes' stroke volume does not plateau: major advantage is diastolic function. Med Sci Sports Exerc 1994;26(9):1116–1121

Häkkinen K, Kallinen M, Izquierdo M, et al. Changes in agonist-antagonist EMG, muscle CSA, and force during strength training in middle-aged and older people. J Appl Physiol (1985) 1998;84(4):1341–1349

Häkkinen K, Kallinen M, Linnamo V, Pastinen UM, Newton RU, Kraemer WJ. Neuromuscular adaptations during bilateral versus unilateral strength training in middle-aged and elderly men and women. Acta Physiol Scand 1996;158(1):77–88

Helgerud J, Ingjer F, Strømme SB. Sex differences in performance-matched marathon runners. Eur J Appl Physiol Occup Physiol 1990;61(5-6):433–439

Herbert RD, Dean C, Gandevia SC. Effects of real and imagined training on voluntary muscle activation during maximal isometric contractions. Acta Physiol Scand 1998;163(4):361–368

Hermansen L, Stensvold I. Production and removal of lactate during exercise in man. Acta Physiol Scand 1972;86(2):191–201

Herzog W, ed. Skeletal Muscle Mechanics. From Mechanisms to Function. Chichester: Wiley; 2000

Hill AV. The series elastic component of muscle. Proc R Soc Lond B Biol Sci 1950;B137:273–280

Kawakami Y, Ichinose Y, Fukunaga T. Architectural and functional features of human triceps surae muscles during contraction. J Appl Physiol (1985) 1998;85(2):398–404

Kernell D. Organization and properties of spinal motoneurons and motor units. Prog Brain Res 1986;64:21–30

Klinke R, Silbernagl P. Lehrbuch der Physiologie. 2nd ed. Stuttgart: Thieme; 1996

Narici MV, Roi GS, Landoni L, Minetti AE, Cerretelli P. Changes in force, cross-sectional area and neural activation during strength training and detraining of the human quadriceps. Eur J Appl Physiol Occup Physiol 1989;59(4):310–319

Ploutz LL, Tesch P, Biro RL, et al. Effect of resistance training on muscle use during exercise. J Appl Physiol (1985) 1994;76(4):1675–1681

Shima N, Ishida K, Katayama K, Morotome Y, Sato Y, Miyamura M. Cross education of muscular strength during unilateral resistance training and detraining. Eur J Appl Physiol 2002;86(4):287–294

Tesch P. Short- and long-term histochemical and biological adaptations in muscle. In: Komi PV, ed. Strength and Power in Sport. Oxford: Blackwell; 1992:361–373

Tillmann B. Binde- und Stützgewebe des Bewegungsapparates. In: Tillmann B, Töndury G, eds. Rauber/Kopsch, Anatomie des Menschen; Band 1. Bewegungsapparat. 2nd ed. Stuttgart: Thieme; 1998:13–48

Zajac FE. Muscle and tendon: properties, models, scaling, and application to biomechanics and motor control. Crit Rev Biomed Eng 1989;17(4):359–411

Zhou B, Conlee RK, Jensen R, Fellingham GW, George JD, Fisher AG. Stroke volume does not plateau during graded exercise in elite male distance runners. Med Sci Sports Exerc 2001;33(11):1849–1854

10 Mechanical Aspects of Skin

Skin has several important functions for the body; some of these are mechanical. Apart from forces acting on the teeth, external forces on the locomotor system are transmitted exclusively via the skin. Strain and deformation of the skin distribute the effect of these forces over larger areas of contact and attenuate peak forces. The ability of the skin to be readily elongated is extremely important to the functioning of joints. Any noticeable force required to elongate the skin on the convex aspect of a joint would make joint movement strenuous and decrease the range of motion. One example is the limited range of motion experienced in a case of a swollen joint. Here the skin is already strained by the swelling and tolerates only minor additional elongation. Another example is the decreased range of motion in the presence of scars close to a joint, as scar tissue is less extensible than normal skin.

Grasping and holding objects effects relatively high pressures and shear forces on the palm of the hand. A pressure distribution with peak pressure values in characteristic locations also exists under the sole of the foot. When a person is sitting or lying down, the skin is subjected to less pressure, because the gravitational force acts on a larger area of contact. In contrast to hand and foot, where we usually experience pressurization and unloading in rapid succession, the pressure on skin when sitting or lying may persist for longer periods. This may have undesirable consequences. Knowledge of the effects of pressure, tension, and shear on the skin is required for the construction and fitting of prostheses and orthoses. Deformation characteristics of the skin are of interest when planning surgical incisions and optimizing wound closure.

In addition to its mechanical functions, skin has a protective function. First and foremost, its external layer, the stratum corneum, acts as a microbial and chemical barrier. Receptors in the skin register touch, pressure, strain, and temperature. Strain effects a sensation of tension; above a certain limit, this sensation is transformed into pain. Skin plays an important role in maintaining the correct body temperature by controlling the blood flow in the skin and by regulating the production of sweat.

10.1 Anatomical Basics

Skin is composed of several distinct layers: epidermis, dermis, and subdermis (**Fig. 10.1**). The epidermis is an avascular cellular layer. Its thickness at different locations of the body is typically 0.1 mm; on the palms of the hands or the soles of the feet a thickness of up to 1.0 mm may be encountered. Cells originate at the basement membrane, at the borderline between epidermis and dermis. Within a period of approximately 1 month these cells migrate towards the skin surface. In the course of the migration they gradually assume a flat form, lose their nuclei, and finally die.

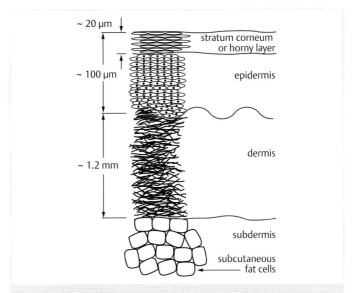

Fig. 10.1 Schematic cross section through skin, depicting the epidermis and its external stratum corneum layer, the dermis, and the subdermis. Typical thicknesses are quoted; at certain locations the thickness of one or more layers may be substantially higher. (Adapted, with permission, from Payne.[1])

During the migration the cells synthesize keratin, a fibrous protein. The keratin from the dead cells, reinforced by additional chemical bonding, remains at the surface of the skin and forms the stratum corneum (horny layer). At body locations which are only rarely loaded, if at all, the horny layer has a thickness in the order of 0.02 mm; at frequently and highly loaded locations the thickness can be substantially greater. During everyday life the surface of the stratum corneum is subject to continuous wear and tear. The fact that its thickness is maintained in the long run is clear proof of the continuous cellular renewal of the epidermis.

The primary function of the dermis is to provide nourishment and mechanical support to the epidermis, as its thin cellular layer is of limited mechanical strength. In terms of volume, the dermis is composed of approximately 35% collagen, 0.5% elastin, and 65% water, with small admixtures of cells and intercellular substances. The collagen fibers are identical with the tension-resistant fibers employed in tendons and ligaments. The collagen fibers form a two-dimensional mesh; in part they are arranged in preferred directions. In the unloaded state, the fibers are not straight but assume a spiral, wavy form. The form of the fibers and their arrangement in the mesh determine the elongation properties and tensile strength of the dermis. The fibers of the elastin form a second mesh. It is hypothesized that the elastin mesh is responsible for the elongation properties of skin under low stress. The intercellular substances are held responsible for the viscoelastic properties of skin.

10.2   Mechanical Properties

10.2.1 Modulus of Elasticity

Fig. 10.2 shows the stress–strain diagram of a skin sample in vitro. Starting from the unloaded state, the sample is elongated by more than 50% of its initial length under tensile stress of small magnitude (region A). After a transitional zone (region B), the strain exhibits only a small further increase in relation to the steep increase in stress (region C). When the strain approaches the value 1.0 (that is, 100% elongation with respect to the initial length), the probe eventually ruptures.

The shape of the stress–strain curve in **Fig. 10.2** is qualitatively explained by the fact that in region A of **Fig. 10.3** the wavy, unordered collagen fibers offer virtually no resistance to elongation.[2] In the transitional region B, the fibers straighten out and become more and more aligned in the direction of the tensile force. The more the fibers are straightened and aligned, the steeper is the slope of the stress–strain curve: that is, the higher is the modulus of elasticity. With all fibers aligned, the strain can increase only by a small amount before rupture occurs. In regions B and C, the stress–strain curve of skin resembles stress–strain curves of tendons. Tendons, however, do not exhibit the large initial strain under low stress (region A), which is characteristic of skin.

Fig. 10.4 shows the initial part of the stress–strain curve of **Fig. 10.2** drawn to a stress scale enlarged by a factor of approximately 100. It can be noted that, in the strain range between $\varepsilon = 0$ and $\varepsilon = 0.4$, there

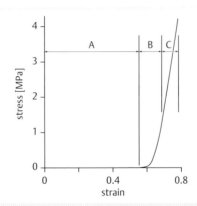

Fig. 10.2 Stress–strain curve of an abdominal skin sample in vitro. A, region of high strain under comparatively low tensile stress, that is, low-stiffness region. Between the origin of the diagram and a strain equal to approx. 0.6, the stress increases, though only by a small amount. This increase is so small that in this graph the curve seems to coincide with the horizontal axis. B, transitional region; C, high-stress region exhibiting high stiffness. (Adapted from Daly.[2])

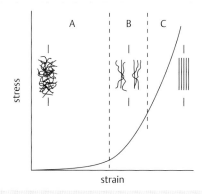

Fig. 10.3 Qualitative explanation for the shape of the stress–strain curve depicted in **Fig. 10.2**. (Adapted from Daly.[2])

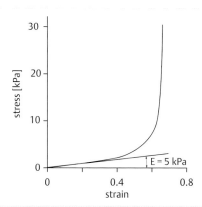

Fig. 10.4 Initial portion of the stress–strain curve depicted in **Fig. 10.2**, though enlarged with respect to the stress scale by a factor of 100. Between zero strain and a strain equal to 0.4 there is a linear relation between stress and strain. The modulus of elasticity (E; slope of the curve) amounts typically to 5 kPa. (Adapted from Daly.[2])

is a virtually linear relation between stress and strain. In this region the modulus of elasticity of skin (the slope of the curve) typically amounts to 5 kPa.[2] This modulus is approximately 100 times lower than that of soft rubber. The elastic behavior of skin in the initial region of large strain is assumed to be determined not by the collagen but by the elastin mesh. In this region, where the collagen fibers are completely relaxed, the elastin is responsible for the mechanical properties of skin. The stress at the rupture limit, on the other hand, is not influenced by the elastin.[3] The elastin mesh disintegrates with age. Without elastin, deformations caused by tensile stress do not entirely return to their initial state when the stress returns to zero, and this is regarded as responsible for the formation of wrinkles.

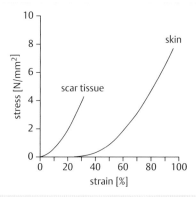

Fig. 10.5 Comparison of the stress–strain curves of skin and hypertrophic scar tissue. In contrast to skin, hypertrophic scar tissue exhibits only low strain under low stress. At higher stress values the moduli of elasticity are virtually identical. (Adapted from Dunn et al.[4])

Scar tissue contains a much higher proportion of collagen fibers than normal skin.[4,5] Qualitatively, scar tissue is characterized by its hardness and red color. **Fig. 10.5** shows the stress–strain diagram of hypertrophic scar tissue compared with normal skin. So-called hypertrophic scars develop at deep wounds, especially burns. The initial region of high strain under low stress, which is characteristic of normal skin, is absent in scar tissue. The maximum strain of scar tissue is thus less than that of normal skin. The maximum stiffness (the slope of the curves in their end region) exhibits no difference between scar tissue and skin. It is assumed that in scar tissue the collagen fibers are already aligned preferentially in the longitudinal direction of the scar. For this reason, an initial region of the stress–strain curve, where the collagen fibers align, is absent. Under high stress, the collagen fibers determine the shape of the curve, both for scar tissue and for skin.

A test which subjects a skin sample only to a single tensile force (uniaxial test) can describe the mechanical properties of skin only approximately. Since collagen forms a planar mesh, and since the strains imposed are high, a precise description of the properties of skin requires loading of the sample in two directions simultaneously (biaxial test) and documenting the strain in both directions.[6–8] Such research helps in the solving of practical problems: for example, which procedure is best adapted to close a skin defect? Pulling the edges together? Performing additional cuts in the vicinity? Or is a transplant required?

To characterize the in vivo mechanical properties of skin, landmarks are glued on the skin.[9] The force required to increase the distance between the landmarks is measured, or perhaps the moment required to twist the landmarks against one another. Such measurements provide only qualitative data, however; specific mechanical parameters cannot be derived from them. The thickness of the tissue layer placed under strain is indeterminate; the tensile or shear stress is not uniform, and any prestress remains unaccounted for.

The so-called compression test observes the time-dependent indentation of a probe into the skin. This protocol resembles the Shore measurement of hardness employed for characterizing technical materials.

Skin is viscoelastic. If the strain of a sample of skin is kept constant, the stress will decrease in time (*stress relaxation*). If the stress is kept constant, the strain will increase in time (*creep deformation*). The viscoelastic properties of skin are assumed to be regulated by the ground substance of the dermis. The ground substance influences the internal friction between the collagen fibers and the potential shift of fluid within the dermis.

10.2.2 Friction Properties

The coefficient of friction of skin depends markedly on the moistness of the surface. Dry skin has a low coefficient of friction. Moistening of the skin increases the adhesion between the callus and external surfaces, while at a still higher wetting the superficial fluid film reduces the coefficient of friction again.

Prostheses are fixed to the body essentially by forces of friction. High friction between the skin and the material of the prosthesis surface would be advantageous for stable fixation, but on the other hand a high friction coefficient could result in high shear forces acting on the skin, and from this point of view a low friction coefficient would be advantageous to avoid damage to the skin due to shear. Thus, the choice of the materials employed for lining prostheses represents a compromise between securing fixation and preventing skin injuries. **Table 10.1** lists coefficients of friction between skin, materials employed for lining prostheses, and woolen socks.[10]

	Skin	Woolen sock
Plastazote, normal	0.75	0.62
Plastazote, hard	0.80	0.64
Pelite, medium	0.73	0.60
Woolen sock	0.53	–

Table 10.1 Coefficients of friction between skin, woolen socks, and materials used for the lining of prostheses

Source: Data from Sanders et al.[10]

10.3 Reaction of the Skin to Mechanical Loading

Skin reacts to chronic pressure and shear forces by thickening the stratum corneum. This thickening, called callus or callosity, is easily observable on the palms of highly stressed hands or the plantar surface of the feet of people who go barefoot, and should be regarded as a protective mechanism rather than a medical condition.[11,12] Sweating can continue through a thickened callus layer because the openings of the sweat glands pass through the callus. This is of importance not only for the friction properties of the skin, but

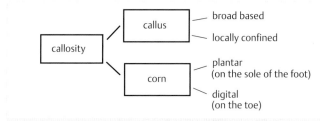

Fig. 10.6 Clinical presentations of hyperkeratosis on the sole of the foot. (Adapted, with permission, from Singh et al.[13])

because the wetting keeps the keratin ductile and pliable. Dry (dehydrated) callus is brittle and has a tendency to crack.

Very thick callosities (hyperkeratosis), however, can induce discomfort. **Fig. 10.6** shows the classification of callosities of the foot. Tight or badly fitting shoes and deformations of the toes are considered as causes of diffuse plantar callosities, which are not observed in people who habitually go barefoot. Measurements show that the pressure under plantar callosities is greater than in the surrounding area of the sole[14]; this can promote further callus formation. On the other hand, shear deformation in loosely fitting shoes or shoes open in the rear can lead to callus formation at the margins of regions under strain, for example at the edge of the heel.[13]

10.4 Injury to the Skin Caused by Mechanical Loading

10.4.1 Injury Caused by Pressure

If the pressure on the skin exceeds the blood pressure in the arteries of the skin, the flow of blood is reduced or completely stopped (*ischemia*). The consequences are oxygen insufficiency (*hypoxia*) and accumulation of metabolites in the tissue. If the blood flow is stopped for too long, the outcome is tissue necrosis. If the blood flow was inhibited by excessive pressure, after decompression all the vessels open and swelling results. If the recovery time before the next pressure episode is too short, the tolerance limit of the skin reduces. In this way, repeated compressive loading at short intervals can lead to a state of "zero tolerance." This can be observed in cases of badly fitted splints, orthoses, or shoes, which patients make repeated efforts to wear, each attempt lasting shorter than the preceding one, before abandoning them altogether.[15]

Accumulation of metabolites, which cannot be removed when the blood flow is stopped, causes pain. This pain signals a need to change the position of the body or to improve or make changes to splints, orthoses, or shoes. Persons with reduced or complete lack of sensitivity of the skin are especially at risk because the physiological warning mechanism does not take effect. This is the case with diabetes patients with reduced sensitivity of the plantar skin,[16,17] or paraplegic or tetraplegic individuals with complete

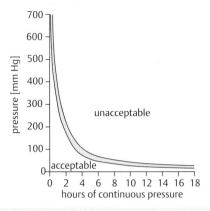

Fig. 10.7 Tolerance limit of skin under bony prominences with respect to pressure magnitude and duration of pressure application. High pressures are tolerated only for short periods; low pressures are acceptable for longer periods. The shaded area indicates individual variability. (Adapted from Reswick and Rogers.[18])

absence of skin sensitivity. Persons with reduced muscular strength are at risk as well, as they may perceive the physiological warning signals but are unable to react appropriately. In elderly persons, lying motionless during sleep—which may be exacerbated by excessive administration of sleep-inducing drugs—increases the risk that pressure ulcers will develop in the region of the back and the pelvis.

The skin's tolerance of ischemia—that is, the length of time for which the blood flow can be interrupted without permanent damage resulting—depends on the magnitude of the pressure and for how long it is applied. High pressure is tolerated only for short periods, lower pressure for longer periods. The study by Reswick and Rogers[18] gives an impression of the tolerance limits for skin areas over bony prominences (**Fig. 10.7**). The authors hypothesize that where there is a thicker layer of soft tissue, for example at the thigh, the tolerance limit will be higher. For example, the arterial pressure in the skin of the back ranges between 20 and 40 mmHg, whereas in the skin of the sole of the foot it ranges between 110 and 130 mmHg during upright standing. Depending on magnitude and duration, compressive stress can also cause direct, mechanical destruction of the skin and underlying muscle right down to the bones.[19] Observations from animal studies (**Fig. 10.8**) suggest that, depending on the *pressure dose* (the product of pressure times duration), the risk of injury to muscle may exceed the risk of injury to the skin.

10.4.2 Injury Caused by Shear

Shear deformation of the skin occurs at the edge of an area loaded in compression or by a force acting parallel to the skin's surface. In shear deformation, the layers of the skin are shifted relative to one another.

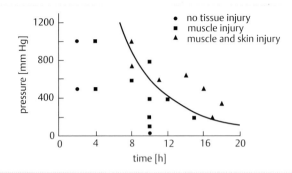

Fig. 10.8 Injury to skin and underlying muscles as a function of the pressure dose (pressure times time) observed in animal experiments. Under low compressive load (region below the curve) predominantly muscle injury is observed. Under higher load, skin injury is also observed. (Adapted from Daniel et al.[19])

Too high or too frequent shear deformation injures predominantly the epidermis and the dermis. With repeated deformation, the skin reddens and parts of the stratum corneum start to peel away, until eventually the epidermis ruptures, accompanied by a biting pain.

If a pressure pad is pressed on the skin, the tissue under the central part of the pad is subject to compressive stress (**Fig. 10.9**). Due to the indentation of the pad into the surface, the tissue at the edge of the pad is also subjected to tensile and shear stress. In **Fig. 10.9** this is visualized by the deformation of the rectangular volume elements into trapezoids. If an object exerting pressure in this way has insufficiently rounded edges, especially high shear deformation will result. Shear stress will occur equally from an internally acting or an externally acting compressive load; for example, a sharp bony prominence under the plantar skin may well produce similar effects to those of a small stone in the shoe. In addition, shear deformation compromises the blood supply because the vessels are constricted.[20] In **Fig. 10.9** this is visualized by the change in the cross-sectional area of blood vessels within the volume subject to shear deformation.

A shear force may originate from static friction or from kinetic friction between the skin and the environment. For example, there is static friction between the skin and the handle of a screwdriver. Static or kinetic friction exists between the skin of the buttocks and the surface of a seat. Kinetic friction exists between the hindfoot and the heel pad of a shoe. Under simultaneous action of a compressive force F_n and a force **F** directed parallel to the skin surface (**Fig. 10.10**), the friction force F_f causes deformation of the soft tissue at the edges of the area under compressive load. At one edge a bulge with compressive stress will develop, while at the other edge tensile stress will develop which can lead to rupture of the tissue. An example of this is the shaft of a prosthesis, which subjects the thigh to compressive stress while at the same

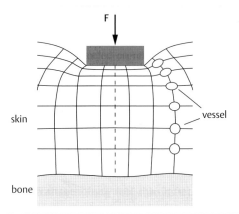

Fig. 10.9 Deformation of the skin below a pressure pad and in the region of its edges under load from a force **F**. Below the central part of the pad the tissue is compressed. This is indicated (in exaggerated fashion) by the reduced height of the tissue volume elements. Because of the indentation of the tissue by the pad, the tissue is subject to tensile stress and shear deformation in the region of the edges of the pad. This is illustrated by the trapezoid deformation of the volume elements in the edge region as well as by the deformation of a circular cross section (representing a vessel) into a narrow, elliptic one in the edge region. (Adapted from Brand and Hollister.[15])

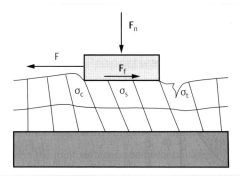

Fig. 10.10 Simultaneous application of a compressive force F_n and a shear force **F** gives rise to a friction force F_f, generating shear stress σ_s, compressive stress σ_c, and tensile stress σ_t.

time the body weight is transmitted from the stump to the shaft by shear forces. Rounding the edges of the loading surfaces decreases the risk of soft tissue damage. Sharp-edged components are avoided in the design of splints, orthoses, or truss pads, for the same reason. In skin areas with a thin stratum corneum, kinetic friction mostly causes open wounds. As an alternative reaction to kinetic friction, blisters may form, and this is seen predominantly in areas with a relatively thick stratum corneum—for example, the hands or the feet. The tendency to develop blisters varies greatly between individuals. Wetted skin is more disposed to form blisters than dry skin. This may be because (moderate) wetting leads to an increase of the coefficient of friction between the skin and the surface of work tools, allowing the exertion of a greater moment on the grip of the screwdriver or the handle of the shovel, with correspondingly higher shear deformation of the tissues.

References

1. Payne PA. Measurement of properties and function of skin. Clin Phys Physiol Meas 1991;12(2):105–129

2. Daly CH. Biomechanical properties of dermis. J Invest Dermatol 1982;79(Suppl 1):17s–20s

3. Oxlund H, Manschot J, Viidik A. The role of elastin in the mechanical properties of skin. J Biomech 1988;21(3):213–218

4. Dunn MG, Silver FH, Swann DA. Mechanical analysis of hypertrophic scar tissue: structural basis for apparent increased rigidity. J Invest Dermatol 1985;84(1):9–13

5. Clark JA, Cheng JCY, Leung KS. Mechanical properties of normal skin and hypertrophic scars. Burns 1996;22(6):443–446

6. Schneider DC, Davidson TM, Nahum AM. In vitro biaxial stress-strain response of human skin. Arch Otolaryngol 1984;110(5):329–333

7. Reihsner R, Menzel EJ. On the orthogonal anisotropy of human skin as a function of anatomical region. Connect Tissue Res 1996;34(2):145–160

8. Shang X, Yen MRT, Gaber MW. Studies of biaxial mechanical properties and nonlinear finite element modeling of skin. Mol Cell Biomech 2010;7(2):93–104

9. Edwards C, Marks R. Evaluation of biomechanical properties of human skin. Clin Dermatol 1995;13(4):375–380

10. Sanders JE, Greve JM, Mitchell SB, Zachariah SG. Material properties of commonly-used interface materials and their static coefficients of friction with skin and socks. J Rehabil Res Dev 1998;35(2):161–176

11. Schuh H, Hönle W. Hyperkeratosen: Wegcremen, abhobeln oder vereisen? MMW 2007;149:42

12. Freeman DB. Corns and calluses resulting from mechanical hyperkeratosis. Am Fam Physician 2002;65(11):2277–2280

13. Menz HB, Zammit GV, Munteanu SE. Plantar pressures are higher under callused regions of the foot in older people. Clin Exp Dermatol 2007;32(4):375–380

14. Singh D, Bentley G, Trevino SG. Callosities, corns, and calluses. BMJ 1996;312(7043):1403–1406

15. Brand PW, Hollister AM, eds. Clinical Mechanics of the Hand. 3rd ed. St. Louis: Mosby; 1999

16. Murray HJ, Young MJ, Hollis S, Boulton AJM. The association between callus formation, high pressures and neuropathy in diabetic foot ulceration. Diabet Med 1996;13(11):979–982

17. Pavicic T, Korting HC. Xerosis and callus formation as a key to the diabetic foot syndrome: dermatologic view of the problem and its management. J Dtsch Dermatol Ges 2006;4(11):935–941

18. Reswick JB, Rogers JE. Experience at Rancho Los Amigos hospital with devices and techniques to prevent pressure sores. In: Kenedi RM, Cowden JM, Scales JT, eds. Bed Sore Biomechanics. London: Macmillan; 1976:301–310

19. Daniel RK, Priest DL, Wheatley DC. Etiologic factors in pressure sores: an experimental model. Arch Phys Med Rehabil 1981;62(10):492–498

20. Bennett L, Kavner D, Lee BK, Trainor FA. Shear vs pressure as causative factors in skin blood flow occlusion. Arch Phys Med Rehabil 1979;60(7):309–314

11 Dimensions, Mass, Location of the Center of Mass, and Moment of Inertia of the Segments of the Human Body

To describe the effect of gravity on the human body, and to derive moments and joint forces from observations of the moving body, the body is conceptualized as composed of individual segments connected by joints: for example, head, arm, trunk, thigh, lower leg, and foot. Depending on the problem under investigation, further subdivision may be appropriate. The arm, for example, can be subdivided into upper arm, lower arm, and hand. The body segments are conceptualized as rigid bodies, but this is only an approximation. In vivo the segments may change shape passively under external forces or actively through activation of the muscles. In addition, it is often impossible to define the boundary between segments precisely. Where exactly, for example, does the trunk end and the thigh begin?

Some reference values published in the scientific literature are based on measurements taken from only a small number of subjects. The reason is that some values have to be determined in vitro from autopsy specimens, which may not be available in large numbers. For this reason, the numbers cited below for the mass, dimension, location of the center of mass, and moment of inertia of body segments are not representative of both sexes and all age groups. They are to be regarded as estimates. They are approximately correct, but in the individual case deviations due to sex, age, and physique may occur. For simplicity, the reference values are often given not in absolute units but in relative units, per meter of height or per kilogram of body mass. This saves having to list values separately for persons of different height or body mass; however, individual variations in physique are ignored. Uncertainties in the values affect all investigations which use these data as input values, for example gait analysis. If high precision is required in the results, the individuals concerned have to be measured beforehand.

11.1 Determination of the Location of the Center of Mass and the Moment of Inertia

11.1.1 Center of Mass

To describe the effect of a gravitational or inertial force on a body in a simple fashion, a point in space can be defined where the total mass m of the body is presumed to be concentrated. The gravitational or inertial force acts at this point, the so-called *center of mass*. (The term *center of gravity* is sometimes used as a synonym for *center of mass*. This is not strictly correct, since the centers of mass and gravity do not coincide if the gravitational force is different on different parts of a body, but such effects can be neglected in orthopedic biomechanics.) It must be pointed out that the center of mass is only a fictitious point; it

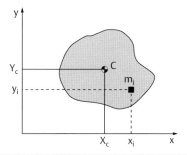

Fig. 11.1 Calculation of the location of the center of mass (C) of a plane plate. The plate is imagined as subdivided into small quadratic elements of masses m_i. The coordinates of the center of mass in an (arbitrarily oriented) coordinate system are obtained by summation (or integration) extended over all mass elements multiplied by their distances from the axes and divided by the total mass of the plate.

does not have to coincide with an actual, material point in the body. The center of mass of an annulus, for example, is located at the center of the circle, a point where no mass is present.

A three-dimensional body can be subdivided into n small volume elements with masses m_i ($i = 1, 2, ...$ n). The gravitational or inertial force acts on each of these volume elements. **Fig. 11.1** illustrates the calculation of the location of the center of mass using the example of a plane plate. For the purposes of calculation the plate is subdivided into n small quadratic elements with masses m_i. The x- and y-coordinates of the center of mass X_c and Y_c are calculated as

(11.1)
$$X_c = \Sigma m_i x_i / m$$
$$Y_c = \Sigma m_i y_i / m$$

where x_i and y_i are the coordinates of the elements with masses m_i; m is the total mass of the plate. Σ is the mathematical summation symbol and implies that the sum is to be extended over all masses m_i from $i = 1$ to $i = n$. Explicitly, the formula for X_c reads

(11.2)
$$X_c = (m_1 x_1 + m_2 x_2 + m_3 x_3 + \cdots m_n x_n) / m$$

If the location of the center of mass of a three-dimensional body is to be calculated, we imagine the body as subdivided into small cubes. X_c and Y_c are then calculated as given above. The z-coordinate Z_c of the center of mass is obtained from

(11.3)
$$Z_c = \Sigma m_i z_i / m$$

It can be shown (the proof is not given here) that the calculated location of the center of mass does not depend on the choice of xyz-coordinate system. Irrespective of the position and orientation of the coordinate system, the same physical location always results.

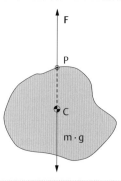

Fig. 11.2 Experimental determination of the location of the center of mass of a plane plate. The plate is suspended by a thread. In static equilibrium the magnitude F of the tensile force of the thread and the magnitude m · g of the gravitational force of the plate are opposite and equal; the center of mass is located below the suspension point P, some-where along the dashed line. Suspending the plate from a second point allows the center of mass to be located.

The segments of the human body have geometrically irregular shapes. In calculating the location of their center of mass, therefore, one may obtain an approximation by substituting simple geometric shapes. For example, the head could be modeled by a sphere or the lower arm by a cylinder, and a uniform density assumed. More refined models adjust the geometric shapes more closely to the body, and take account of density distributions within the segments (see, for example, Hatze[1]).

Fig. 11.2 illustrates an experimental procedure for locating the center of mass of a plane plate. If the plate is suspended by a thread attached to an arbitrary point P on its rim, one knows that in static equilibrium its center of mass is located perpendicularly below point P. (If this were not the case, the plate would oscillate back and forth and a resting position would not be attained.) If the plate is suspended from two different points, the location of the center of mass is given by the intersection of the perpendiculars through the suspension points. The center of mass of a three-dimensional body can be obtained by suspending the body from three noncollinear points (points that are not in a line).

Alternatively, the location of the center of mass can be measured from the support reactions of a two-point support, each support instrumented with a force transducer (**Fig. 11.3**). In equilibrium of moments, force transducer 1 on the right-hand side of the setup measures the force as

(11.4)
$$F_1 = \frac{m \cdot g \cdot (L - L_1)}{L}$$

This equation is obtained by summing all moments in relation to support 2 on the left-hand side. In the formula m designates the mass of the body, g is the gravitational acceleration, L is the distance between

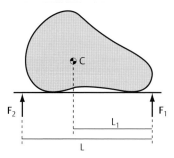

Fig. 11.3 Experimental determination of the location of the center of mass by measuring the support reaction on a two-point support, each support instrumented with a force transducer. If one reaction force, the mass of the object, and the distance between the supports are known, the distance L_1 of the center of mass from the support can be calculated.

the supports, and L_1 is the distance of the center of mass from support 1. By solving the equation for L_1, the distance of the center of mass from support 1 is obtained. To obtain the other two coordinates of the center of mass, the measurement is carried out twice more with the body rotated by 90° each time.

If the mass of a segment of the human body is known, it is possible to determine the location of its center of mass in vivo. **Fig. 11.4** illustrates the procedure for the example of the segment consisting of the lower leg and foot. The body is positioned on a base supported by two force transducers. The mass of the lower leg and foot is designated by m. The magnitude of force $\mathbf{F}_1$ on transducer 1 is measured in the initial state i (knee flexed 90°) and in the final state f (knee extended). Related to the point of application of force $\mathbf{F}_2$, the sums of the moments (all forces designated by their magnitudes) read

(11.5)
$$L_3 \cdot F_3 + L_i \cdot m \cdot g - L \cdot F_{1i} = 0$$
$$L_3 \cdot F_3 + L_f \cdot m \cdot g - L \cdot F_{1f} = 0$$

Subtraction results in

(11.6)
$$(L_f - L_i) \cdot m \cdot g - L \cdot (F_{1f} - F_{1i}) = 0$$

The distance L_c from the center of mass of the lower leg to the knee's axis of rotation is given by

(11.7)
$$L_c = L_f - L_i = L \cdot (F_{1f} - F_{1i}) / m \cdot g$$

If the location of the center of mass is known, the method can also be employed to determine the mass of the segment. To do this, Eq. 11.7 has to be solved for m.

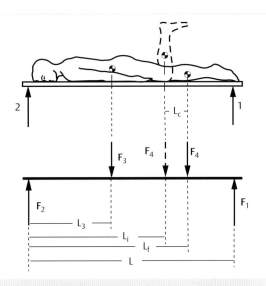

Fig. 11.4 Example of in vivo determination of the location of the center of mass of a body segment. If the mass of the lower leg and foot is known, the location of the center of mass of this body segment can be calculated from the support reactions measured with the knee bent at 90° (initial state i) and with the knee extended (final state f). Alternatively, if the location of the center of mass is known, the mass of the segment can be obtained.

11.1.2 Moment of Inertia

A point mass at distance L from an axis of rotation has the moment of inertia I

(11.8)
$$I = m \cdot L^2$$

The moment of inertia has the dimension [kg · m²]. A three-dimensional body can be imagined as subdivided into small volume elements, each contributing to the total moment of inertia. If the body is subdivided into n cube-shaped elements with masses m_i (**Fig. 11.5**), the moment of inertia is calculated as

(11.9)
$$I = \sum_{i=1}^{i=n} L_i^2 \cdot m_i$$

where L_i designates the distance of the i-th volume element from the axis of rotation. The sum is to be extended over all volume elements. If the mass is continuously distributed within the volume, Eq. 11.9 is written in form of an integral to be extended over the whole volume V:

(11.10)
$$I = \int_V L^2 \, dm$$

It follows from the definition that a moment of inertia is always related to a specific axis of rotation. If the axis is changed, the moment of inertia changes as well. Since the number of axes is unlimited, an

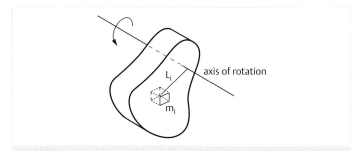

Fig. 11.5 To calculate the moment of inertia, the body is imagined as composed of small volume elements of mass m_i. The moment of inertia is obtained by summation over all masses m_i multiplied by the square of their distance L_i from the axis of rotation.

unlimited number of moments of inertia also exist. If, however, one confines the discussion to axes running through the center of mass, this multiplicity of axes can be reduced to three *principal moments of inertia*. The principal moments are moments in relation to three mutually perpendicular axes running through the center of mass: the principal axes. It can be shown (the proof is not given here) that the moment of inertia about any axis that runs through the center of mass can be calculated if the three principal moments are known. For bodies such as spheres, cylinders, or cuboids, which are symmetrical in relation to certain axes, the principal axes coincide with the axes of symmetry. As an example, **Fig. 11.6** shows the direction of the principal axes and the respective principal moments of inertia, obtained by integration, for a sphere and a cylinder with uniform mass distribution.

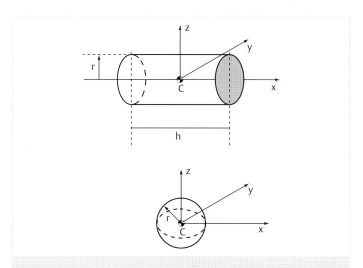

Fig. 11.6 Coordinate systems employed for specifying the moments of inertia of a solid cylinder and solid sphere of uniform density ρ. These simple geometric shapes can be used as models for body segments.

For a cylinder of density ρ, mass m, and moments of inertia I_x, I_y, I_z about the x-, y-, and z-axes, it holds that

(11.11)

$$m = \rho \cdot \pi \cdot r^2 \cdot h$$
$$I_x = \frac{m \cdot r^2}{2}$$
$$I_y = I_z = \frac{m}{12} \cdot (3r^2 + h^2)$$

For a solid sphere of density ρ, mass m, and moments of inertia I_x, I_y, I_z about the x-, y-, and z-axes, it holds that

(11.12)

$$m = \frac{4}{3} \rho \cdot \pi \cdot r^2$$
$$I_x = I_y = I_z = \frac{2}{5} m \cdot r^2$$

Further examples of principal axes and moments for geometrically simple shapes are given in mechanics textbooks and formula collections.

If the moment of inertia of a body in relation to an axis through its center of mass is known, the moment in relation to any other axis parallel to this axis can easily be obtained. The parallel axis theorem states that "the moment of inertia about an arbitrary axis is equal to the moment about a parallel axis running through the center of mass plus the moment of the total mass m, concentrated at the center of mass, about the arbitrary axis" (**Fig. 11.7**).

(11.13)

$$I = I_c + m \cdot L^2$$

where I denotes the moment of inertia about the arbitrary axis, I_c the moment about the parallel axis through the center of mass, m the mass of the body, and L the distance of the axis from the center of mass.

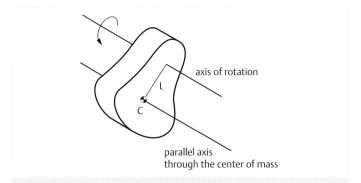

Fig. 11.7 Parallel axis theorem. The moment of inertia about an arbitrary axis is equal to the moment I_c about a parallel axis through the center of mass plus the moment of inertia $m \cdot L^2$, where m is the mass of the body and L the distance of the center of mass from the axis of rotation.

As we have said, the segments of the human body (head, trunk, thigh, lower leg, etc.) are irregularly shaped. To calculate approximate values of their moments of inertia, the true shapes may be replaced by simple geometric shapes of comparable dimensions, for example the head by a sphere or the lower arm by a cylinder. A refined model may substitute an ellipsoid for the head, a hemisphere for the shoulder, or a truncated cone for the thigh. Another requirement for finer modeling is knowledge of the density distribution. Knowledge of the density distribution within human body segments is incomplete, but as an approximation, a uniform density between that of bone and soft tissue may be chosen.

Alternatively, the moment of inertia of a body about a given axis can be obtained experimentally by setting up the body to swing about that axis and observing it. In the setup shown in **Fig. 11.7**, the body oscillates about an axis located at a distance L from the center of mass. The angular frequency of an undamped physical pendulum (see textbooks of physics) is given by

$$(11.14) \qquad \omega = \frac{2\pi}{T} = \sqrt{\frac{m \cdot g \cdot L}{I}} = \sqrt{\frac{m \cdot g \cdot L}{I_c + m \cdot L^2}}$$

where ω is the observed angular frequency, T the oscillation period, m the mass of the body, g the gravitational acceleration, L the distance of the axis from the center of mass, I the moment of inertia about the axis of oscillation, and I_c the moment about a parallel axis through the center of mass. If the mass of the body and the location of its center of mass in relation to the axis of oscillation are known and the oscillation period T is measured, the moments I and I_c can be calculated.

If in the setup shown in **Fig. 11.7** the axis of rotation were to pass through the center of mass (L = zero), the pendulum would not oscillate. If, however, the body is suspended from a torsion spring, for example from a thin elastic wire, which deforms in torsion, any deflection from the idle state will generate a moment. The body will then execute a rotary oscillation with a frequency

$$(11.15) \qquad \omega = \frac{2\pi}{T} = \sqrt{\frac{D}{I_c}}$$

where D denotes the torsion coefficient of the torsion spring and I_c the moment of inertia related to an axis which passes through the center of mass. By using the measured period of oscillation T, the moment of inertia I_c can be calculated. (In this experiment, the torsion coefficient D of the torsion spring is determined beforehand by observation of the oscillation of a body with a known moment of inertia.) Moments of inertia of segments of the human body have been determined in vitro using both the physical pendulum and the torsional pendulum method. In vivo, too, the moments of inertia of an arm or a leg have been measured by observing free oscillations of these body segments about anatomical joint axes (physical pendulum method). However, such experiments require that the muscles crossing the joints should be completely relaxed and that the surrounding soft tissue should not damp the oscillation too much.

Moments of inertia of segments of the human body (head, arms, trunk, etc.) are usually not cited in units of kilograms per square meter [kg · m²]. Instead, the *radius of gyration* i is given in meters [m]. From the radius of gyration i and the mass m_s of the segment, the moment of inertia I can be calculated as

(11.16) $$I = i^2 \cdot m_s$$

Stating the radius of gyration has the advantage that the variations in body segment weight can be accounted for in a simple fashion. This presumes that body segments of persons of differing body mass are geometrically similar. In reality this is only approximately true—think, for example, of the differences in the shape of the thigh in different individuals. Occasionally, the *relative radius of gyration* i_{rel} is stated; this is equal to the radius of gyration divided by the length of the segment. Stating the relative radius of gyration has the advantage that, for every body segment, a single number suffices to quantify the moment of inertia in persons of differing body height.

11.2 Mass, Density, and Dimensions of Body Segments

The mass of the whole body can be determined by weighing. Individual segments cannot be weighed in vivo; prepared specimens must be used. Alternatively, mass can be determined in vivo from the absorption of gamma or X-rays (see, for example, Zatsiorsky and Seluyanov,[2] Wicke et al[3,4]); this requires knowledge of the coefficient of absorption for the type of radiation employed. Another way to obtain the mass of a segment is to measure its volume and multiply the volume by the mean density. The volume of a segment can be obtained by immersing it in a water bath and measuring the amount of fluid displaced, or by three-dimensional, optical surface measurement. The term *mean density* is employed because body segments are made up of tissues with different densities. For a reference value, the mean density of the whole body (body mass divided by body volume) is employed, or else the densities of bone, muscles, and fat are used and assumptions made about the percentages of the segment volume made up of these three tissue types.

Table 11.1 lists reference values for the mean density of the whole body and of the three main tissue types. The mean density of the body as a whole varies according to the relative proportion of bone, muscle, and fat that is present. For bone, the *apparent density* is stated (mass divided by volume including all voids). Trabecular bone filled with body fluid or bone marrow has a density close to 1.0 g/cm³.

The numbers in **Table 11.2** give an impression of the variations in mean density between the different segments of the body. The density of segments with a large proportion of bone, such as the lower arm, is higher than the mean density of the whole body. The reverse is true for segments with a low proportion of bone or a larger proportion of fat, such as the trunk.

Table 11.3 presents results for the masses of the segments of the human body as a percentage of whole body mass, as determined by various authors. Variations in the data are due to differences in the cohorts

Tissue	Density [g/cm³]
Whole body	Approx. 1.04–1.10
Trabecular or cortical bone, depending on porosity	0.1 to > 1.5
Muscle	Approx. 1.05
Fat	Approx. 0.95

Table 11.1 Reference values for mean density of the tissues of the human body

Segment	Density [g/cm³]
Head, neck, trunk	1.03
Upper arm	1.04
Lower arm	1.09
Hand	1.12
Thigh	1.04
Lower leg	1.04
Foot	1.08

Table 11.2 Mean density of the segments of the male human body, measured from specimens

Source: Data from Webb Associates.[5]

Segment	Mass [% body mass]			
	Dempster[6] (adults)	Zatsiorsky and Seluyanov[2] (adults)	Clauser et al,[7] cited in Nigg[8] (adults)	Jensen[9] (adolescents[a])
Head	7.9	6.9	7.3	10.1
Trunk	48.6	43.5	50.7	41.7
Upper arm	2.7	2.7	2.6	3.2
Lower arm	1.6	1.6	1.6	1.7
Hand	0.6	0.6	0.7	0.9
Thigh	9.7	14.2	10.3	11.0
Lower leg	4.5	4.3	4.0	5.3
Foot	1.4	1.4	1.5	2.1

Table 11.3 Mass of the segments of the human body as a percentage of body mass in adults and adolescents

[a] Age 12 years.

investigated and in the experimental procedures employed. (Probably due to rounding errors, the numbers reported by Dempster[6] and Clauser et al[7] do not add up exactly to 100%.)

Table 11.4 lists reference values for the volume of the segments of the body, determined by the immersion method. The average volume of the whole body is around 70 L. In the individual case, a good estimate of body volume is obtained by dividing body mass by mean whole body density (**Table 11.1**).

The lengths of the segments were determined by Drillis and Contini.[10] **Table 11.5** contains the measured relative heights of distinctive landmarks or joints above the floor in persons standing upright with

Segment	Volume [% of body volume]
Head and neck	7.2
Trunk	47.2
Upper arm	3.4
Lower arm	1.6
Hand	0.6
Thigh	11.5
Lower leg	4.5
Foot	1.4

Table 11.4 Volume of the segments of the human body as a percentage of body volume, determined in vivo

Source: Data from Webb Associates.[5]

Landmark or joint	Relative height[a]
Vertex	1.0
Chin	0.870
Shoulder	0.818
Elbow joint	0.630
Wrist	0.485
Fingertips	0.377
Hip joint	0.530
Knee joint	0.285
Ankle joint	0.039

Table 11.5 Height of distinctive landmarks or joints, measured in upright stance with arms hanging vertically downwards

Source: Data from Drillis and Contini,[10] cited by Winter.[11]

[a] Height of landmark or joint divided by body height.

Body segment	Relative width/length[a]
Shoulder	0.259
Pelvis	0.191
Foot (width)	0.055
Foot (length)	0.152

Table 11.6 Width of shoulders and pelvis, and width and length of the foot

Source: Data from Drillis and Contini,[10] cited by Winter.[11]

[a] Width or length divided by body height.

arms hanging vertically downwards. The lengths of individual segments were determined from these data by subtraction. For some segments, the width (measured horizontally) is also reported (**Table 11.6**). Additional reference values for dimensions of the human body will be found in textbooks of ergonomics.

11.3 Center of Mass of Body Segments

Table 11.7 lists results of various studies reporting the location of the center of mass of body segments of adult subjects. If one restricts the analysis of postures or motions in the sagittal plane, knowledge of one coordinate suffices. The numbers quoted in **Table 11.7** are the distance of the segment's center of mass from the proximal joint; in the case of head and trunk the distance quoted is from the vertex, and in the case of the three subsections of the trunk[2] the distances quoted are measured from the C7 vertebra, the lower margin of the ribcage (labeled *xyphion* by Zatsiorsky and Seluyanov[2]), and the upper rim of the iliac bones (labeled *omphalion* by Zatsiorsky and Seluyanov[2]), given as a percentage of the segment length. De Leva[12] published corrections to the data of Zatsiorsky and Seluyanov,[2] which resulted from different choices for the landmarks when determining segment length.

The differences between the various studies are the result of differences in the cohorts investigated and in the measurement methods (variations in the definitions of segment boundaries; in vitro measurements of specimens vs. in vivo measurements using irradiation or optical surface measurement). The location of body segment centers of mass in young persons differ only slightly from those cited in **Table 11.7**.[9,13] What the values in these tables show is the usefulness of simple geometrical modeling of the human body. If all body segments were described as cylinders of spherical or elliptical cross section, their centers of mass would be in the middle of those cylinders—that is, at 50% of their length. The numbers in **Table 11.7** are

Segment	Distance from proximal joint [% segment length]		
	Dempster[6]	**Clauser et al,[7] cited in Nigg[8]**	**Zatsiorsky and Seluyanov[2]**
Head and trunk[a]	60.4	–	–
Trunk, T1–T12	62.7	–	–
Trunk, L1–hip joint	59.9	–	–
Trunk, upper part[b]	–	–	50.7
Trunk, middle part[c]	–	–	45.0
Trunk, lower part[d]	–	–	35.4
Upper arm	43.6	51.3	55.0
Lower arm	43.0	39.0	57.3
Hand	50.6	–	63.1
Thigh	43.3	37.2	45.5
Lower leg	43.3	37.1	40.5
Foot	42.9	44.9	55.8

Table 11.7 Location of the center of mass of body segments, measured as a percentage of segment length

[a] Measured from the vertex.

[b] Measured from the C7 vertebra to the lower margin of the rib cage.

[c] Measured from the lower margin of the rib cage to the upper rim of the iliac bones.

[d] Measured from the upper rim of the iliac bones to the upper rim of the thighs.

indeed not far from 50%, thus showing that modeling body segments with simple geometric shapes produces a good approximation.

11.4 Moment of Inertia of Body Segments

Table 11.8 lists the radius of gyration of the body segments about axes that are perpendicular to the sagittal plane and run through the segment's center of mass. These moments of inertia are of particular importance in orthopedic biomechanics, because walking or running are often modeled in a simplified fashion as plane motion in the sagittal plane. (In the analysis of athletic exercises, such an assumption would not be permissible.) The table quotes the radius of gyration in relative units, related to segment length. This allows the radius of gyration to be converted for individual body height. Differences between studies are due to differences in the cohorts investigated and the measurement methods employed.

The numerical data reported by Winter[11] derive from measurements carried out by Dempster[6] on specimens from eight adults, employing the pendulum method. To achieve this, the segment masses (given by Dempster) were used to convert the moments, given by Dempster in units of $g \cdot cm^2$, into radii of gyration.[6] The known body heights[6] and relative segment lengths[10] (see **Table 11.5**) were then used to calculate the relative radii of gyration. Zatsiorsky and Seluyanov[2] determined distributions of mass in adults in vivo using an irradiation method, and from these they derived the radii of gyration. The radii of gyration of young persons are very similar to those of adults.[9,13]

As an example of how to use the tables, here is the calculation for the moment of inertia of the lower leg of an adult of height 1.70 m, body weight 60 kg. According to **Table 11.3** (data from Clauser et al[7]) the lower leg has a mass of 4% of body weight, equal in this case to 2.4 kg. For the lower leg, **Table 11.5** yields a relative segment length of $0.285 - 0.039 = 0.246$. For a body height of 1.70 m, it follows that the lower leg has a length of $0.246 \cdot 1.70 = 0.418$ m. With a relative radius of gyration of 3.02 (**Table 11.8**, data from Winter[11]), the moment of inertia about its center of mass is calculated as $(0.302 \cdot 0.418)^2 \cdot 2.4 = 0.0382 \ [kg \cdot m^2]$.

Segment	Relative radius of gyration [m/m]	
	Winter,[11] as derived from Dempster[6]	**Zatsiorsky and Seluyanov[2]**
Head, trunk, and arms	0.503	—
Trunk	0.496	—
Upper arm	0.322	0.310
Lower arm	0.303	0.284
Hand	0.297	0.230
Thigh	0.323	0.267
Lower leg	0.302	0.275
Foot	0.475	0.245

Table 11.8 Relative radii of gyration of the body segments about axes perpendicular to the sagittal plane and running through the segment's center of mass

References

1. Hatze H. A mathematical model for the computational determination of parameter values of anthropomorphic segments. J Biomech 1980;13(10):833–843

2. Zatsiorsky V, Seluyanov V. The mass and inertia characteristics of the main segments of the human body. In: Matsui H, Kobayashi K, eds. Biomechanics VIII-B. Champaign, IL: Human Kinetics; 1986:1152–1159

3. Wicke J, Dumas GA, Costigan PA. Trunk density profile estimates from dual X-ray absorptiometry. J Biomech 2008;41(4):861–867

4. Wicke J, Dumas GA, Costigan PA. A comparison between a new model and current models for estimating trunk segment inertial parameters. J Biomech 2009;42(1):55–60

5. Webb Associates. Anthropometric Source Book. Vol 1: Anthropometry for Designers. Washington, DC: National Aeronautics and Space Administration, Scientific and Technical Information Office; 1978. NASA Reference Publication 1024

6. Dempster WT. Space Requirements of the Seated Operator. Geometrical, Kinematic and Mechanical Aspects of the Body with Special Reference to the Limbs. Wright-Patterson Air Force Base, Ohio: Wright Air Development Center; 1955. WADC Technical Report 55-159

7. Clauser CE, McConville JV, Young JW. Weight, volume and center of mass of segments of the human body. AMRL Technical Report TR 69–70. Wright-Patterson Air Force Base, Ohio, 1969

8. Nigg BM. Inertial properties of the human or animal body. In: Nigg BM, Herzog W, eds. Biomechanics of the Musculo-Skeletal System. Chichester: Wiley; 1994:337–364

9. Jensen RK. Body segment mass, radius and radius of gyration proportions of children. J Biomech 1986;19(5):359–368

10. Drillis R, Contini R. Body Segment Parameters. New York: Office of Vocational Rehabilitation, Department of Health, Education and Welfare. 1966. Report 1163-03

11. Winter DA. Biomechanics and Motor Control of Human Movement. 3rd ed. Hoboken, NJ: Wiley; 2005

12. de Leva P. Adjustments to Zatsiorsky-Seluyanov's segment inertia parameters. J Biomech 1996;29(9):1223–1230

13. Jensen RK. Changes in segment inertia proportions between 4 and 20 years. J Biomech 1989;22(6-7):529–536

12 Determination of Joint Load in a Model Calculation

Joint load is the name given to the force acting between the articulating bones. A knowledge of this force is of great practical importance to understanding the etiology of disorders, planning rehabilitation measures appropriately, and developing joint prostheses. In a few cases, joint loads have been measured directly by means of instrumented joint prostheses. In the majority of cases, however, one has to rely on biomechanical model calculations to gain an impression of the magnitude of a joint load. The use of the term *model* points to the fact that these calculations always require assumptions and simplifications to be made, the validity and justification of which will always be a matter of debate. This chapter outlines how to calculate joint loads and illustrates the method by simple examples. To limit the calculations required, only the two-dimensional case (that is, posture or motion in a plane) will be considered. The two-dimensional case is often a valid approximation, for example when calculating the load on the lumbar spine during forward bending of the trunk. Forward bending combined with axial torsion, however, cannot be treated as a two-dimensional case. Such cases require a three-dimensional approach which takes account of the three-dimensional architecture of bones, muscles, and tendons.

12.1 Mechanical Equilibrium

Static model calculations are based on a state of *static mechanical equilibrium*. The conditions of static mechanical equilibrium read: "a body is in static equilibrium if it experiences no accelerated linear motion (translation) and no accelerated rotation." In static equilibrium the sum of all external forces and the sum of all external moments is equal to zero.

(12.1)
$$\sum \mathbf{F}_i = 0$$
$$\sum \mathbf{M}_i = 0$$

The symbol Σ in these equations is the mathematical sum sign. The vector sums are to be extended over all forces $\mathbf{F}_1$, $\mathbf{F}_2$, $\mathbf{F}_3$, ... and all moments $\mathbf{M}_1$, $\mathbf{M}_2$, $\mathbf{M}_3$, ... acting on the body. If in the two-dimensional case a moment is defined as "the product of the magnitude of the distance from the center of rotation times the magnitude of the force," the equilibrium condition for moments can be formulated as

(12.2)
$$\sum \mathbf{M}_i = \pm L_1 F_1 \pm L_2 F_2 \pm L_3 F_3 \cdots = 0$$

The designations "±" in this formula indicate that the signs of the moments have to be chosen in accordance with the sign rule for moments, that is, in dependence on the direction of rotation (clockwise or counterclockwise).

The validity of these equations can be seen immediately. If the sum of all forces were not equal to zero, a resultant force (unequal to zero) would act on the body. The body would then be linearly accelerated and, in contrast to the assumption, not be in static equilibrium. The analogous argument holds for the sum of the moments. If the sum of all moments were not equal to zero, a resultant moment (unequal to zero) would act on the body. The body would then undergo an accelerated rotation and would thus not be in static equilibrium. It follows that if a body is seen to perform no accelerated translation or rotation (in the simplest case: if the body is at rest), the sum of all forces and the sum of all moments must be zero. Additionally, in the dynamic case, when accelerated translations and/or rotations occur, the conditions of mechanical equilibrium remain valid if the sum of the forces (Eq. 12.1) is extended over the inertial force $m \cdot (-\mathbf{a})$ and the sum of the moments (Eq. 12.2) over the moment of inertia $I \cdot (-\alpha)$.

Fig. 12.1 illustrates a state of mechanical equilibrium. The force from the hand onto the tray is opposite and equal to the weight of the drink and the burger (the tray is neglected); that is, the sum of the forces is equal to zero. The support provided by the hand is placed in such a way that the moment of the weight of the drink (in the case shown here, the drink is heavier than the burger) is opposite and equal to the moment of the weight of the burger. The sum of the moments equals zero as well.

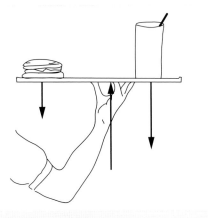

Fig. 12.1 Balancing a meal tray in mechanical equilibrium. (Adapted from Roberts and Falkenburg.[1])

In a state of mechanical equilibrium, two unknowns can be determined by using Eq. 12.1. **Fig. 12.2** illustrates the calculation of an unknown moment with the example of a beam allowed to rotate about a center of rotation. Vectors $\mathbf{F}_1$ and $\mathbf{F}_2$ represent the forces exerted on the beam; F_1 and F_2 are their magnitudes. The xy-coordinate system is oriented so that both forces point in the y-direction. L_1 and L_2 are the perpendicular distances of the points of force application from the center of rotation, the "moment arms." Initially F_1 is known; F_2 is unknown. In static equilibrium (that is, if no accelerated rotation is observed), the sum of all moments must be equal to zero. It then holds (keeping the sign convention for moments in mind) that

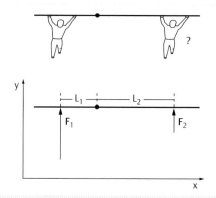

Fig. 12.2 Example of the calculation of an unknown moment $L_2 \cdot F_2$ in a state of mechanical equilibrium.

(12.3)
$$L_1 \cdot F_1 - L_2 \cdot F_2 = 0$$
$$L_2 \cdot F_2 = L_1 \cdot F_1$$

Thus the unknown moment $L_2 \cdot F_2$ is obtained.

Fig. 12.3 illustrates the calculation of an unknown force in a condition of static mechanical equilibrium. Three forces act on a body. F_1 and F_2 are known; the direction and magnitude of F_3 are unknown. In equilibrium the vector sum of all forces must be equal to zero:

(12.4)
$$F_1 + F_2 + F_3 = 0$$

To fulfill this equation, F_3 must be oppositely directed and equal in magnitude to the sum of F_1 and F_2. In the graphical representation, vectors F_1, F_2, and F_3 form a closed triangle. Thus the magnitude and direction of F_3 are unequivocally determined.

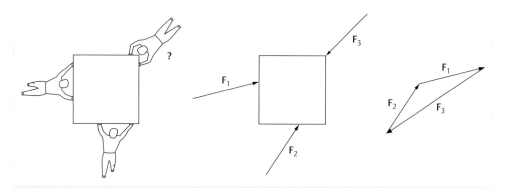

Fig. 12.3 Example of the calculation of an unknown force F_3 in a state of mechanical equilibrium.

12.2 Example: Calculation of the Joint Load of a Beam Balance in Static Equilibrium

To illustrate the principle of calculating joint loads in the human body by using the conditions of equilibrium, the joint load of a simple mechanical instrument, a beam balance, can be calculated (**Fig. 12.4**). For reasons of clarity, the pointer of the beam balance (though essential to the mechanical functioning of the balance) is not shown in the illustration. In the state of static equilibrium the unknown force **F**, which equilibrates a gravitational force of 10 N, and the joint load **G**, which supports the beam at the center of rotation, are to be calculated (**Fig. 12.4a**). In a first step (**Fig. 12.4b**) the magnitude of the force **F** is determined using the condition of equilibrium of moments:

(12.5)
$$2 \cdot 10 - 1 \cdot F = 0 \text{ Ncm}$$
$$F = 20 \text{ N}$$

In a second step (**Fig. 12.4c**) G is calculated from the equilibrium of forces:

(12.6)
$$G - 20 - 10 = 0 \text{ N}$$
$$G = +30 \text{ N}$$

The joint load **G** points in the positive y-direction.

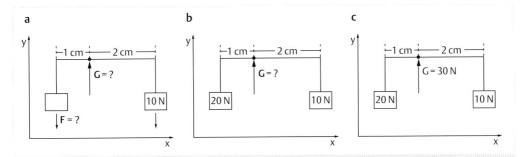

Fig. 12.4a–c Calculation of the joint load **G** of a beam balance loaded on one side by a known weight and on the other side by an initially unknown weight **F**.

a Initial condition with both **F** and **G** unknown.

b Step 1: employing the condition of equilibrium of moments, the magnitude of the weight **F** is calculated as 20 N.

c Step 2: employing the condition of equilibrium of forces, the magnitude of the joint force **G** is calculated as 30 N.

If force **F**, which maintains the equilibrium at the beam, is not directed in the y-direction (**Fig. 12.5**), **F** is decomposed into forces F_x and F_y, and the x- and y-components of force **G** are determined separately. In a second step, the magnitude and direction of **G** are determined from its components G_x and G_y. In the setup shown in **Fig. 12.5** it is assumed that the angle between the line of action of **F** and the beam amounts to 45°. In equilibrium of moments, F_y and G_y equal those calculated already for the setup shown in **Fig. 12.4**.

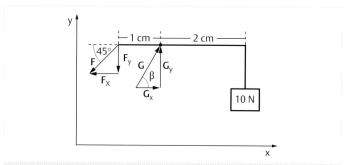

Fig. 12.5 Calculation of the joint load **G** of a beam balance with the forces acting on both sides but in different directions.

(12.7)
$$F_y = -20 \text{ N}$$
$$G_y = +30 \text{ N}$$

The x-component of force **F** effects a moment equal to zero because its line of action passes through the center of rotation of the beam.

Given the angle of force **F** to the x-axis and with knowledge of F_y, vector F_x is determined. To do this, the missing side of the triangle formed by **F**, F_x, and F_y has to be constructed. If the angle (as assumed here) equals 45°, it holds that

(12.8)
$$F_x = F_y / \tan(45°)$$
$$F_x = -20 \text{ N}$$

The magnitude of the force **F** is determined from

(12.9)
$$|\mathbf{F}| = \sqrt{F_x^2 + F_y^2} = \sqrt{20^2 + 20^2} = 28.3 \text{ N}$$

In the state of static equilibrium the sum of the x-components of all forces must be equal to zero. The weight on the right side does not contribute to the sum, because the gravitational force points in the y-direction. With $F_x = -20$ N it follows that

(12.10)
$$F_x + G_x = 0 \text{ N}$$
$$G_x = 20 \text{ N}$$

The vector of the joint load **G** is determined from its components G_x and G_y. Its magnitude is calculated from

(12.11)
$$|\mathbf{G}| = \sqrt{G_x^2 + G_y^2} = \sqrt{30^2 + 20^2} = 36.1 \text{ N}$$

The angle β between the vector of the joint load and the x-axis is determined from

(12.12)
$$\beta = \text{atan}(G_y / G_x)$$

In the case discussed here the angle β is equal to 56.3°.

12.3 Calculation of a Joint Load in the Static Case (Example: The Elbow Joint)

The forearm is held at an angle of 90° with respect to the upper arm (**Fig. 12.6**). The mass of 10 kg held in the hand exerts a gravitational force of 98.1 N on the hand; this value is rounded up to 100 N in the calculation below. For the time being the weight of the forearm is neglected. To maintain equilibrium the biceps muscle is activated. In relation to the xy-coordinate system shown, both external load and muscle force are parallel to the y-direction; the gravitational force **W** and the muscle force **B** have only y-components. The moment arms of the external force and the muscle force are assumed to be 20 cm and 2 cm, respectively (approximately correct, rounded values).

When writing down the equilibrium condition for the moments, attention must be paid to using the correct signs. Then

(12.13) $$-B \cdot 2 + 100 \cdot 20 = 0 \text{ Ncm}$$

This equation yields for the required force of the biceps muscle

(12.14) $$B = 1000 \text{ N}$$

In the state of equilibrium, the (vector) sum of forces must equal zero:

(12.15) $$\mathbf{G} + \mathbf{B} + \mathbf{W} = \mathbf{0}$$

Here the y-component of the weight **W** has a negative sign because the gravitational force points in the negative y-direction. The force of the biceps points in the positive y-direction and has a positive sign.

(12.16) $$G + 1000 - 100 = 0 \text{ N}$$
$$G = -900 \text{ N}$$

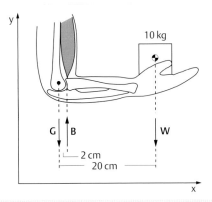

Fig. 12.6 Calculation of the load **G** on the elbow joint exerted by a mass held in the hand. Only the biceps is activated. The weight of the hand and lower arm is neglected.

The joint load **G** has a magnitude of 900 N. The negative sign shows that force **G** points in the negative y-direction. In other words, the humerus is pressed against the ulna with a force of 900 N. It can be seen that the largest contribution to the joint load (1000 N) comes from the muscle force of the biceps.

In the example shown in **Fig. 12.6** equilibrium is established solely by activation of the biceps muscle; antagonistic muscle activation is not taken into account. This is certainly a simplification because experience shows that agonistic and antagonistic muscles are usually activated simultaneously to maintain postures or perform activities. However, consideration of the force **T** of the triceps in addition to the force **B** of the biceps (**Fig. 12.7**) immediately gives rise to the problem that the two equilibrium conditions are insufficient for unambiguous calculation of two unknown muscle forces (biceps and triceps) and the unknown joint load. To obtain an unequivocal solution an additional assumption has to be made. To explore the extent to which the joint load changes if an antagonist is activated, we assume (arbitrarily) that the force developed by the triceps is small and amounts to 25% of the force of the biceps.

To keep the calculation simple, it is further assumed that the force of the triceps is, like the force of the biceps, directed in the positive y-direction. With a moment arm of the triceps of 2 cm (approximate value) and with reference to the sign convention for moments we obtain in equilibrium of moments

(12.17)
$$-B \cdot 2 + 100 \cdot 20 + T \cdot 2 = 0 \text{ Ncm}$$
$$-B \cdot 2 + 100 \cdot 20 + 0.25B \cdot 2 = 0 \text{ Ncm}$$

From these two equations we obtain B and T:

(12.18)
$$B = 1333.3 \text{ N}$$
$$T = 0.25B = 333.3 \text{ N}$$

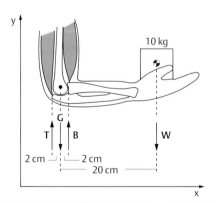

Fig. 12.7 Calculation of the load **G** on the elbow joint by a mass held in the hand. Both biceps and triceps are activated. The weight of the hand and lower arm is neglected.

In equilibrium of forces

(12.19) $$G + B + T + W = 0$$

we obtain for their y-components (digits after the decimal point omitted)

(12.20)
$$G + 1333 + 333 - 100 = 0 \text{ N}$$
$$G = -1566 \text{ N}$$

The joint load now amounts to 1566 N. Again, the negative sign indicates that the humerus is pressed against the ulna. The participation of the antagonist increases the joint load by a considerable amount. The force developed by the antagonist is assumed to be 25% of the force of the agonist; the joint load, however, has increased by 74% (from 900 N to 1566 N). Antagonistic muscle activation may be helpful in stabilizing postures by making them insensitive to small perturbations. If, however, a muscle is forced to carry out a movement against strong resistance from the antagonist, very high joint loading may be expected to result. This could, for example, be seen in spastic patients with overactivation of certain muscles, or in persons with Parkinson disease.

In general, the procedure for determining joint loads in a state of static equilibrium can be summarized as follows (**Fig. 12.8**): magnitudes, directions, and points of application of all forces are marked, in so far as they are known from the outset, on the "free" body (that is, the body imagined as separated from its environment). This diagram is termed the *free body diagram*. In the case discussed above, the initial knowledge comprises the magnitude, direction, and point of application of the external load F_1 and (to complete the description) the gravitational force of forearm and hand F_2. These forces are applied at the centers of mass of the external load and of the forearm, respectively. Regarding the muscle force F_3, only its point of application and its direction are known from anatomical observations. As far as the joint load F_4 is concerned, only its point of application is known: due to the fact that there is only negligible friction between the articulating surfaces, this force is directed through the center of rotation. (The supporting argument for this is that a frictionless joint cannot transmit any moment. If the joint load were not directed through the

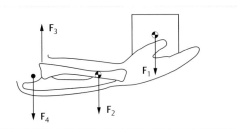

Fig. 12.8 Free body diagram of the lower arm for calculation of the elbow joint load.

center of rotation, a moment, and hence an accelerated rotational movement, would result. Static equilibrium would not exist, in contradiction of the assumption.)

In the first step, the moment of the muscle force and (with a known moment arm of the muscle) the magnitude of the muscle force F_3 are determined from the equilibrium condition of moments. In the second step, the magnitude and direction of the joint load F_4 are determined from the equilibrium condition of forces. The prerequisites for performing this model calculation are: (1) assuming only one muscle to be active, specifically excluding multiple or antagonistic muscle activation, (2) assuming a punctiform application of muscle and tendon forces at the bones (instead of an anatomically correct area of force application), and (3) ignoring the elastic tension of other muscles, joint capsules, or ligaments spanning the joint.

With respect to muscle forces and joint loads, the results obtained at the elbow joint are typical of many joints of the locomotor system:

- The muscle force needed to guarantee equilibrium is, in general, much larger than the external forces acting on the body. This is due to the ratio of the moment arm of the external force compared to the moment arm of the muscles. For the long bones of the extremities it holds as a rule that moment arms of external forces are comparable to the length of the bones while moment arms of the muscles are comparable to the diameter of the bones.
- The magnitude of the joint load is determined essentially by the muscle force; the external force makes only a small additional contribution.
- The absolute minimum of the joint load occurs when only the agonist muscle is activated. Additional activation of antagonistic muscles increases the joint load disproportionately.

The underlying reason for the high muscle forces and joint loads is in the architecture and anatomical function of the muscles (**Fig. 12.9**). Muscles can produce large tensile forces while the change of muscle

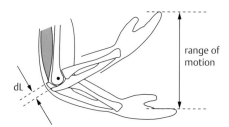

Fig. 12.9 The ability of muscles to increase or decrease their length is limited. For this reason, the line of action of the muscle forces usually lies close to the joint axis. Consequently, the moment arm of the muscle force is small.

length is limited to relatively small values. If the range of motion of a joint is large, the muscle must, for geometrical reasons, be positioned close to the joint. Its length change dL will then be small. In many cases the moment arms of external forces (or of the body weight) are much larger than the moment arms of the muscles. The ratio of the moment arms of muscles to those of the external forces requires a large muscle force to guarantee equilibrium. The large muscle forces cause large joint loads.

12.4 Calculation of the Joint Load in the Dynamic Case (Example: The Ankle Joint)

In the dynamic case, when accelerated linear and rotational movements occur, inertial forces and inertial moments have to be taken into account. For the purpose of calculation, the human body is imagined to be divided into segments at the joints. In detail, the following assumptions are made[2]:

- The mass m of each segment remains constant during the course of the movement.
- The segments are modeled as rigid bodies. Thus, during the course of the movement the location of the center of mass does not change with respect to the anatomical structures (that is, the bones) or to the landmarks located at the surface of a segment.
- The moment of inertia I remains constant throughout the course of the movement.
- The joints are frictionless hinge or ball-and-socket joints.
- The linear movement (translational motion) of a segment is represented by the motion of its center of mass.
- The rotational movement (rotational motion) of a segment is represented by the rotation about its center of mass.

For a movement of a segment of mass m and moment of inertia I in the xy-plane (x-axis pointing horizontally and y-axis pointing vertically upwards) it holds that

$$\sum_{1}^{n} R_{ix} = m \cdot a_x$$

(12.21)
$$\sum_{1}^{n} R_{iy} + S = m \cdot a_y$$

$$\sum_{1}^{n} M_i = I \cdot \alpha$$

The first two equations are known as the scalar equations of plane motion. $\mathbf{R}_i$ and M_i are the reaction forces and reaction moments, which are transmitted from the neighboring segments onto the segment under consideration. The moments are regarded as representing pure moments—that is, moments effected by a force couple. The moments are taken about the center of mass. The lines of action of the forces $\mathbf{R}_i$ pass through the centers of rotation of the joints. The sums are to be extended over all acting moments and forces from i = 1 to i = n. The variables a_x and a_y designate the components of the linear acceleration of the center of mass; α is the angular acceleration about an axis running through the center of mass with normal (perpendicular) orientation to the xy-plane. In the equations the effects of inertia (inertial force and moment of inertia) are explicitly specified on the right-hand side. For this reason, the quantities $m \cdot a_x$ and $I \cdot \alpha$ bear positive signs. The gravitational force points in the negative y-direction. $S = -m \cdot g$ is the y-coordinate of the gravitational force. The reaction forces $\mathbf{R}_i$ transmitted from the neighboring segments are not identical to the joint loads but rather represent the net (the vector sum) force transmitted from one segment to the next. It is shown below that, to calculate joint (bone on bone) loads, a model of the joint has to be established. Such models are derived from anatomical observations and specify the directions, points of application, and moment arms of the relevant muscles and tendons.

Fig. 12.10 illustrates the approach using the example of the lower leg. The leg is imagined to be divided into the three segments—foot, lower leg, and upper leg—linked by hinge joints. The reaction force $\mathbf{R}_2$ with components R_{2x} and R_{2y} and the reaction moment M_2 act on the distal end of the lower leg. The reaction force $\mathbf{R}_3$ with components R_{3x} and R_{3y} and the moment M_3 act on the proximal end of the lower leg. The lower leg has the mass m and (related to the center of mass) the moment of inertia I. The gravitational force acting on the segment amounts to $S = -m \cdot g$. Under these forces and moments the motion of the lower leg occurs in accordance with the above-stated equations of motion. The variables a_x and a_y designate the components of the linear acceleration of the center of mass; α is the angular acceleration around the center of mass.

Calculation of the forces and moments transmitted from one segment to the next is elaborated below with the example of the ankle joint (**Figs. 12.11, 12.12, 12.13, 12.14**). The designations are: m = mass of the foot, I = moment of inertia of the foot related to its center of mass, $m \cdot g$ = gravitational force acting on the foot, a_x and a_y = linear acceleration of the center of mass of the foot, α = angular acceleration of the foot around its center of mass, $\mathbf{R}_{1x}$ and $\mathbf{R}_{1y}$ = components of the reaction force acting distally (on the tip) on the foot, $\mathbf{R}_{2x}$ and $\mathbf{R}_{2y}$ = components of the reaction force acting proximally on the foot segment, M_1 = reaction moment acting distally (this moment is, however, equal to zero because as long as the foot is not glued to the floor, no moment can be transmitted), M_2 = reaction moment acting proximally, L_1 and L_2 = position of the center of rotation of the ankle joint relative to the center of mass, and L_3 and L_4 = point of application of the reaction force acting from the floor on the foot in relation to the center of mass.

To provide clear insight into the calculation and relate it to the calculation of the joint load of the elbow joint described above, reaction forces and moments are determined below for three cases:

- Static case: No force between foot and floor. With reference to this case, the relation between joint loads and reaction forces and moments is discussed.
- Dynamic case: Accelerated motion of the foot, but no force between foot and floor.
- Dynamic case: Accelerated motion of the foot, taking account of a force acting from the floor on the foot.

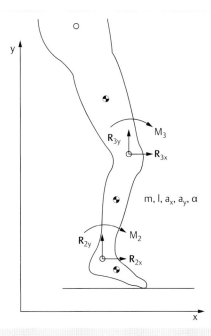

Fig. 12.10 The two-dimensional case. Reaction forces R_2 and R_3 and reaction moments M_2 and M_3 act distally and proximally on the lower leg segment. The linear acceleration a of the center of mass and the angular acceleration α around the center of mass are effected by these forces and moments. The segmented circle designates the center of mass of the segment. The open circles represent the centers of rotation. The segment has the mass m and the moment of inertia I related to an axis through the center of mass and running perpendicular to the plane of motion. In this figure and also in **Figs. 12.11, 12.12, 12.13, 12.14**, the arrows designating the reaction forces R_i and the reaction moments M_i are purely symbolic. They indicate that forces and moments are acting, but convey nothing about their magnitude or sense of direction. Magnitudes and directions are obtained as a result of the calculation.

12.4.1 Case 1: Foot Held Freely, No Motion (**Fig. 12.11**)

The force and the moment acting from the floor on the foot and the linear and angular accelerations are equal to zero. The gravitational force acts on the foot. With a_x, a_y, R_{1x}, R_{1y}, M_1, and α equal to zero we obtain by insertion into the equations of motion for the forces

$$R_{2x} = 0$$
$$R_{2y} - m \cdot g = 0$$
$$R_{2y} = m \cdot g$$

(12.22)

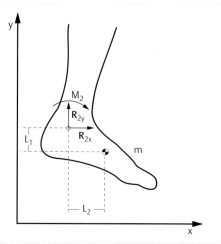

Fig. 12.11 Freely held, motionless foot. Reaction force **R**$_2$ and reaction moment M$_2$ transmitted from the lower leg onto the foot. See also legend to **Fig. 12.10**.

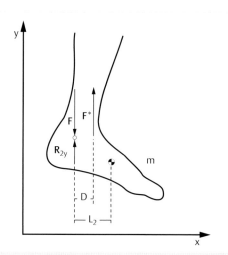

Fig. 12.12 Freely held, motionless foot. Biomechanical model designed to determine the load on the ankle joint. See also legend to **Fig. 12.10**.

and for the moments (moments taken about the center of mass of the foot, signs according to the sign convention for moments), with $R_{2y} = m \cdot g$ as determined above

(12.23)
$$M_2 + L_2 \cdot R_{2y} = 0$$
$$M_2 = -m \cdot g \cdot L_2$$

Determination of Joint Load in a Model Calculation

If it is intended merely to calculate the reaction force $\mathbf{R}_2$ and the reaction moment M_2 from the lower leg on the foot, the problem is thus solved. For reasons of equilibrium, the force and the moment acting from the foot on the lower leg are opposite but equal to $\mathbf{R}_2$ and M_2; that is, the force and moment transmitted from the foot to the lower leg equal $-\mathbf{R}_2$ and $-M_2$.

To provide the link between the reaction force and moment between the foot and lower leg and the load on the ankle joint, we start from $\mathbf{R}_2$ and M_2 and determine the force between tibia and talus. To reach a solution it is necessary to specify which muscle actually provides the moment M_2. An obvious candidate is the tibialis anterior whose tendon effects the dorsiflexion of the foot. We assume that this tendon pulls in the y-direction and at a distance D from the center of rotation (**Fig. 12.12**). The moment $M_2 = -m \cdot g \cdot L_2$, which acts proximally on the foot, is imagined to be generated by a force couple $\mathbf{F}$ and $\mathbf{F}^*$. The force $\mathbf{F}$ is exerted at the center of rotation of the tibiotalar joint. $\mathbf{F}^*$ is the tensile force of the tendon of the tibialis anterior. $\mathbf{F}^*$ points in the positive, and $\mathbf{F}$ in the negative y-direction. $\mathbf{F}$ and $\mathbf{F}^*$ are of equal magnitude.

Expressed by the force couple we write for the moment M_2 (all moments in relation to the center of mass of the foot)

(12.24) $$M_2 = -L_2 \cdot |\mathbf{F}| + (L_2 - D) \cdot |\mathbf{F}^*|$$

According to the sign convention for moments, the moment of $\mathbf{F}$ bears a negative, and the moment of $\mathbf{F}^*$ a positive sign. With

(12.25) $$M_2 = -m \cdot g \cdot L_2$$

we obtain

(12.26) $$-m \cdot g \cdot L_2 = -L_2 \cdot |\mathbf{F}| + (L_2 - D) \cdot |\mathbf{F}^*|$$

With $|\mathbf{F}| = |\mathbf{F}^*|$ it follows that

(12.27) $$|\mathbf{F}| = |\mathbf{F}^*| = m \cdot g \cdot L_2 / D$$

The forces $\mathbf{R}_2$ and $\mathbf{F}$ act between tibia and talus. The load on the ankle joint $\mathbf{G}$ is the sum of the forces $\mathbf{F}$ and $\mathbf{R}_{2y}$. The y-coordinate of the load $\mathbf{G}$ is equal to

(12.28) $$G_y = F + R_{2y}$$
$$G_y = -m \cdot g \cdot L_2 / D + m \cdot g$$

In contrast, the sum of all y-coordinates of the forces acting at the proximal end of the segment "foot" amounts to

(12.29) $$F + F^* + R_{2y} = m \cdot g$$
$$R_{2y} = m \cdot g$$

A comparison of these results reveals that $\mathbf{R}_2$ is the net force transmitted from the lower leg segment to the foot segment. In the case discussed here, the force $\mathbf{R}_2$ is directed opposite to the gravitational force of the mass of the foot. If the foot were to be moved in plantarflexion so that its center of mass was positioned perpendicularly below the center of rotation ($L_2 = 0$), the moment M_2 and the force $\mathbf{F}$ would equal zero, but the reaction force $\mathbf{R}_{2y}$ would still amount to $m \cdot g$. The reaction force would then be equilibrated by tensile forces of the soft tissues surrounding the joint; the force between tibia and talus would be equal to zero.

Readers may convince themselves that the result for the joint load of the foot loaded only by gravity and held in equilibrium by activation of the tibialis anterior muscle is exactly analogous to the result obtained above for the elbow joint with gravity acting on the mass held in the hand. If interest had been confined to the load on the ankle joint, it might have been easier to perform a straightforward calculation employing the conditions of equilibrium (as in the case of the elbow) instead of making a detour via reaction forces and moments. If, on the other hand, the movement of the lower leg and the force and moment transmitted from the lower to the upper leg are focuses of interest, knowledge of the reaction force $\mathbf{R}_2$ and the reaction moment M_2 is indispensable. What is not required in this latter case is knowledge of the load on the ankle joint.

In addition, the equations show that the load G_y on the ankle joint varies in proportion with the moment M_2. An increase in the moment results in an increased joint load; a decrease results in a decreased joint load. This observation is of general validity; specifically, it remains valid even if the muscle and/or tendon forces (and their moment arms) generating equilibrium are not known (in other words: if a biomechanical model of the joint is not established). It has to be pointed out, however, that a proportionality between joint loads and transmitted moments is valid only if identical joint positions are compared. If the joint position is changed, the moment arms of the forces may change as well and a comparison of joint loads can no longer be based on the comparison of moments. It is important to keep this restriction in mind when, for reasons of simplification only the moments of the external forces are determined and conclusions on joint loading are based on these moments (with no effort being taken to establish models of the joints).

12.4.2 Case 2: Foot with Accelerated Motion but No Floor Contact (**Fig. 12.13**)

The reaction force $\mathbf{R}_1$ and the moment M_1 equal zero as the foot is not in contact with the floor. The linear and angular accelerations are not equal to zero. To determine the proximal reaction force and reaction moment, these accelerations must have been measured, for example from video sequences of the moving foot. By insertion into the equations of motion we obtain

(12.30)
$$R_{2x} = m \cdot a_x$$
$$R_{2y} - m \cdot g = m \cdot a_y$$
$$M_2 + L_1 \cdot R_{2x} + L_2 \cdot R_{2y} = I \cdot \alpha$$

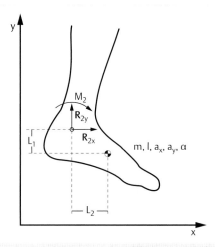

Fig. 12.13 Foot undergoing accelerated motion with no floor contact. See also legend to **Fig. 12.10**.

R_{2x} and R_{2y} can be determined from the first two equations; the third equation then permits M_2 to be determined. If the load on the ankle joint were to be determined in this case too, a joint model would have to be established. The muscle or tendon force generating the moment M_2 would then depend on the sense of direction (dorsi- or plantarflexion) of the foot motion. In other words, the model would have to consider either the tibialis anterior or the Achilles tendon and the appertaining moment arms.

12.4.3 Case 3: Foot with Accelerated Motion and Floor Contact (**Fig. 12.14**)

In this case the reaction force $\mathbf{R}_1$ is not equal to zero. The components $\mathbf{R}_{1x}$ and $\mathbf{R}_{1y}$ are required to be available from measurements, for example by means of a force platform. The reaction moment M_1 is equal to zero as no tensile force is transmitted from the floor onto the foot. After insertion in the equations of motion we obtain

(12.31)
$$R_{1x} + R_{2x} = m \cdot a_x$$
$$R_{1y} + R_{2y} - m \cdot g = m \cdot a_y$$
$$M_2 + L_1 \cdot R_{2x} - L_3 \cdot R_{1x} + L_2 \cdot R_{2y} - L_4 \cdot R_{1y} = I \cdot \alpha$$

The moments are, as always, related to the center of mass of the foot. The minus sign of the moments of the forces R_{1x} and R_{1y} follows from their counterclockwise direction of rotation according to the sign convention for moments. R_{2x} and R_{2y} can be determined from the first two equations; the third equation then permits M_2 to be determined.

The approach used to determine forces and moments from measured translational and rotational motion is termed *inverse dynamics*. An important application of inverse dynamics in orthopedic biomechanics is in the field of gait analysis. The case outlined above—the calculation of forces and moments

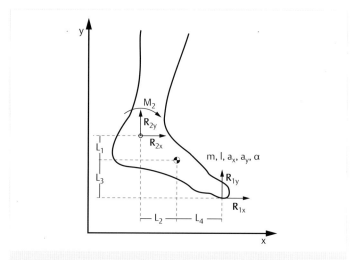

Fig. 12.14 Foot undergoing accelerated motion. Force **R**$_1$ acts from the floor onto the foot. See also legend to **Fig. 12.10**.

transmitted from the foot segment to the lower leg segment—is the first experimental and computational step in determining the loads on the ankle, knee, and hip joints. Modern gait analysis measures and calculates three-dimensionally.

12.5 Calculation of the Joint Load When More Than One Active Muscle Spans the Joint

If more than one single muscle force has to be taken into account, the equilibrium conditions do not suffice to determine all unknowns. In this case we have an "indeterminate" mechanical system. For an indeterminate system there are usually many possible solutions. Additional information and/or selection criteria are required to select one single solution from this multitude.

If several muscles spanning a joint could in principle participate in generating the required moment, it is up to our neuromuscular control to decide which muscle(s) will actually be activated. Will only the muscle with the largest moment arm be activated? Only the strongest muscle? Only the muscle with the highest resistance to fatigue? Will all the muscles be activated, and if so, what proportion of the required moment is generated by each of the individual muscles?

Unfortunately, the strategy underlying the muscle activation pattern is unknown. To reach solutions in biomechanical model calculations despite this gap in our knowledge, various paths are followed:

1. If electromyography (EMG) measurements show that in certain phases of a motion some muscles are activated only weakly or not at all, these muscles can be neglected and the number of muscles to be taken into account can (as an approximation) be reduced to one. This eliminates the indeterminacy.

2. In a preparatory step an attempt can be made to calibrate muscle force against the EMG signal. The EMG amplitudes measured can then be converted into muscle forces. Alternatively, it can be postulated that muscle force is proportional to the physiological cross-sectional area of the muscle. This also permits unequivocal solutions.

3. General constraints such as "joint loading should take a minimum value" or "muscle stress (force/cross section) should be equal for all muscles" also eliminate indeterminacy.

These different approaches are briefly summarized below.

12.5.1 Reducing the Number of Muscles Included in a Calculation by Measuring Muscle Activity

If several muscles might in principle participate in the generation of the required moment, measuring the muscle activity by EMG may serve to decide whether all these muscles are in fact active in a given phase of the movement under investigation. If only one muscle proves to remain active at certain instants of time or, alternatively, if forces from small muscles are negligible so that only one active muscle remains, the indeterminate system is reduced to a determinate system and an unequivocal solution is feasible. This procedure was applied in the first experiments aimed at determining the load on the joints of the lower extremity from gait analysis. In his pioneering work on the loading of the knee joint when walking, Morrison[3] assumed that at each phase of the movement either only the flexor or the extensor muscles (treated as one muscle in each case) were active; forces in the ligaments were ignored.

12.5.2 EMG-Supported Model Calculation

EMG-supported model calculations are based on muscle force data derived from electromyographic measurements. For this purpose, a relation between the EMG signal and the muscle force has first to be established. In a posture where only one single muscle is loaded isometrically, the amplitude of the EMG signal can be calibrated against the moment and (with knowledge of the moment arm) the force of the muscle in an individual test subject. In subsequent postures or movements the EMG signal is recorded; the calibration procedure then yields the muscle force (see for example Dolan and Adams[4] and Lloyd and Besier[5]). The difficulty is that only in rare cases is it possible to load a single muscle isometrically in order to perform the required calibration. In each case, correction factors taking account of changes in muscle length or contraction velocity have to be introduced into the model calculation because length change and contraction velocity influence the relation between EMG amplitude and force. EMG-supported model calculations claim to have the advantage that individual activation patterns can be taken into account. However, this advantage is not valid for the more deeply located muscles, as their EMG cannot be reliably recorded by surface electrodes.

Alternatively, muscle cross-sectional areas are measured from magnetic resonance images, and the amplitude of the EMG signal as well as the muscle force are assumed to be proportional to the cross-sectional area (see, for example, Granata and Marras[6]). Measuring muscle cross sections by magnetic resonance is not as easy as it may appear at first sight, because cross sections change with posture; furthermore, cross-sectional areas are different in vitro and in vivo (see, for example, Gatton et al[7]). The factor by which a given signal amplitude for a given cross section of the muscle can be converted into the muscle force is known only imprecisely and may vary interindividually. Furthermore, such a factor will probably depend on the muscle length and contraction velocity.

12.5.3 Hypotheses on the Co-activation of Several Muscles

Mathematically, the solution of a set of equations containing more unknowns than equations is indeterminate. Introducing additional assumptions or constraints allows a unique solution to be enforced. The constraint may imply selection, from the multitude of possible solutions, of one single solution for which a specified function ("cost function" or "objective function") takes an extreme (maximum or minimum) value. It might, for example, be assumed that muscles generate force in such a way that the joint load is minimized. It would follow from this assumption (the proof is not given here) that only the muscles with the largest moment arm were active at any given time while all other muscles with smaller moment arms were inactive. Experience shows, however, that this assumption is not compatible with physiological observations and EMG measurements.

Alternatively, it can be assumed that the sum of the squares of the muscle stresses or the sum of the muscle stresses raised to the third power will take a minimum value (see, for example, Bean et al[8]). It can be postulated in addition that the tensile stress of individual muscles may not exceed certain physiological limits. Muscle stress is defined as the muscle force divided by the cross-sectional area of the muscle. Estimates for the maximum stress are around $50\ \mathrm{N/cm^2}$. These assumptions are supported by physiologically based arguments, but the arguments are not compelling. Postulating that the sum of the squares of the muscle stresses takes a minimum value, this will result in the stress being evenly distributed over all the muscles in question. If the sum of the muscle stresses raised to the third power takes a minimum value, this will result in high muscle forces, which may lead to rapid fatigue, being avoided. However, other task-specific strategies for the cooperation of several muscles are conceivable. Praagman et al[9] propose employing the energy consumption of the muscles, as characterized by their oxygen consumption, as a criterion.

If a choice between various hypotheses remains after exclusion of the obviously incorrect hypotheses, an attempt can be made to compare the results of model calculations performed under different assumptions with each other or with measured data of joint loading. Such a study has been performed by Glitsch and Baumann[10] for the lower extremity. The authors showed that results for joint loads for hip and knee obtained under different assumptions exhibited only minor differences. Compared with data on the load of the hip joint measured in vivo, the calculations produced higher joint loads. For the knee joint, comparison of calculated and measured data was not possible as no in vivo experiments with instrumented knee joint replacements had yet been published. As alternative to these different assumptions, one can also specify an activation pattern of the muscles and compare the resulting motion of the body with measured motion data (so-called *forward dynamics*; see, for example, Erdemir et al[11]).

Not being able to decide which objective function to choose for a particular type of motion merely reflects our fragmentary knowledge of the underlying strategy of the neuromuscular control system. There is no doubt that our control system always adheres to a specific strategy (see, for example, Hatze[12] and Rasmussen et al[13]). The observation that certain motions can be repeated with high precision gives support to this assumption. In other words, for any intended motion or posture, our control system does not have to solve the mathematically indeterminate problem of which muscles, out of a number of potential contributors, to activate in a specific situation. In reality, there is no indeterminacy problem to be solved.

Examples of model calculations which rely on the three-dimensional architecture of muscles and tendons and make use of different hypotheses on the activation patterns include (this is not a comprehensive list): for the lower extremity, White et al,[14] Glitsch and Baumann,[10] and Menegaldo et al[15]; for the knee, Pandy et al[16] and McLean et al[17]; for the shoulder, van der Helm[18]; for the upper extremity, Garner and Pandy,[19] Langenderfer et al,[20] and Chadwick et al[21]; for the elbow and wrist, Ramsay et al[22]; for the cervical spine, Netto et al[23]; and for the lumbar spine, Schultz et al.[24]

References

1. Roberts SL, Falkenburg SA. Biomechanics: Problem Solving for Functional Activity. St. Louis: Mosby; 1992

2. Winter DA. Biomechanics and Motor Control of Human Movement. 3rd ed. New York: Wiley; 2005

3. Morrison JB. Bioengineering analysis of force actions transmitted by the knee joint. Biomed Eng 1968;3:164–170

4. Dolan P, Adams MA. Repetitive lifting tasks fatigue the back muscles and increase the bending moment acting on the lumbar spine. J Biomech 1998;31(8):713–721

5. Lloyd DG, Besier TF. An EMG-driven musculoskeletal model to estimate muscle forces and knee joint moments in vivo. J Biomech 2003;36(6):765–776

6. Granata KP, Marras WS. An EMG-assisted model of loads on the lumbar spine during asymmetric trunk extensions. J Biomech 1993;26(12):1429–1438

7. Gatton ML, Pearcy MJ, Pettet GJ. Difficulties in estimating muscle forces from muscle cross-sectional area. An example using the psoas major muscle. Spine 1999;24(14):1487–1493

8. Bean JC, Chaffin DB, Schultz AB. Biomechanical model calculation of muscle contraction forces: a double linear programming method. J Biomech 1988;21(1):59–66

9. Praagman M, Chadwick EKJ, van der Helm FCT, Veeger HEJ. The relationship between two different mechanical cost functions and muscle oxygen consumption. J Biomech 2006;39(4):758–765

10. Glitsch U, Baumann W. The three-dimensional determination of internal loads in the lower extremity. J Biomech 1997;30(11-12):1123–1131

11. Erdemir A, McLean S, Herzog W, van den Bogert AJ. Model-based estimation of muscle forces exerted during movements. Clin Biomech (Bristol, Avon) 2007;22(2):131–154

12. Hatze H. Neuromusculoskeletal control systems modeling - a critical survey of recent developments. IEEE Trans Automat Contr 1980;25:375–385

13. Rasmussen J, Damsgaard M, Voigt M. Muscle recruitment by the min/max criterion — a comparative numerical study. J Biomech 2001;34(3):409–415

14. White SC, Yack HJ, Winter DA. A three-dimensional musculoskeletal model for gait analysis. Anatomical variability estimates. J Biomech 1989;22(8-9):885–893

15. Menegaldo LL, de Toledo Fleury A, Weber HI. Moment arms and musculotendon lengths estimation for a three-dimensional lower-limb model. J Biomech 2004;37(9):1447–1453

16. Pandy MG, Sasaki K, Kim S. A three-dimensional musculoskeletal model of the human knee joint. Part 1: Theoretical construct. Comput Methods Biomech Biomed Engin 1998;1(2):87–108

17. McLean SG, Su A, van den Bogert AJ. Development and validation of a 3-D model to predict knee joint loading during dynamic movement. J Biomech Eng 2003;125(6):864–874

18. van der Helm FCT. A finite element musculoskeletal model of the shoulder mechanism. J Biomech 1994;27(5):551–569

19. Garner BA, Pandy MG. Musculoskeletal model of the upper limb based on the visible human male dataset. Comput Methods Biomech Biomed Engin 2001;4(2):93–126

20. Langenderfer J, LaScalza S, Mell A, Carpenter JE, Kuhn JE, Hughes RE. An EMG-driven model of the upper extremity and estimation of long head biceps force. Comput Biol Med 2005;35(1):25–39

21. Chadwick EK, Blana D, van den Bogert AJ, Kirsch RF. A real-time, 3-D musculoskeletal model for dynamic simulation of arm movements. IEEE Trans Biomed Eng 2009;56(4):941–948

22. Ramsay JW, Hunter BV, Gonzalez RV. Muscle moment arm and normalized moment contributions as reference data for musculoskeletal elbow and wrist joint models. J Biomech 2009;42(4):463–473

23. Netto KJ, Burnett AF, Green JP, Rodrigues JP. Validation of an EMG-driven, graphically based isometric musculoskeletal model of the cervical spine. J Biomech Eng 2008;130(3):031014

24. Schultz AB, Andersson GB, Haderspeck K, Ortengren R, Nordin M, Björk R. Analysis and measurement of lumbar trunk loads in tasks involving bends and twists. J Biomech 1982;15(9):669–675

Further Reading

Hatze H. Comments on 'theoretical considerations on cocontraction of sets of agonistic and antagonistic muscles'. J Biomech 2001;34(7):975–978

Tsirakos D, Baltzopoulos V, Bartlett R. Inverse optimization: functional and physiological considerations related to the force-sharing problem. Crit Rev Biomed Eng 1997;25(4-5):371–407

Zatsiorski VM. Kinetics of Human Motion. Champaign: Human Kinetics; 2002

13   Mechanical Aspects of the Hip Joint

Healthy human beings take between one hundred thousand and several million steps per year, and peak values of the load on the hip joint, corresponding to a multiple of the weight of the whole body, occur in the heel-strike and toe-off phases of every one of them. The hip joint seems to be adapted to this high, repetitive loading. Even in old age, in the majority of people the function of the hip joint is only slightly restricted, if at all. This finding is not inconsistent with the regular finding of age-related alteration (*degeneration*) of the joint cartilage as well as changes in bone density and trabecular architecture. Severe alterations, leading to clinical symptoms and a restriction of joint function, are encountered in only a minority of individuals. However, in persons showing significant deviations from the normal geometric configuration of the femoral head and acetabulum, premature destruction of the joint may be observed. The magnitude and repetition rate of the load on the hip joint suggest that primary mechanical causes may be responsible for the development and progress of osteoarthritis.

Interest in the mechanical aspects of the hip joint has been substantially encouraged by the pioneering work of Pauwels.[1] This chapter outlines how to determine the load on the hip joint in the stance phase of slow gait by means of a biomechanical model calculation. Within the framework of this simplified model, the question of how the joint load may be influenced by pathologic gait, walking aids, or surgical interventions is discussed, with examples. Detailed information on hip joint loading is obtained from gait analysis as well as from direct measurements employing instrumented joint replacements. Knowledge of the joint load is a prerequisite for determining the pressure on the joint surface and to forming hypotheses on mechanical factors in the etiology of osteoarthritis of the joint.

13.1   Load on the Hip Joint in the Stance Phase of Slow Gait

The load on the hip joint is analyzed in the stance phase of slow gait on the basis that this phase may be regarded as typical of everyday activities. In the stance phase, one foot is on the floor while the other is lifted off the floor with the leg being swung forward through the frontal plane. The designation "slow" indicates that the inertial forces resulting from slowing down and accelerating the body segments during each step are assumed to be negligibly small.

The simplistic model calculation (**Fig. 13.1**) takes into account only three forces acting on the pelvis in the frontal plane. **W** is the gravitational force ("weight") of the body mass less the mass of the standing leg. The point of force application is the center of mass of the body less the standing leg: that is, the center of mass of the head, arms, trunk, and swinging leg. The gravitational force points vertically downwards. **F** is the force of the abductor muscles, which balance the moment of the gravitational force. The vector **F** represents the forces of all muscles that may effect an abduction of the standing leg. The direction of **F** is

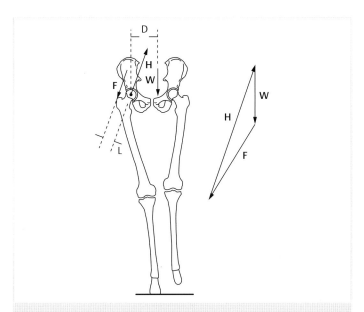

Fig. 13.1 Load **H** on the hip joint in the stance phase of slow gait. The model calculation is based on the condition of equilibrium of the pelvis. The gravitational force **W**, the force of the abductor muscles **F**, and the force **H** transmitted from the femoral head onto the acetabulum act on the pelvis. L denotes the moment arm of the abductor muscles. D denotes the moment arm of the force **W**. In mechanical equilibrium, the vector sum of **W**, **F**, and **H** equals zero.

chosen along the direction of the gluteus medius muscle. The points of force application of **F** are the centers of the insertion areas of the gluteus medius at the iliac bone and at the major trochanter. All additional muscle forces that may be active in stabilizing the hip joint during the stance phase with respect to flexion and extension are disregarded. The hip joint is assumed to be a perfect, friction-free ball-and-socket joint. Thus, the joint force **H**, acting from the femoral head onto the acetabulum, runs through the center of the femoral head. (The rationale is as follows: In a state of static equilibrium a friction-free joint cannot transmit a moment. If the vector of the joint load did not pass through the center of the femoral head, it would generate a moment with respect to the center and the joint would start moving.)

With knowledge of the magnitude of **W**, its point of application (that is, the location of the center of mass of the body less the standing leg), and the direction and points of application of the muscle force **F**, the magnitude of **F** can be obtained from the equilibrium condition of moments. The equilibrium condition of forces requires the vector sum of **W**, **F**, and **H** to be equal to zero. As result the direction and magnitude of **H** can be determined.

To determine **H**, it is advantageous to determine the components H_x and H_y separately (**Figs. 13.2 and 13.3**). The coordinate system is oriented so that the x-axis points in the horizontal direction and the y-axis in the vertical direction. Since the gravitational force **W** is aligned vertically and the muscle force **F** almost vertically, we expect the load on the hip joint to be determined essentially by the y-components of these forces; the x-components will make only a small additional contribution.

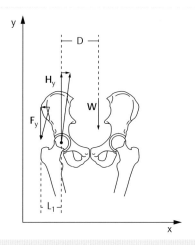

Fig. 13.2 Calculation of the y-components $\mathbf{F}_y$ and $\mathbf{H}_y$ of the forces **F** and **H** in mechanical equilibrium. D designates the moment arm of the gravitational force $\mathbf{W}_y$; L_1 designates the moment arm of the muscle force $\mathbf{F}_y$.

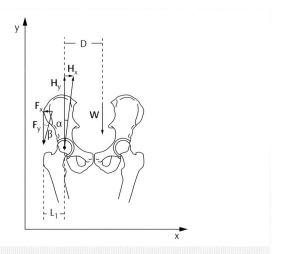

Fig. 13.3 With knowledge of the direction of the muscle force **F** (angle β with respect to the y-axis) and knowledge of $\mathbf{F}_y$, the component $\mathbf{F}_x$ can be obtained (see Eq. 13.9).

It is assumed that the mass of one leg equals approximately 20% of the body mass. Under this assumption, we obtain for the y-component of the gravitational force **W**

(13.1)
$$|W_y| = 0.8 \cdot \text{body mass} \cdot \text{gravitational acceleration} = 0.8 \cdot m \cdot g$$

In good approximation, the center of mass of the whole body is positioned above the symphysis (as the architecture of our body is, broadly, right–left symmetrical). The center of mass of the body regardless of the standing leg is shifted to the side of the swinging leg. For the relationship between the moment arm D of the gravitational force and the moment arm L_1 of the y-component of the muscle force we assume

(13.2)
$$D = 2.0 \cdot L_1$$

Under these assumptions (and in accordance with the sign convention for moments) we obtain in equilibrium of moments

(13.3)
$$-F_y \cdot L_1 + W_y \cdot D = 0$$

and for the y-coordinates of the forces

(13.4)
$$F_y = 2.0 \cdot W_y$$

In static equilibrium it holds for the y-components of the forces that

(13.5)
$$\mathbf{H_y + F_y + W_y = 0}$$

and, for their y-coordinates when inserting F_y from Eq. 13.4

(13.6)
$$H_y = -2.0 \cdot W_y - W_y$$
$$H_y = -3.0 \cdot W_y$$

W_y points in the negative y-direction. W_y is thus equal to $-0.8 \cdot m \cdot g$. After insertion into Eq. 13.6 we obtain

(13.7)
$$H_y = 2.4 \cdot m \cdot g$$

In other words: the y-component of the force transmitted from the femoral head onto the acetabulum has a magnitude 2.4 times the weight of the whole body. The positive value of H_y indicates that this force points in the positive y-direction; the femoral head exerts a compressive force on the acetabulum.

In equilibrium of forces it holds for the x-components of the hip joint load and the muscle force (**Fig. 13.3**) that

(13.8)
$$\mathbf{H_x + F_x = 0}$$

This equation contains only two addends as the x-component of the gravitational force equals zero. With β as the angle between the vertical and the direction of the muscle force **F**, we obtain for the x-coordinate F_x of the muscle force

(13.9) $$F_x = F_y \cdot \tan\beta$$

and in equilibrium with $F_y = 2.0 \cdot W_y$ we obtain

(13.10)
$$H_x = -F_y \cdot \tan\beta$$
$$H_x = 2.0 \cdot 0.8 \cdot m \cdot g \cdot \tan\beta$$
$$H_x = 1.6 \cdot m \cdot g \cdot \tan\beta$$

The angle β is approximately $15°$; the tangent of $15°$ is 0.27. Thus H_x is much smaller than H_y. With knowledge of H_x and H_y the magnitude of the total hip joint load H is calculated as

(13.11) $$H = \sqrt{H_x^2 + H_y^2}$$

The angle α between the vector of the hip joint load **H** and the vertical is calculated as

(13.12)
$$\tan\alpha = H_x / H_y$$
$$\tan\alpha = 0.27 \cdot 2 \cdot W_y / 3 \cdot W_y$$
$$\alpha = 10.2°$$

13.2 Influence of Gait Technique, Walking Aids, or Surgical Intervention on the Hip Joint Load

The model calculation of the hip joint load in the stance phase of slow gait can be used to visualize the effects on the joint load of gait techniques, the use of walking aids, or changes to bone geometry through surgical intervention.

13.2.1 Gait Technique

A gait anomaly termed "Duchenne limp" is illustrated in **Fig. 13.4**. In this type of gait, the center of mass of the body is shifted to the side of the standing leg. This shift reduces the moment arm D_1 of the gravitational force **W** with respect to the moment arm D during normal gait. Consequently the force **F** of the abductor muscles required for equilibrium will decrease. This results in a decrease of the load H on the hip joint. In the limiting case, when the center of mass of the body less the standing leg is positioned perpendicularly above the hip joint and the moment arm D_1 assumes a value of zero, a very substantial load decrease results. The Duchenne limp is, however, unsuitable for long-term reduction of the load on the hip joint because the accompanying bending of the lumbar spine to the side cannot be tolerated over long periods.

In practice a Duchenne limp may indicate an attempt by an individual to reduce the load on an already impaired joint, or it may indicate weakness of the abductor muscles. The implications for therapy in these two cases would be quite different.

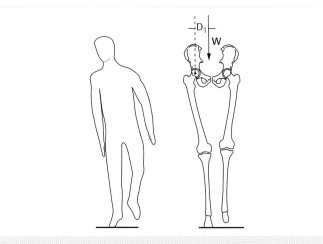

Fig. 13.4 Effect of the Duchenne limp on the loading of the hip joint. Shifting the body mass to the side of the standing leg decreases the moment arm D_1 of the gravitational force **W**.

13.2.2 Cane

Fig. 13.5 shows the pelvis again in the stance phase of slow gait. A cane is employed contralaterally to the standing leg. For brevity, we consider here only the y-components of the forces. **S** is the force from the cane onto the hand. S_y is the y-component of this force; it points in the positive y-direction. For calculation of the joint load, the assumptions on the moment arm of the body weight and the magnitude of the gravitational force are left unchanged:

(13.13)
$$|W_y| = 0.8 \cdot m \cdot g$$
$$D = 2.0 \cdot L_1$$

In addition, we assume the moment arm E of the cane force **S** to amount to twice the moment arm D and thus to four times the moment arm of the of the abductor muscles:

(13.14)
$$E = 4.0 \cdot L_1$$

With these assumptions we obtain from the equilibrium condition of moments (in accordance with the sign convention for moments)

(13.15)
$$-F_y \cdot L_1 + W_y \cdot D - S_y \cdot E = 0$$
$$F_y = 2.0 \cdot W_y - 4.0 \cdot S_y$$

Using the cane reduces the magnitude of the required muscle force F_y by an amount equal to four times the magnitude of the cane force S_y.

In equilibrium of forces it holds for the y-coordinates of the forces that

(13.16)
$$H_y + F_y + W_y + S_y = 0$$

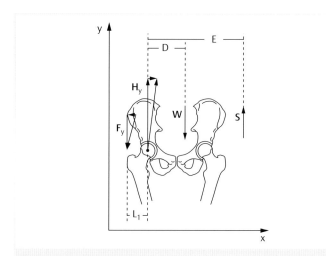

Fig. 13.5 Influence of the use of a cane on hip joint load in the stance phase of slow gait (only the y-components of the forces are discussed). **S** designates the force from the cane on the hand, E designates the moment arm of the force **S**, other designations as in **Figs. 13.1** and **13.2**.

The addends in this equation can assume positive or negative values, depending on whether the forces point in the positive or the negative y-direction. For the coordinates of the forces **W** and **S** it holds in equilibrium of moments that

$$(13.17) \qquad F_y = 2.0 \cdot W_y + 4.0 \cdot S_y$$

(Note: As Eq. 13.16 deals with the coordinates of the forces and not with their magnitudes, inserting $F_y = 2.0 \cdot W_y - 4.0 \cdot S_y$ from Eq. 13.15 would be incorrect. It should be pointed out that W_y is a negative number and S_y a positive number. Eq. 13.17 implies that the magnitude of F_y is lessened by four times the magnitude of S_y.) It then follows for **H** that

$$(13.18) \qquad \begin{aligned} H_y &= -2.0 \cdot W_y - 4.0 \cdot S_y - W_y - S_y \\ H_y &= -3.0 \cdot W_y - 5.0 \cdot S_y \end{aligned}$$

and with insertion of $W_y = -0.8 \cdot m \cdot g$

$$(13.19) \qquad H_y = 2.4 \cdot m \cdot g - 5.0 \cdot S_y$$

Using a cane reduces the y-component of the load on the hip joint by an amount equal to five times the force between the cane and the hand. The effect can be illustrated with an example. Given a body mass of 60 kg, the gravitational force W amounts to approximately 600 N. The y-coordinate of the load on the hip joint then amounts to (Eq. 13.6)

$$(13.20) \qquad H_y = 2.4 \cdot 600 = 1440 \text{ N}$$

Using a cane and assuming a force of $S_y = +50$ N between hand and cane, we obtain

(13.21) $$H_y = 1440 - 250 = 1190 \text{ N}$$

Using the cane reduces the joint load by about 20%. It must be stressed that the reduction in joint load can be achieved only if the cane is used contralaterally to the hip joint in question. Using the cane ipsilaterally would increase the load on the hip joint. Alternatively, a reduction in body mass might be considered in order to decrease the hip joint load. In principle this is a valid idea as the joint load H_y depends directly on the body mass m. To achieve a reduction in load comparable to that when a cane is used, however, the body mass must be reduced by approximately 20%. In many cases this will probably be difficult to achieve.

13.2.3 Surgical Intervention

Surgical interventions can alter the geometry of the bony skeleton and thus change the moment arms of muscles. **Fig. 13.6** shows the example of a varisation osteotomy, where a bone wedge is excised from the intertrochanteric region. Geometrically this intervention effects a decrease in the angle between the femoral neck and the femur and lateralization of the greater trochanter. Postoperatively the moment arm L_1 of the abductor muscle can be about 15% larger than the preoperative moment arm L. Because the moment arm is larger, the required muscle force becomes proportionally smaller (change from F to F_1), and accordingly so does the joint load. In addition, the psoas muscle has become shorter. The subsequent reduction in the stress of this muscle will induce a further reduction of the load on the hip joint. For a quantitative estimate of this effect, information on the passive stiffness of the muscle is required; this is not precisely known.

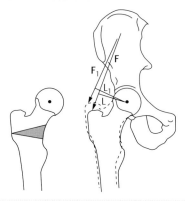

Fig. 13.6 Example of the influence of surgical intervention on the load on the hip joint. Removal of a wedge between the greater and lesser trochanter (intertrochanteric varisation osteotomy) effects lateralization of the greater trochanter and an increase in the moment arm of the abductor muscles from L to L_1.

A further effect of the surgical intervention illustrated in **Fig. 13.6** is the rotation of the femoral head with respect to the acetabulum. This results in relocation (relative to each other) of those parts of the surface areas of the head and acetabulum that are subjected to compressive stress.

13.3 Determination of Hip Joint Load by Gait Analysis

If accelerated linear or rotational motions of the body segments occur, influences of inertial forces and inertial moments must be taken into account when determining the load on the hip joint. To illustrate the effect of inertial forces, we start by discussing a simple, intuitively accessible example. The posture shown in **Fig. 13.7** is not to be interpreted as the stance phase in slow gait but as the posture assumed when hitting the ground with the right foot after jumping from a low wall. On landing, the velocity of the body mass cranial to the hip joint must be slowed down (decelerated) from its initial value to zero. The variable a designates the magnitude of the acceleration involved. The magnitude of the inertial force $\mathbf{F}_{in}$ amounts to

(13.22) $$|\mathbf{F}_{in}| = 0.8 \cdot m \cdot a$$

Regarding the sign of the inertial force: when the person hits the ground, the velocity points in the negative y-direction; the change in velocity (the acceleration) points in the positive y-direction. The inertial force $\mathbf{F}_{in}$ is opposite to the acceleration and thus in the negative y-direction—that is, in the same direction as the gravitational force.

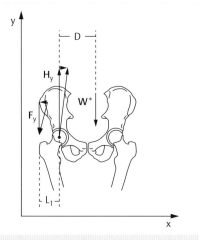

Fig. 13.7 If the body is accelerated in the vertical direction, an inertial force acts in addition to the gravitational force. The magnitude of the inertial force and thus the load on the hip joint depend on the magnitude of the acceleration.

The load on the hip joint can now be estimated using formulae almost identical to those in the stance phase of slow gait. The only difference is that instead of the gravitational force $\mathbf{W}_y$ the sum of the gravitational and inertial forces has to be inserted. In **Fig. 13.7** this sum is designated by $\mathbf{W}^*$.

$$(13.23) \qquad \qquad W_y + F_{in} = -(0.8 \cdot m \cdot g + 0.8 \cdot m \cdot a)$$

For the magnitude of the y-component of the hip joint load we obtain

$$(13.24) \qquad \qquad |\mathbf{H}_y| = 2.4 \cdot m \cdot (g + a)$$

In this example the inertial force acts as if the body weight were momentarily increased by an amount equal to $2.4 \cdot m \cdot a$. The numerical value of this increase depends on the magnitude of the acceleration a. If the change from the initial velocity to zero takes place within a short time interval (for example, when landing with the legs straight), the acceleration will have a high value. If the change in velocity can be extended over a longer time interval (for example, by bending the knees and thus providing a soft impact), the acceleration will assume a lower value.

The load on the hip joint can be determined in a model calculation if a person's anthropometric data (dimension and mass of body segments) are known and kinematic (motion) and kinetic data (forces between the feet and the ground) are measured in the course of a gait cycle. Gait analysis supplies important information on hip joint loading far beyond what can be obtained by looking at simple models such as the stance phase of slow gait. For the purpose of calculation, the standing leg is regarded as a free body (**Fig. 13.8**). The masses, locations of the centers of mass, and moments of inertia about the centers of mass of the segments foot, lower leg, and thigh must be known. The course over time of the linear acceleration of the centers of mass of the segments, the angular acceleration of the segments about their centers of mass, and the force $\mathbf{R}_F$ from the floor onto the foot are measured during walking. Starting from the foot, one after another the forces and moments on the ankle joint, knee joint, and hip joint can now be calculated (see Chapter 12). To determine the load on the hip joint, a model of the joint must be established that accurately describes its geometry and the lines of action and moment arms of the muscles that cross the joint. If more than a single muscle is active at a particular instant in time, additional assumptions are required in order to obtain an unequivocal solution.

As an example, **Fig. 13.9** shows a result from the pioneering experiments of Paul.[2] At that time, measurement and calculation could be performed only for the time interval when the foot was in contact with the floor. For this reason, the curves end at about 60% of the gait cycle. Maximum values of the hip joint load occur after heel-strike and before toe-off. These peak loads are caused by the deceleration and acceleration of the body mass. The peak loads rise with increasing gait velocity, because the accelerations increase and hence so do the inertial forces.

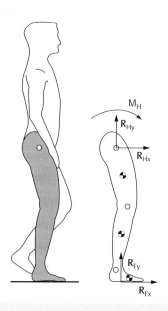

Fig. 13.8 Determination of the load on the hip joint from gait analysis. The lower extremity is regarded as a free body. Proximally the reaction force **R**$_H$ and the reaction moment M$_H$ and distally the reaction force **R**$_F$ act on this body. The lower extremity is subdivided into the segments foot, lower leg, and upper leg, interlinked by hinge joints. The reaction force **R**$_F$ as well as the linear and angular accelerations (related to the centers of mass, segmented circles) are measured. From these measured data together with anthropometric data, **R**$_H$ and M$_H$ can be calculated.

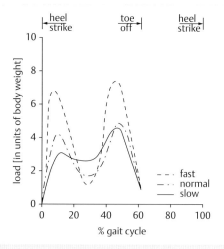

Fig. 13.9 Load on the hip joint in relation to gait velocity. The interval from 0% to 100% designates one full gait cycle. (Adapted from Paul.[2])

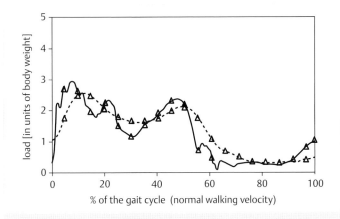

Fig. 13.10 Load on the hip when walking. Solid line: data from gait analysis; dashed line: simultaneous measurement by means of an instrumented artificial hip joint. (Adapted, with permission, from Stansfield et al.[3])

Fig. 13.10 illustrates the result of a gait analysis.[3] It also shows the result of a direct measurement of hip joint loading employing an instrumented joint prosthesis (see below, Section 13.4). The agreement between the calculated and the measured magnitude of the peak loads and the time points at which they occur is excellent. (The "waviness" of the load curve computed from the gait analysis is due to the underlying algorithm, which takes several muscle groups into account; for details, see the original paper.)

13.4 Determination of the Load on the Hip Joint by Means of an Instrumented Joint Prosthesis

If an artificial hip joint replacement is equipped with force transducers and the transducer signals are transmitted telemetrically to the outside of the body, the load on the hip joint can be determined directly in vivo, free from the numerous restrictions that have to be considered in model calculations. Interpretation of the measured data requires no theoretical assumptions on the co-activation of the muscles crossing the joint. Specifically, antagonistic muscle activity does not have to be excluded. Contributions to the joint load originating from the elastic tension of muscles, tendons, or joint capsules are automatically included in the measured results.

Comprehensive data on the loading of the hip joint, measured by instrumented joint prostheses, have been published by Bergmann et al[4-9] and Damm et al.[10] A complete dataset from the Bergmann team is available on CD.[11] For the first time, these data facilitate comparisons between model calculations and direct measurements. In addition, load data are presented for loading modes inaccessible to model calculations.

The results are of eminent importance for the further development of artificial joint replacements and for the insight they give into bone growth and remodeling around implants. The results are helpful for developing guidelines for postoperative physical therapy and give general advice regarding the physical activity of patients with joint replacements.

Activity	Hip joint load [% body weight]
Symmetrical stance on both legs	70
Walking, 4 km/h	250
Walking, fast	350
Jogging	500
Stumbling (unintentional)	800
Walking up stairs	250
Walking down stairs	300
Lifting the pelvis while lying supine	300
Lifting the leg against resistance while lying supine	250
Bicycling	80% of the load when walking
Walking, using a cane	25% load reduction

Table 13.1 Maximum values of the load on the hip joint measured during a number of postures and activities

Source: Measurements by Bergmann and coworkers. To provide an overview, numbers have been rounded. For details, see Bergmann et al.[4–9]

Table 13.1, extracted from the work of the Bergmann team, lists the maximum values of the load on the hip joint measured during a number of postures and activities. The fact that in symmetrical stance on both legs the hip joint load amounts to roughly 70% of body weight may at first sight seem surprising. As the mass of head, arms, and trunk amounts to about 60% of body mass, one might (naively) expect a hip joint load of $0.5 \cdot 60\% = 30\%$ of body weight in symmetrical stance. In reality the value corresponds to roughly 70% of body weight due to the muscle tension still active in relaxed standing and the elastic tension of all tissues (muscles, ligaments, etc.) that cross the joint. The agreement between the hip joint loads measured during walking and the corresponding results from simple model calculations (Section 13.1) is fair, and as we have seen, the agreement between the results of direct measurements and the results of gait analysis based on complex muscle models is excellent (see **Fig. 13.10**).

The measured data also allow important questions relating to the postoperative rehabilitation of patients with artificial hip joints to be answered. For example, lifting the leg while lying supine loads the hip joint more than standing erect on two legs. Also, interestingly, it appears that when a leg is moved against gravity or against external resistance, the joint load of the contralateral hip rises to approximately equal values. Evidently, active exercises by one leg involuntarily activate the muscles of the other leg as well. If hip joint loads are not to exceed certain limiting values, it follows from the measurements of Bergmann and coworkers that bedridden patients should not lift their pelvis actively to allow a bedpan to be placed, but should lift it only with support from the nursing staff.

As the instrumented joint prosthesis measures the three components of the joint load separately, not only the magnitude but also the direction of the load vector is obtained. It has been shown that, for the femoral head, the point of force application varies within only a small area, whereas for the acetabulum it varies greatly depending on the orientation of the leg. This is intuitively understandable. The load on the hip joint is essentially determined by muscle forces, and these muscles course in approximately the same direction as the long axis of the femur. Therefore, the vector sum of the muscle forces points in approximately the same direction as the long axis of the femur. Knowledge of the load vector allows the bending and torsional moment exerted on the shaft of the prosthesis and the surrounding bone to be estimated. These data are important for the design of prostheses and for assessing the stability of their fixation in the surrounding bone.

13.5 Calculation of the Pressure Distribution on the Surface of the Hip Joint

Mechanical factors directly influencing the tissues of the joints are the pressure (stress) on the joint surface and the stress within the cartilage and the underlying trabecular bone. Both the pressure and the stress depend on the direction and magnitude of the force transmitted by the joint. In addition, pressure and stress depend on the shape and fit (congruency) of the articulating bones and on the mechanical properties of bone and cartilage. Knowledge of the stress distribution at the joint surface and within the tissues is not only of academic interest in understanding the function of the locomotor system. With better insight, it is hoped that primary mechanical causes of the destruction of joints may be recognized and helpful suggestions obtained for the construction of artificial joint replacements. The following remarks on the pressure distribution on the hip joint may serve also as example for other spherical or cylindrical joints in the body.

An initial estimate of the magnitude of the pressure on the surface of the hip joint can be achieved by calculating the mean pressure. For this purpose the magnitude and direction of the force **H** on the hip joint must be known. The mean pressure is given by

(13.25)
$$p_{mean} = H / A$$

where A denotes the projected area of the joint (that is, the area seen when looking along the direction of the force vector onto the joint) (**Fig. 13.11**). If (for reasons of simplification) we disregard the fact that the femoral head is not fully covered by the acetabulum, the area A is a circle with the radius of the femoral head. With a radius of 2.5 cm, a body mass of 60 kg, and a load on the hip joint of three times body weight (typical load when walking), we obtain for the mean pressure

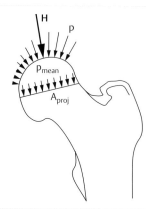

Fig. 13.11 Estimate of the pressure on the surface of the femoral head by calculation of the mean pressure p_{mean} from the joint load **H** and the projected area A_{proj}.

$$(13.26) \qquad p_{mean} = \frac{3 \cdot 600}{\pi \cdot 2.5^2} = 91.7 \, \text{N} / \text{cm}^2 = 0.917 \, \text{MPa}$$

Further information on the pressure distribution on the hip joint is obtained from model calculations based on measurements of the shape of the articulating surface and assumptions about the elastic properties of articular cartilage. As the femoral head has the shape of a sphere, concentrically positioned in the spherical shell of the acetabulum, the articulating surface of the head and acetabulum can be determined from an anteroposterior radiograph of the hip (**Fig. 13.12**). This shows us the image of an incompletely

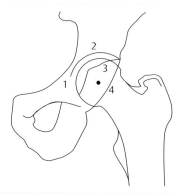

Fig. 13.12 Contours of the hip joint visible in an anteroposterior radiographic view. Solid circle: center of rotation of the joint; 1: contour of the bony femoral head; 2: cranial contour of the bony acetabulum; 3: contour of the anterior rim of the acetabulum; 4: contour of the posterior rim of the acetabulum. The actual joint surface is located approximately halfway between contours 1 and 2.

covered ball-and-socket joint with irregularly shaped rims that are different anteriorly and posteriorly. The circular contour of the femoral head can be easily recognized. Starting from the lateral rim of the iliac bone, the anterior rim of the acetabulum can be followed for some distance; the posterior rim is usually visible for its whole length. The gap between the circular contours of the head and the acetabulum is filled with articular cartilage; the joint surface is located approximately midway between these contours. Measurement of the rim of the acetabulum makes it possible to reconstruct the three-dimensional shape of the articulating surface: each point of the rim has a clear relation to a point on the spherical shell that, as we have said, is concentric to the center of the hip joint.

Pressure can be transmitted, not by the whole area where the surfaces of acetabulum and femoral head are in contact, but only by the part of the contact area that is "seen" by looking along the direction of the load vector onto the joint. To be precise: pressure is transmitted only by the part of the surface of the sphere that is bounded either by the rim of the acetabulum or, at most, by a great circle (circle with the diameter of the femoral head) in a plane perpendicular to the load vector. The reason why the pressure-transmitting surface is restricted is that joint surfaces cannot transmit tensile stress, only compressive stress. In a spherical joint that was completely covered by the socket, the bearing surface would correspond to a hemisphere. Because of the irregular shape of the acetabular rim, the bearing surface of the hip joint is smaller than a hemisphere.

The type of pressure distribution that can be expected in an incompletely covered ball-and-socket joint will now be discussed with reference to the model shown in **Fig. 13.13**. In a joint consisting of a rigid hemi-sphere and a rigid hemispherical socket separated by an intermediate layer of soft material, the maximum

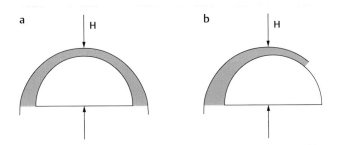

Fig. 13.13a, b Model employed to derive the pressure distribution on the surface of a ball-and-socket joint. If the socket covers the ball symmetrically in relation to the point of application of the force **H** (**a**), we expect maximum pressure at the point of force application and zero pressure at the rim of the socket. If the socket covers the ball incompletely and asymmetrically (**b**), we expect the point of maximum pressure to shift in the direction of the rim of the socket. (Adapted from Brinckmann et al.[12])

compression of the intermediate layer, and thus the maximum pressure, is expected to occur at the point where the force vector **H** intersects the joint surface. Since the articulating surfaces merely glide across each other at the rim of the hemisphere, it is reasonable to assume that the pressure falls to zero at the rim. In an incompletely covered joint we expect the site of maximum compression, and hence of maximum pressure, to be shifted towards the rim of the socket. Because of the right–left asymmetry of the socket and the consequent asymmetry of the counterpressure exerted by the socket on the head, the head has a tendency to "escape" sideways out of the socket. This tendency will increase as coverage of the sphere by the socket decreases. In the limiting case of coverage just up to the point of force application, the loaded sphere would immediately jump out of the socket. Dislocation of the femoral head out of the acetabulum is indeed observed in vivo in individuals in whom the acetabulum gives little or no cover laterally to the femoral head (hip luxation associated with dysplastic acetabulum).

The pressure distribution on the surface of the femoral head is determined from the equilibrium condition of forces in the incompletely covered, spherical joint (**Fig. 13.14**). Since friction between the

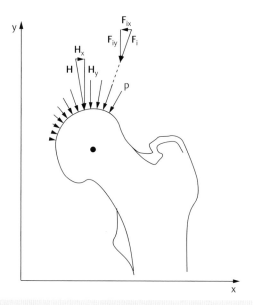

Fig. 13.14 Equilibrium of forces at the hip joint. The sum of the individual forces $\mathbf{F}_i$, calculated as a product of the locally effective pressure and the area elements dA_i, must be equal to the joint load **H**. Because the coverage of the head by the acetabulum is incomplete laterally, the pressure and thus the forces $\mathbf{F}_i$ in the region of the lateral acetabular rim must take on high values in order to satisfy the equilibrium condition for the x-components of all forces.

articulating surfaces is virtually zero, force transmission between head and acetabulum can only occur perpendicular to the cartilaginous surface. If we imagine the surface area of the head to be subdivided into many small area elements of size dA, the sum of the forces $\mathbf{F}_i$, defined as the product of local pressure and the related area dA_i, must (in equilibrium) be equal to the hip joint load $\mathbf{H}$. For the sums of the x- and y-components it holds that

(13.27)
$$\mathbf{F}_{1x} + \mathbf{F}_{2x} + \cdots \mathbf{F}_{nx} = \mathbf{H}_x$$
$$\mathbf{F}_{1y} + \mathbf{F}_{2y} + \cdots \mathbf{F}_{ny} = \mathbf{H}_y$$

To satisfy the equilibrium condition for the y-components, the pressure distribution can vary within wide limits. Even a uniform pressure distribution can satisfy this condition. Satisfying the equilibrium condition for the x-components requires the pressure (and thus the forces) to be much larger laterally than medially from the point of application of the vector $\mathbf{H}$. Otherwise, because the articulating area between head and acetabulum is smaller laterally than medially, and because the laterally located articulating area is inclined by only a small angle with respect to the x-axis, the summed x-components $\mathbf{F}_{ix}$ would be too small to balance the component $\mathbf{H}_x$ of the joint load.

The outcome of this discussion is the model of the hip joint shown in **Fig. 13.15**. The joint is a ball-and-socket joint with an irregularly shaped rim of the socket. Only part A of the articulating surface transmits pressure. The pressure distribution is not uniform. Depending on the location of the rim of the socket with respect to the point of application of the vector $\mathbf{H}$, the point of maximum pressure p_{max} is located somewhere between the rim and the point of force application. While the pressure medially from the

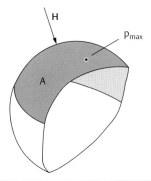

Fig. 13.15 Model of the hip joint; left hip, seen from the front. The loaded area of the femoral head is enclosed by the anterior and posterior rim of the acetabulum. The point of maximum pressure p_{max} is shifted from the point of application of the load vector $\mathbf{H}$ in the direction of the lateral rim of the acetabulum. (Adapted from Brinckmann et al.[12])

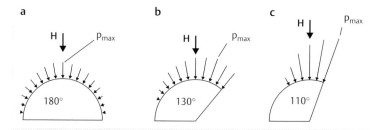

Fig. 13.16a–c Result of a model calculation of the pressure distribution on the surface of a completely (**a**) and an incompletely (**b, c**) covered ball-and-socket joint. The figure illustrates the magnitude and distribution of the pressure under the identical load **H**. (Adapted from Brinckmann et al.[14])

point of force application falls to zero, the pressure at the lateral rim of the socket is not equal to zero. The maximum pressure value depends on the magnitude of the load vector, the radius of the sphere, and the position of the load vector **H** relative to the rim of the socket.

For a congruent ball-and-socket joint (or for an initially incongruent joint that becomes congruent under load) we may assume as an initial approximation that the pressure distribution on the sphere follows a cosine distribution.[12–14] In a cosine distribution the pressure decreases from a specified point (designated as the pole of the distribution) with the cosine of the angle between the pole and a point on the sphere. Under this model assumption, Brinckmann et al[14] calculated the pressure distribution in relation to the coverage of the head by the acetabulum (**Fig. 13.16**). In the case of a sphere covered by the acetabulum over 180° (which is approximately true for mammals walking on four legs) the pressure takes its maximum value at the point of application of the force vector **H**. In the case of a sphere covered by 130° (corresponding roughly to the normal shape of human hip joints), the site of the point of maximum pressure is shifted towards the rim of the socket; the value of the maximum pressure is higher than in the case of the symmetrically covered joint. If the sphere is covered only by 110° (a model of a dysplastic acetabulum), the maximum pressure value increases again and the maximum pressure occurs at the lateral rim of the socket.

Yoshida et al[15] measured the articulating surface of the hip joint. Using the data of Bergmann et al[5,7] on the magnitude and direction of the load vector, they determined the magnitude of the pressure and the location of its maximum (**Fig. 13.17**) in several normal daily activities. **Table 13.2** shows that high pressure values are encountered when, because of the position of the femur, only a small section of the acetabulum is employed for the transmission of pressure. The magnitude of the joint load is higher during walking down stairs than during walking up stairs (see **Table 13.1**), but because the pressure-transmitting area is larger, the pressure during walking down stairs is *lower* than it is during walking up stairs.

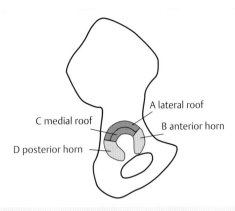

C medial roof

A lateral roof

B anterior horn

D posterior horn

Fig. 13.17 Regions of the acetabulum which are differently loaded during different activities (see **Table 13.2**). (Adapted, with permission, from Yoshida et al.[15])

Physical activity	Peak pressure [MPa]	Location of peak pressure	% of joint surface used
Fast walking	3.28	A	78.7
Normal walking	3.26	A	76.3
Slow walking	2.87	A	81.2
Rising from a chair	8.97	D	19.7
Sitting down	9.36	D	17.6
Squatting	3.65	D	51.6
Going up stairs	5.71	A	52.1
Going down stairs	3.77	A	80.6

Table 13.2 Peak pressures, sector of the acetabulum where they occur (see **Fig. 13.17**), and percentage of the joint surface (acetabular dome) used for pressure transmission, measured during various activities of daily living

Abbreviations: A, lateral roof of acetabulum; D, posterior horn of acetabulum.
Source: Data from Yoshida et al.[15]
Note: Body weight is assumed to be 700 N.

The numerous assumptions and approximations required in the model calculations determining pressure distribution on the hip joint make comparisons with direct experimental data desirable. Pressure sensitive foils have been developed for measuring pressure distributions over planar surfaces (or surfaces that can be unrolled into planar surfaces). These foils change color depending on the pressure exerted. Unfortunately the pressure distribution on the hip joint cannot be measured by means of these foils because planar foils cannot be fitted to the spherical femoral head without wrinkling or rippling.

Rushfeldt et al[16,17] employed an ultrasound probe for the measurement of the surface geometry and cartilage thickness of human hip joint specimens. These authors found that the cartilaginous surface of the acetabulum deviated by less than 0.15 mm from an ideal spherical shape. The underlying bone surface was not precisely spherical. With respect to its mean value, the thickness of the cartilage exhibited deviations of ± 0.5 mm. Subsequently, pressure distribution was measured, using the head of an artificial hip joint replacement instrumented with miniature pressure transducers. Along an anteroposterior path the measured distribution showed some resemblance to a cosine distribution; along a mediolateral path, however, the experimental distribution was definitely narrower than a cosine distribution. The extension of the area subject to pressure and the magnitude of the maximum pressure depended very strongly on the diameter of the instrumented artificial joint head. Even when the diameter of the instrumented head was selected to be as close as possible to that of the anatomic specimen acetabulum, it was not the whole area of the acetabulum that was subjected to pressure.

Brown and Shaw[18] instrumented specimens of femoral heads with 24 miniature pressure transducers mounted flush with the cartilaginous surface of the head. The femoral heads were then loaded via the corresponding acetabula. In the specimens investigated, the maximum of the pressure distribution was found within a cone of 30° with respect to the direction of the load vector. The site of maximum pressure appeared to shift randomly along an anteroposterior or mediolateral path.

A problem inherent in instrumented specimens is that the stiffness of the miniature pressure transducers is markedly different from that of trabecular bone and cartilage. We thus have to expect a transducer that has been inserted flush with the joint surface in an unloaded state to project from the surface in a loaded state, because the transducer material (which is metal) is stiffer than bone or cartilage. The measurements of Brown and Shaw show that the pressure distributions under prolonged loading vary over time due to the viscoelastic deformation of cartilage and trabecular bone.[18] For the same reason, we expect the magnitude of the pressure on the hip joint and the shape of the pressure distribution in vivo to vary in relation to the duration of the loading.

13.6 Mechanical Factors as a Primary Cause of Osteoarthritis of the Hip Joint

Several hypotheses have been put forward that relate mechanical factors to the development of osteoarthritis. Individually, these proposals offer some convincing arguments, but unfortunately there are some marked contradictions between them. A short overview follows.

Harrison et al[19] investigated degenerative changes in the cartilage of hip joint specimens. They found the first signs of degeneration of the cartilage, interpreted as signs of incipient osteoarthritis, in those parts of the joint surface that are expected to be subject to pressure only rarely, if at all. In erect stance, for example, these parts are the mediocaudal surface of the femoral head and, laterally, that portion of the surface of the head not in contact with the acetabulum. The authors concluded that too little pressure on the cartilage will trigger (or at least promote) degeneration of the cartilage.

Pauwels[1] hypothesized that osteoarthritis of the hip joint is caused by excessive pressure on certain parts of the joint surface, specifically in the region of the lateral rim of the acetabulum. Indeed, on radiographs of subjects with a less-than-normal lateral extension of the acetabulum, increased bone density can regularly be discerned in the region of the lateral aspect of the acetabulum. This increased density, which is seen even in young subjects, is interpreted as a reaction of the cartilage and the underlying bone to the excessively high mechanical stress. Pauwels showed that such signs of (incipient) joint damage regress after surgical interventions performed to relieve the load on the joint.

Radin et al[20,21] investigated the damping of peak forces using hip joint specimens. They found that damping is effected, not by the cartilage, but almost exclusively by the underlying trabecular bone. They hypothesized that, in vivo, short episodes of overloading damage primarily the trabecular bone. When the resulting microfractures are healed, the bone is stiffer. With less damping because of the increased bone stiffness, the cartilage is now more subject to mechanical damage by subsequent overloading episodes. According to this hypothesis, osteoarthritis begins not in the cartilage but in the bone. In accordance with this hypothesis, Brandt et al[22] have conjectured that osteoarthritis develops because of an imbalance between mechanical overloading and the physiological repair processes of joints.

Ganz et al[23] argue that not only a small acetabulum, but also an abnormally extended one may be responsible for damage to the joint. In certain orientations of the femur, bony contact may occur between the femoral neck and the acetabular rim. This results in stress concentrations at the point of contact and also at the opposite rim—because the resulting moment tends to lever the femoral head out of the acetabulum. In addition, these authors suggest that subtle deviations from normal joint geometry that may be present even at a young age—for example, small deviations from sphericity of the head, or local irregularities in cartilage thickness—may lead to osteoarthritis in later life.

Many important issues remain unresolved at present. While osteoarthritis probably does not develop as a result of a single episode of overloading, how the biological impact of repeated load cycles "adds up" is still unknown. For example, does a pressure of 2 MPa exerted 50 times on a particular region of cartilage have the same biological impact as a pressure of 1 MPa exerted 100 times? At what magnitude and temporal sequence of overloading episodes can the physiological repair processes no longer keep up with the damage produced? Such questions can only be answered by longitudinal in vivo observation. It may be the case that increased bone density contributes to the development of osteoarthritis—but bone density is affected by physical activity. As osteoarthritis progresses, pain reduces activity, and for this reason no conclusions about the etiology of osteoarthritis can be drawn on the basis of observations of bone density in individuals who already have the disease.[24] This is a question that can only be answered by measuring bone density in healthy persons and relating this to the incidence of osteoarthritis in the same population at a later date (see Yoshida et al[15]).

An increased prevalence of osteoarthritis of the hip and knee joint is observed in persons with physically demanding occupations (see, for example, Lievense et al[25] and Rossignol et al[26]). This suggests that high joint loads may cause the disease. On the other hand, it is quite possible that mechanical factors merely accelerate progression of the disease and/or aggravate its clinical symptoms. There is no conclusive evidence that athletic activities affect the development of osteoarthritis.[27] Obesity, defined as body mass index > 25, is associated with only a small increase in the incidence of osteoarthritis.[28]

In different orientations of the femur, the point of application of the load vector shows only a small variation relative to the femoral head. As mentioned above, this is because the relevant muscles course in approximately the same direction as the long axis of the femur, and thus their force vectors move with the femur. In relation to the acetabulum, however, the point of force application shows a large variation. In flexion of the hip joint, the point of force application is located in the posterior region; in extension it is located in the anterior region. The point of maximum pressure on the femoral head, then, is always in more or less the same place, whereas the point of maximum pressure on the acetabulum migrates over the entire contact area (see Yoshida et al[15]). If mechanical factors were primarily responsible for the development of osteoarthritis, one would expect to see overload damage in the femoral head first, not in the acetabulum. This seems not to be the case.

References

1. Pauwels F. Gesammelte Abhandlungen zur funktionellen Anatomie des Bewegungsapparates. Heidelberg: Springer; 1965

2. Paul JP. Force actions transmitted by joints in the human body. Proc R Soc Lond B Biol Sci 1976;192(1107):163–172

3. Stansfield BW, Nicol AC, Paul JP, Kelly IG, Graichen F, Bergmann G. Direct comparison of calculated hip joint contact forces with those measured using instrumented implants. An evaluation of a three-dimensional mathematical model of the lower limb. J Biomech 2003;36(7):929–936

4. Bergmann G. In-vivo-Messung der Belastung von Hüftimplantaten. Berlin: Köster; 1997. Wissenschaftliche Schriftenreihe Biomechanik; Band 2

5. Bergmann G, Deuretzbacher G, Heller M, et al. Hip contact forces and gait patterns from routine activities. J Biomech 2001;34(7):859–871

6. Bergmann G, Graichen F, Rohlmann A. Hip joint contact forces during stumbling. Langenbecks Arch Surg 2004;389(1):53–59

7. Bergmann G, Graichen F, Rohlmann A. Hip joint loading during walking and running, measured in two patients. J Biomech 1993;26(8):969–990

8. Bergmann G, Kniggendorf H, Graichen F, Rohlmann A. Influence of shoes and heel strike on the loading of the hip joint. J Biomech 1995;28(7):817–827

9. Bergmann G, Rohlmann A, Graichen F. In vivo Messung der Hüftgelenkbelastung. 1. Teil: Krankengymnastik. Z Orthop Ihre Grenzgeb 1989;127(6):672–679

10. Damm P, Graichen F, Rohlmann A, Bender A, Bergmann G. Total hip joint prosthesis for in vivo measurement of forces and moments. Med Eng Phys 2010;32(1):95–100

11. Bergmann G, Ed. Hip98: Loading of the Hip Joint [CD-ROM]. Berlin: Freie Universtät Berlin; 2001

12. Brinckmann P, Frobin W, Hierholzer E. Stress on the articular surface of the hip joint in healthy adults and persons with idiopathic osteoarthrosis of the hip joint. J Biomech 1981;14(3):149–156

13. Greenwald AS, O'Connor JJ. The transmission of load through the human hip joint. J Biomech 1971;4(6):507–528

14. Brinckmann P, Frobin W, Hierholzer E. Belastete Gelenkfläche und Beanspruchung des Hüftgelenks. Z Orthop Ihre Grenzgeb 1980;118(1):107–115

15. Yoshida H, Faust A, Wilckens J, Kitagawa M, Fetto J, Chao EY. Three-dimensional dynamic hip contact area and pressure distribution during activities of daily living. J Biomech 2006;39(11):1996–2004

16. Rushfeldt PD, Mann RW, Harris WH. Improved techniques for measuring in vitro the geometry and pressure distribution in the human acetabulum. I Ultrasonic measurement of acetabular surfaces, sphericity and cartilage thickness. J Biomech 1981;14(4):253–260

17. Rushfeldt PD, Mann RW, Harris WH. Improved techniques for measuring in vitro the geometry and pressure distribution in the human acetabulum. II Instrumented endoprosthesis measurement of articular surface pressure distribution. J Biomech 1981;14(5):315–323

18. Brown TD, Shaw DT. In vitro contact stress distributions in the natural human hip. J Biomech 1983;16(6):373–384

19. Harrison MH, Schajowicz F, Trueta J. Osteoarthritis of the hip: a study of the nature and evolution of the disease. J Bone Joint Surg Br 1953;35-B(4):598–626

20. Radin EL, Paul IL, Rose RM. Role of mechanical factors in pathogenesis of primary osteoarthritis. Lancet 1972;1(7749):519–522

21. Radin EL, Parker HG, Pugh JW, Steinberg RS, Paul IL, Rose RM. Response of joints to impact loading. 3. Relationship between trabecular microfractures and cartilage degeneration. J Biomech 1973;6(1):51–57

22. Brandt KD, Dieppe P, Radin EL. Etiopathogenesis of osteoarthritis. Rheum Dis Clin North Am 2008;34(3):531–559

23. Ganz R, Leunig M, Leunig-Ganz K, Harris WH. The etiology of osteoarthritis of the hip: an integrated mechanical concept. Clin Orthop Relat Res 2008;466(2):264–272

24. Hurwitz DE, Sumner DR, Block JA. Bone density, dynamic joint loading and joint degeneration. Cells Tissues Organs 2001;169(3):201–209

25. Lievense A, Bierma-Zeinstra S, Verhagen A, Verhaar J, Koes B. Influence of work on the development of osteoarthritis of the hip: a systematic review. J Rheumatol 2001;28(11):2520–2528

26. Rossignol M, Leclerc A, Allaert FA, et al. Primary osteoarthritis of hip, knee, and hand in relation to occupational exposure. Occup Environ Med 2005;62(11):772–777

27. Lievense AM, Bierma-Zeinstra SM, Verhagen AP, Bernsen RM, Verhaar JA, Koes BW. Influence of sporting activities on the development of osteoarthritis of the hip: a systematic review. Arthritis Rheum 2003;49(2):228–236

28. Lievense AM, Bierma-Zeinstra SM, Verhagen AP, van Baar ME, Verhaar JA, Koes BW. Influence of obesity on the development of osteoarthritis of the hip: a systematic review. Rheumatology (Oxford) 2002;41(10):1155–1162

14 Mechanical Aspects of the Knee Joint

14.1 Features Common to All Joints: The Example of the Knee Joint

Irrespective of the diversity of their outward appearance, the movable joints (diarthroses) of the locomotor system possess several common properties with respect to their architecture and mechanical function. These properties can be well demonstrated using the example of the knee joint.

14.1.1 Incongruency of the Articulating Bones

When examining the architecture of a "typical" joint, one is immediately aware that the surface shapes of the articulating bones do not match: the articulating surfaces are incongruent. In the knee joint (**Fig. 14.1**) neither the surfaces of the femur and tibia nor those of the femur and patella match exactly. Far from it: in fact, the shapes of their articulating surfaces are grossly different. This characteristic incongruency is common to virtually all joints of the body: think only of the joints of the hand, or the skeleton of the foot, or the vertebral joints. The hip joint, with its matching spherical head and spherical acetabular dome, seems to be an exception—though the academic discussion as to whether the head and acetabulum in the hip match precisely, or whether they start out incongruent and only develop congruency under load is not yet settled.

Contact between rigid bodies with incongruent surface shapes can occur only at points or along lines. In the joints of the human body, these points develop into contact areas between the articulating bones through the deformation of cartilage and bone under load. Nevertheless, these contact areas are usually small, so the pressure on them is accordingly high. In some highly loaded joints—between femur and tibia, for instance, and between vertebral bodies—nature considered it advantageous to place soft tissue (menisci, intervertebral disks) between the articulating bones to increase the articulating (pressure-transmitting) area and thus limit the magnitude of the pressure.

14.1.2 Architecture of the Bones in the Vicinity of a Joint

The dimensions of all bones are greater near the joints than in the mid-section of the bones. Like all long bones and like the vertebral bodies, the femur and tibia exhibit the typical waisted shape. However, the larger surface area thus created at the ends of the bones is not utilized as a whole for force transmission; because of the incongruency of the articulating surfaces, and depending on the position of the articulating bones, usually only a fraction of this area is placed under pressure. In the femur and tibia, the cortical bone beneath the articulating cartilage is very thin. The cortical bone in the mid-section of both these bones may well exceed 1 cm in thickness. Close to the joint, both femur and tibia are filled with

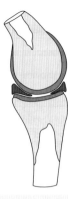

Fig. 14.1 Typical architecture of a joint: the femorotibial joint as an example. Note the increase in bone diameter in the vicinity of the joint, the incongruency of the articulating bones, the increase in pressure-transmitting area resulting from the insertion of soft tissue (dark gray) into the joint space, the coverage of the joint surfaces with cartilage (medium gray), and the subchondral trabecular bone (light gray) filling the bone volume below the articulating surface. (Adapted from Frost.[1])

trabecular bone; in their mid-portion they are practically hollow. These observations are broadly valid for the other long bones, too. (The only reason why vertebral bodies are completely filled with trabecular bone is because of their small height.) The thin layer of cortical bone and the trabecular bone beneath the surface of the joint are more easily deformable than a thicker layer of cortical bone. The resulting deformation under load effectively damps short peak forces, while at the same time it momentarily increases the pressure-transmitting area, further reducing the pressure on the joint surface.

14.1.3 Force-Transmitting Area

It seems that nature has "designed" all joints to tolerate high localized pressure. At the same time, during joint motion the loaded area shifts and so alternating loading and unloading occur. It is assumed that the resulting variation in pressure is of importance both for maintaining the friction properties of the joint and for cartilage metabolism. **Fig. 14.2** shows data on the contact area between the femur and the tibia measured with and without menisci. As stated above, even with intact menisci the contact area between femur and tibia never extends over the entire tibial plateau. The pressure-loaded area is seen to shift with the motion of the joint. As flexion increases, the contact area shifts from anterior to posterior. When menisci are missing, the contact area is reduced by a factor of 2 to 3. In the femoropatellar joint (**Fig. 14.3**) the patella, despite the great thickness of its cartilage, never comes into complete contact with the femoral condyles. The shifting of the contact area between patella and femur with knee flexion is clearly visible.

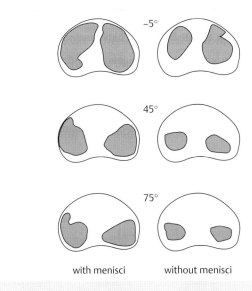

Fig. 14.2 Size and location of the contact area between the femur and the tibia with and without menisci, related to the flexion angle of the knee joint. (Adapted from Maquet.[2])

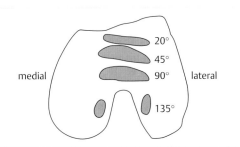

Fig. 14.3 Size and location of the contact area between the femur and the patella. (Adapted from Seedholm et al.[3])

14.1.4 Friction Properties of Joint Surfaces

The coefficients of static and kinetic friction between cartilage surfaces wetted by synovial fluid are very small. The coefficient of static friction between cartilage surfaces amounts (depending on test conditions) to between 0.001 and 0.005.[4,5] In broad terms, therefore, we may regard the knee joint, and all other joints with cartilage surfaces, as friction-free. As high forces are transmitted through the joints, low friction is of extreme importance to their mechanical functioning. If friction in the joints was at any appreciable level, the joints would become virtually immobile and thus useless under high load, due to the high moment exerted by the friction force. In a moving joint shear forces act on the joint surfaces. If shear forces were to become too high, due to a large coefficient of friction, the cartilage could be damaged.

14.1.5 Guidance of the Joint Motion by Ligaments

The integrity of the joints, the guidance of their motion, and the restriction of the range of motion is brought about by ligaments. If the ligaments are torn or destroyed, the joints "fall apart" and their range of motion is no longer controlled. These observations are likewise valid for the cruciate and collateral ligaments of the knee as well as, for example, for the ligaments of the hand skeleton or the spinal ligaments. The guidance of motion by the shape of the articulating bones (as seen in the hip joint) or solely by muscles (as between the scapula and the thorax) are exceptions to the general rule.

14.2 Motion of the Knee Joint

The architecture of the knee joint and the description of its motion have fascinated many researchers. Some examples from the large number of studies in the field, which describe the motion of the joint from different points of view, are discussed below. The descriptions and interpretations range from the greatly simplified to the mathematically complex. Which description one chooses depends on its intended use.

14.2.1 Knee Joint Modeled as a Pure Hinge Joint

If the knee joint is modeled as a hinge joint with its axis of rotation oriented perpendicular to the sagittal plane, the location of the axis can be determined from measurements on specimens (see Chapter 6). With the tibia held in a fixed position, two small metallic markers (easily visible in a radiograph) are placed on the femur (**Fig. 14.4**). Radiographs are taken with the joint in extension and in flexion. Under

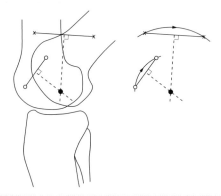

Fig. 14.4 Protocol for measuring the location of the center of rotation of the knee joint. Two markers are placed on the femur of a knee joint specimen. As the joint is moved while the tibia is held in a fixed position, the markers move in concentric circles around the center of rotation. The center of rotation is given by the point of intersection of the perpendicular bisectors of the lines connecting the locations of the two markers.

the assumptions of the model of a hinge, during the change from extension to flexion the marks move in concentric circles about the center of rotation. The radiographs do not show the trajectories of the movement, only its start and end points. The common center of the circles, the center of rotation, is given by the intersection of the perpendicular bisectors of the chords.

If, however, the joint is moved in small angular intervals, and if the procedure depicted in **Fig. 14.4** is repeated for each of these intervals, it turns out that the location of the center of rotation determined in this way shifts by a few millimeters as a function of the joint angle. This observation is an indicator that the hinge model of the joint gives only an approximate description of the joint's true motion. If one disregards this detail, the center of rotation of the knee joint is located in the posterior third of the femoral condyle and approximately 2.5 cm above the tibial plateau. This specification suffices for the determination of moment arms of muscles or external loads for the purposes of estimating the load on the femorotibial joint.

14.2.2 Motion of the Knee Seen as Guided by the Cruciate Ligaments

Menschik[6] described the motion of the knee guided by the cruciate ligaments by a surprisingly simple model. If we assume that the length of the cruciate ligaments remains unchanged in the course of the flexion–extension motion, the cruciates guide the motion of the femur relative to the tibia like a four-bar linkage. The four bars of this linkage are formed by the two cruciates and the lines connecting their points of insertion into the femur and tibia. Under the assumptions of this model, the instantaneous center of rotation is located at the point of intersection of the cruciates (**Fig. 14.5**). The rationale for this is that, in the case of a finite motion of the tibia with respect to the femur, the center of rotation C_1 is constructed as the intersection of the perpendicular bisectors of the lines $B_1–B'_1$ and $A_1–A'_1$. In the case of a very small

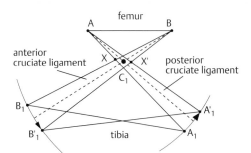

Fig. 14.5 Description of the motion of the knee joint using the model of a four-bar linkage. It is assumed that the bars do not change their length in the course of the movement. The instantaneous center of rotation is located at the point of intersection of the two bars representing the cruciate ligaments. (Adapted from Müller.[7])

(infinitesimal) motion, the points of intersection X and X_1 of the cruciates coincide with the point C_1. If the joint is flexed, the location of the center of rotation constructed thus is shifted posteriorly and proximally (**Fig. 14.6**). If the path of the collateral ligaments is viewed in addition (**Fig. 14.7**), these ligaments are found to cross in a region close to the instantaneous center of rotation. Crossing the center of rotation

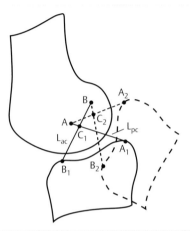

Fig. 14.6 Shift in the location of the center of rotation in relation to the flexion angle under the assumptions of the model of the four-bar linkage. L_{ac} and L_{pc}, anterior and posterior cruciate ligaments.

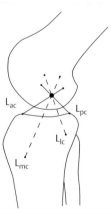

Fig. 14.7 The collateral ligaments cross close to the intersection of the cruciate ligaments—that is, in the region of the instantaneous center of rotation of the knee joint. L_{mc} and L_{lc}, medial and lateral collateral ligaments; L_{ac} and L_{pc}, anterior and posterior cruciate ligaments. (Adapted from Menschik.[6])

ensures that the change in the length of the collateral ligaments during flexion or extension of the knee remains small.

Contrary to the assumptions of Menschik's model,[6] the diameters of the two femoral condyles are not equal, and some fiber bundles of the cruciate ligaments do actually change their length during flexion and extension.[8–10] Fuss[9] showed that over the whole range of motion only a fraction of the fibers of the cruciate ligaments are continuously under tension. Due to the extended (rather than punctiform) area of insertion of the cruciates, a constant tensile stress on all fiber bundles is impossible for geometrical reasons alone. The fibers under tension guide the motion and limit the posteroanterior translation of the tibia relative to the femur. At the end points of motion, however, all fibers are under tension.

14.2.3 Interpretation of Knee Motion Based on the Shape of the Condyles

Freeman and Pinskerova[11] pointed out that the contour of the femoral condyles can be subdivided into three regions (**Fig. 14.8**). In region 1, the region of contact in maximum extension (approximately −5° to 20°), the contour may be approximated by a circle with a midpoint Z_1 and a radius slightly greater than 30 mm. In region 2, representing normal, active motion from about 20° to 120° of flexion, the contour more or less circular with a midpoint at Z_2 and a radius slightly greater than 20 mm. In region 3, the region of maximum active and passive flexion (approximately 120° to 140°), the radius of the medial condyle is somewhat smaller than in region 2. Taken together, the three circular contours combine to form an approximately elliptical shape.

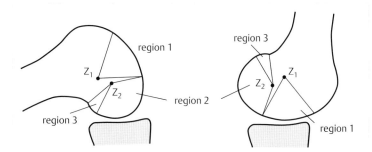

Fig. 14.8 Regions of joint contact in the femorotibial joint. Region 1: region of maximum extension; region 2: region used for normal activities; region 3: region of maximum flexion. (Adapted, with permission, from Freeman and Pinskerova.[11])

In the region of normal, active motion between 20° and 120° of flexion, the joint rotates about an axis through Z_2. In this region, rotation of the tibia about its longitudinal axis is also possible, but is not rigidly coupled with the flexion motion. In this region the medial condyle approximates a spherical joint, because in the frontal plane the curvature of the lateral condyle is smaller than the curvature of the

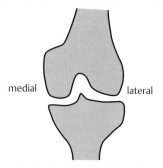

Fig. 14.9 Difference in the contours of the femoral condyles in the frontal plane. (Adapted, with permission, from Freeman and Pinskerova.[11])

medial condyle (**Fig. 14.9**). The lateral condyle slides and rolls in the posterior and anterior directions, thus enabling the rotation of the tibia about its long axis.[12] Some studies, in specimens as well as in vivo, have demonstrated obligatory coupling between extension and external rotation in the region of maximum extension between 20° and −5° (see, for example, Moro-oka et al[13]). This coupled motion is termed *screw home motion*. This external rotation, which is in the order of 15°, is hypothesized to be due to an asymmetry of the femoral condyles in region 1 or to the anterior cruciate ligament. Other studies were unable to confirm the existence of a screw home motion. Apparently considerable interindividual differences exist in respect of this motion, or it may be possible that measurement errors could simulate its existence.[14]

14.2.4 Description of Knee Motion in Terms of a Helical Axis

Combining flexion and extension, external and internal rotation, and medial and lateral translation of the femur and tibia, the motion of the knee joint is motion in three-dimensional space. This motion can be described as rotation about and simultaneous translation along an axis oriented in space, termed a *helical axis* (see Chapter 7). Blankevoort et al[15] determined the location and orientation of the helical axis in knee joint specimens by measuring flexion motion carried out in small steps combined with a moment effecting internal or external rotation about the tibia. (The additional moment was used to obtain reproducible data for the helical axes. Without this moment, minor adjustment errors or uncontrollable forces exerted by the experimental setup would cause wide scatter of the results.) Metallic markers were placed on the femur and tibia of the specimens and the position of the markers was measured with high precision by stereoradiography. The location and orientation of the helical axis was computed from the relative motion of the tibial and femoral markers. Since the motion was performed in steps of approximately 4°, the axis determined in this way is referred to as a *finite* helical axis. This in contrast to the *instantaneous* helical axis

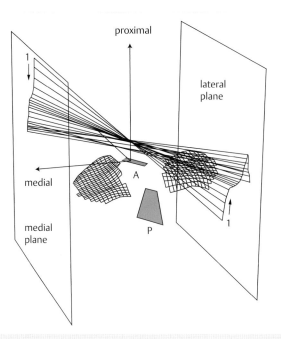

Fig. 14.10 Finite helical axis of the knee joint, determined in 4° increments from full extension to 95° flexion (with additional internal rotation of the tibia). 1: axis for full extension. A and P designate the areas of insertion of the anterior and posterior cruciate ligaments on the tibia. (Adapted, with permission, from Blankevoort et al.[15])

which would have been obtained from the observation of infinitesimal steps of motion. After the motion had been observed, the specimens were dissected. After placement of additional markers, stereoradiography was then used again to map the articulating surfaces and the insertion areas of the cruciate ligaments and relate them to the three-dimensional coordinate systems fixed to the tibia and the femur.

For pure flexion and extension in the sagittal plane one would intuitively expect the orientation of the helical axis to be horizontal. For a pure internal or external rotation of the tibia one would expect it to be vertical. For a motion combining flexion and rotation we would thus expect the axis to be oriented obliquely. **Fig. 14.10** shows as an example the helical axis in the coordinate system of the tibia. The measurements were performed in increments of approximately 4° from full extension to 95° flexion. In the example shown, a moment effecting internal rotation acted on the tibia. The authors observed that in almost all cases the helical axes they determined crossed the space between the insertion areas of the cruciate ligaments. In this respect their findings are qualitatively consistent with the Menschik model,[6] which predicts a center of rotation at the intersection of the cruciate ligaments.

14.2.5 So-called Compromise Axis of the Knee Joint

Ideally the axis of rotation of an orthosis should coincide with the anatomical axis of rotation of the knee, because a rotation cannot occur simultaneously about two different axes. Commonly orthoses for the knee joint are equipped with pure hinge joints because of their simple construction and reliable functioning. Experience does also show that persons with a total knee replacement of the hinge joint type can walk without problems. We thus expect that having knee joint motion guided by an orthosis with a pure hinge joint should not result in major functional constraints. It might well be possible to devise joints for orthoses that are better adapted to the anatomical motion, but to do this properly would require determining the location and orientation of the axis of rotation of the anatomical joint in the individual patient. In practice this cannot be done, because when markers are placed externally, the movement of the soft tissues makes it impossible to measure the motion of the femur and tibia precisely. Measurement employing radiography is ruled out because of the radiation exposure.

From radiographs of specimens of the knee joint, Nietert[16] reconstructed the point where the rotational axis for plane flexion and extension intersected with the sagittal plane. He observed that the location of this point (the center of rotation) varied only within a very small area (**Fig. 14.11**). A fixed axis running through the center of this region is called a *compromise axis*, as it disregards the details of the shifting of the true axis during the motion. We may assume that this axis coincides approximately with the axes resulting from Menschik's[6] or Freeman's[11] models discussed above. Nietert[16] proposed adjusting the axis of an orthosis as shown in **Fig. 14.12**. To do this, the external diameter D of the knee is measured and the location of the joint line is palpated. An orthosis fitted as shown here will not noticeably interfere with the physiological motion of the joint. Any unavoidable remaining divergences between the axes of the

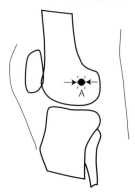

Fig. 14.11 Reconstruction of the axis of rotation of the knee from radiographs. A, area where the axes intersect the sagittal plane. (Adapted from Nietert.[16])

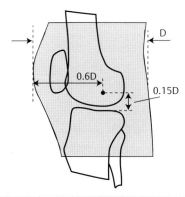

Fig. 14.12 How to locate the "compromise axis" of the knee joint, based on measurement of the outer dimension of the knee and palpation of the joint space. (Adapted from Nietert.[16])

orthosis and the anatomical knee will result in tilting and translation of the orthosis relative to the thigh and lower leg, but experience shows that small amounts of tilting and translation are easily absorbed by the soft tissues.

14.3 Load on the Femorotibial and Femoropatellar Joint

Fig. 14.13 depicts the forces of the quadriceps, hamstrings, and gastrocnemius muscles which serve to balance external moments acting in the sagittal plane. As an example of estimating the load on the femorotibial joint, we will take a static posture with an upright trunk and bent knee (**Fig. 14.14**). The distance between the center of mass of the body, where the gravitational force acts, and the support

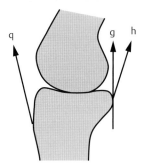

Fig. 14.13 The quadriceps (q), gastrocnemius (g), and hamstring muscles (h) cross the knee joint. (Adapted, with permission, from Schipplein and Andriacchi.[17])

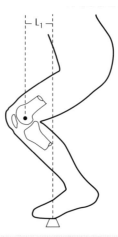

Fig. 14.14 In static equilibrium the center of mass of a body is located perpendicularly above the area of support; that is, above the heads of the metatarsal bones. L_1 is the moment arm of the gravitational force of the body mass (less the mass of the lower leg and foot) in relation to the center of rotation of the knee joint.

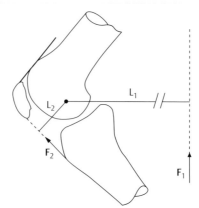

Fig. 14.15 Moment arm L_1 of the force $\mathbf{F}_1$ exerted by the floor on the leg and moment arm L_2 of the force $\mathbf{F}_2$ of the patellar tendon in relation to the center of rotation of the knee.

under the metatarsals is equal to L_1 (because in a static stable posture the center of mass must be located perpendicularly above the base of support). The force $\mathbf{F}_1$ is exerted by the floor on the foot (**Fig. 14.15**). Equilibrium is maintained by the force $\mathbf{F}_2$ of the patella tendon which has the moment arm L_2. The magnitude of force $\mathbf{F}_2$ thus amounts to $F_2 = F_1 \cdot L_1/L_2$. The posture shown in **Fig. 14.14** is similar to that adopted when walking up stairs. When standing on one leg, the magnitude of force $\mathbf{F}_1$ is approximately equal to

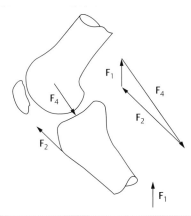

Fig. 14.16 Equilibrium of forces at the tibia if only three forces are assumed to be active. F_1 is the force exerted by the floor on the foot, F_2 the force of the patellar tendon, and F_4 the force exerted by the femur on the tibia. It can be seen from the diagram that the femorotibial force is greater than the force of the patellar tendon.

the body weight (disregarding the weight of the lower leg and foot). The greater the height (rise) of the stair—and, therefore, the greater the bending angle of the knee—the greater moment arm L_1 will be; in consequence, the magnitude of force F_2 can equate to several times the body weight. Looking at the equilibrium of forces at the tibia (ignoring the forces of other muscles and of the cruciate ligaments) (**Fig. 14.16**), it can be seen that the force F_4 exerted by the femur on the tibia is greater than the force F_2 of the patellar tendon. It follows that if, in a given posture, the patellar tendon is loaded by several times the body weight, the same will be true of the force between the femur and the tibia.

With bending angles greater than about 120°, the situation changes.[18] When the knee is deeply bent, there is contact and thus transmission of force between the thigh and the lower leg. The force F_L on the lower leg (**Fig. 14.17**) exerts a moment on the knee in the opposite direction to the moment of the force F_1 exerted by the floor on the foot. This results in a reduction of the force of the patellar tendon. If there is contact between the knee and the floor, force F_1 is further reduced because a fraction F_C of the gravitational force is now transmitted directly by the knee. This results in a reduction of the moment acting on the knee and consequently in a reduction of the force of the patellar tendon.

In one-legged stance and static equilibrium, the center of mass of the body is located vertically above the sole of the foot (**Fig. 14.18**). As the femur and tibia are not aligned exactly to the vertical, the ground reaction force F_1 creates a moment in the frontal plane with respect to the center of rotation of the knee. This moment must be balanced by a moment of the muscle force F_6, which represents the force of the gluteus maximus and tensor fasciae latae. If force F_6 is not sufficient to maintain equilibrium, the lateral

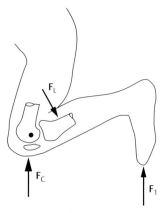

Fig. 14.17 In a deep kneel a fraction of the body weight F_L will be transmitted directly from the thigh onto the lower leg. If contact is made between the knee and the floor, the gravitational force of the body is redistributed to the forces F_C and F_1.

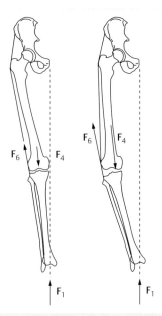

Fig. 14.18 Equilibrium of forces on the tibia in the frontal plane when standing on one leg. Active forces: force F_1 from the floor onto the foot (opposite and equal to the gravitational force of the body mass), the femorotibial force F_4, and force F_6 designating the combined force of the gluteus maximus muscle and the tensor fasciae latae. The line of action of F_1 passes medial and the line of action of F_6 lateral to the knee joint. Where there is a varus deformity, the moment arm of force F_1 increases.

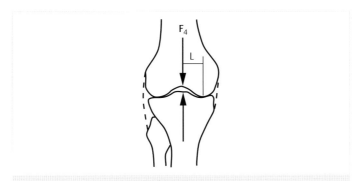

Fig. 14.19 The moment $L \cdot F_4$ acts in the opposite direction to an adduction moment on the tibia. (Adapted, with permission, from Schipplein and Andriacchi.[17])

collateral ligament must generate a part of the moment. This ligament is then loaded in tension and strained. The femorotibial joint opens laterally and the load is shifted onto the medial part of the joint. The result is a varus malalignment of the leg. Normally, the femorotibial load F_4 is oriented perpendicular to the joint surface of the tibia and runs through the center of the knee (**Fig. 14.19**). In relation to the contact point of the medial condyle, this force exerts a moment $L \cdot F_4$ in the opposite direction to an adduction moment acting on the tibia. Thus, in a healthy joint both condyles are under approximately equal load. This is the reasoning behind the proposal to respond to a malalignment by increasing the force F_4 through antagonistic activation of the quadriceps and hamstrings, to counteract any lateral opening of the joint. An alternative proposal is to make use of a laterally wedged sole or insole to shift the point of application of force F_1 laterally in order to reduce the moment of this force on the knee.

The dynamic load on the knee joint can be determined from gait analysis. Input data for the calculation are the mass, location of the center of mass, and moment of inertia of the foot and lower leg, the measured temporal course of the location, velocity, and acceleration of these segments, and the force between the floor and the foot. It is then possible to calculate the reaction force and the reaction moment transmitted from the upper to the lower leg. Employing a model of the knee joint—that is, with knowledge of the directions and moment arms of all the muscles and ligaments involved—the load on the knee joint can then be determined. Due to the complex architecture of the knee joint, there are initially more unknowns than equilibrium equations. Morrison[19] and Paul[20] reduced the indeterminate system to a determinate one by representing the forces of several muscles and ligaments by a single force and by neglecting (on the basis of electromyography measurements) certain forces in specific phases of the gait cycle. For example, in flexion or extension of the knee only the quadriceps or only the gastrocnemius or only the hamstrings were taken into consideration. Later studies have been based on detailed models of the architecture of muscles, tendons, and ligaments. Shelburne et al,[21] for example, included 13 muscle and 14 ligament forces. To solve

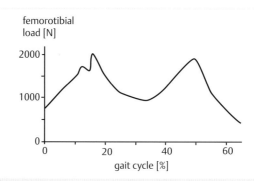

Fig. 14.20 Femorotibial load during gait, calculated for a subject of 700 N body weight. (Adapted from Shelburne et al.[21])

the indeterminate model calculation, energy consumption when walking was chosen as an additional constraint. **Fig. 14.20** shows the femorotibial force in the course of a step calculated in this way.

Heinlein et al[22] developed a total knee prosthesis that was instrumented for direct measurement of the force vector acting from the femur onto the tibia. The measured results do not depend on model assumptions of architecture, activation, and load sharing between muscles and ligaments. They demonstrate the magnitude of the forces to which artificial joint replacements are exposed in the body. **Table 14.1** reports force components in the direction of the longitudinal axis of the tibia as measured in two patients.

Activity	Load [× body weight]
Walking on level ground	2.5
Walking up stairs	3.0
Walking down stairs	3.5

Table 14.1 Maximum values (rounded) of the load on the femorotibial joint: components of the load in the direction of the longitudinal axis of the tibia

Source: Data from Heinlein et al.[22]

The menisci between the femur and tibia serve to increase the force-transmitting area of the joint surface. In the loaded joint the menisci are squeezed toward the periphery of the joint; this results in tensile stress both in the volume of the menisci and at their insertions (**Fig. 14.21**). It is hypothesized that this tensile straining of the menisci may contribute to the damping of peak forces on the knee. The contact area of the femorotibial joint amounts to about 20 cm² if the knee is fully extended.[2,23] Roughly one half of the joint load is then transmitted by the menisci.[24] As can be seen from **Fig. 14.2**, if menisci are missing, the force-transmitting area decreases by about 50%, and consequently the pressure rises to about twice its

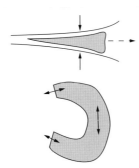

Fig. 14.21 Tensile stress in a meniscus in a loaded knee joint.

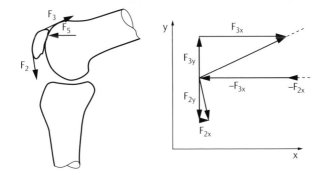

Fig. 14.22 Equilibrium of forces at the patella. On the patella act the force F_2 of the patellar tendon, the force F_3 of the quadriceps tendon and the femoropatellar force F_5. The directions of F_2 and F_3 are given by the anatomical directions of the tendons; F_5 is oriented perpendicularly to the contact area of patella and femur (modeled as a plane).

original value.[25] The high pressure to be anticipated where menisci are missing is believed to be responsible for premature development of arthritis in the joint (see, for example, Rath and Richmond[26]).

For calculation of the force between femur and patella, the equilibrium of forces at the patella is considered (**Fig. 14.22**). Three forces act on the patella, the force F_3 of the quadriceps tendon, the force F_2 of the patellar tendon, and the force F_5 between the femur and the patella. In static equilibrium the sum of these forces must be equal to zero. The directions of force F_2 of the patellar tendon and of force F_3 of the quadriceps tendon are taken from anatomical or radiographic measurements. The magnitude of force F_2 of the patellar tendon is determined from the equilibrium condition of moments (see example in **Fig. 14.15**). Since the friction between femur and patella is negligible, force F_5 between the femur and the patella is directed perpendicular to the (approximately plane) area of contact between these bones. The x-axis of the xy-coordinate system is set parallel to the direction of $\mathbf{F}_5$. Equilibrium of the y-components of forces $\mathbf{F}_2$ and $\mathbf{F}_3$ ($\mathbf{F}_5$ has no y-component) results in

(14.1)
$$\mathbf{F}_{3y} = -\mathbf{F}_{2y}$$

As the direction of $\mathbf{F}_3$ is known, we may now construct the x-component of the quadriceps force. In equilibrium it holds for the x-components of the forces $\mathbf{F}_2$, $\mathbf{F}_3$, and $\mathbf{F}_5$ that

(14.2)
$$\mathbf{F}_{5x} = -\mathbf{F}_{2x} - \mathbf{F}_{3x}$$
$$\mathbf{F}_{5y} = 0$$

As a result, the force $\mathbf{F}_5$ (equal to $\mathbf{F}_{5x}$) between femur and patella is known.

If the equilibrium of forces is inspected at other angles of flexion, the magnitude of the force $\mathbf{F}_2$ of the patellar tendon may take on different values. In addition, the direction of the forces $\mathbf{F}_2$ and $\mathbf{F}_3$ of the quadriceps and patellar tendons will change. **Fig. 14.23** shows the numerical results of the calculation of the loading of the femoropatellar joint in relation to the angle of flexion of the knee, here in one-legged stance for a person of 85 kg body mass. The steep increase in load with the angle of flexion can be seen. This is why persons whose bone strength has been reduced by osteoporosis are advised against performing deep knee bends during quadriceps strength training or when lifting objects up off the floor. **Fig. 14.24** shows the load on the femoropatellar joint during gait calculated for a person of 70 kg body mass using a model calculation.[21] Cohen et al[28] investigated the load on the femoropatellar joint in both open- and closed-chain

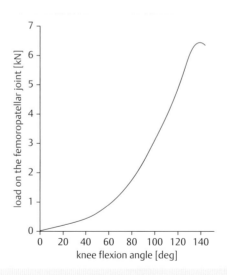

Fig. 14.23 Load on the femoropatellar joint in relation to the flexion angle. Data refer to a body mass of 85 kg and a knee bend on one leg. (Adapted from Reilly and Martens.[27])

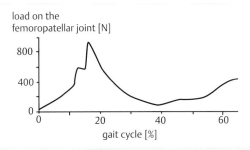

Fig. 14.24 Load on the femoropatellar joint during gait, calculated using a model for a person of 700 N body weight. (Adapted from Shelburne et al.[21])

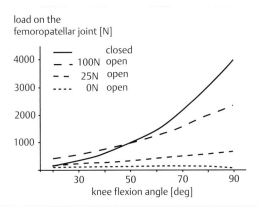

Fig. 14.25 Load on the femoropatellar joint during closed-chain flexion (squat) and open-chain flexion with additional resistance acting at the ankle. (Adapted from Cohen et al.[28])

exercises, during performance of knee bends, and during active extension of the knee against the gravitational force of the lower leg and foot as well as with additional loads of 25 N and 100 N. **Fig. 14.25** shows that the loads on the femoropatellar joint during knee bends and during active extension with additional load are of comparable magnitude.

The pressure distribution in the femoropatellar joint can be measured by means of pressure-sensitive foils. Unlike in joints with strongly curved surfaces, this measuring method can be applied here because the contact area between the femur and the patella is practically plane. Huberti and Hayes[29] showed that the pressure on the articulating surface is near-enough uniform. In specimens with pathologic changes such as chondromalacia patellae, Huberti and Hayes[30] observed nonuniform pressure distributions.

The etiology of retropatellar afflictions is still a matter of debate (see for example Selfe[31]). As these afflictions occur predominantly in postures where the knees are flexed (stair climbing, prolonged sitting), some observers hypothesize that an unphysiologic position and/or orientation of the patella with respect to the femur causes high local pressure on the joint surface (see for example Brechter and Powers[32]). Various treatment protocols thus aim to achieve a better geometrical fit between patella and femur so as to bring about an increase in contact area with a subsequent decrease in peak pressure. The methods of treatment are (1) specific training of the vastus medialis obliquus, medialis, and lateralis; (2) a bandage exerting a medially directed force on the patella; (3) orthoses for the knee joint; and (4) laterally wedged soles or insoles applied to bring about internal rotation of the tibia about its long axis.

14.4   Loading of the Cruciate Ligaments

The cruciate ligaments guide the motion of femur and tibia; in addition they limit the range of motion in flexion and extension. Furthermore, the cruciates balance shear forces in the plane of the tibial plateau that are generated by the muscles spanning the knee joint or by external forces. An anteriorly directed shear force acting on the tibia stresses the anterior cruciate ligament; a posteriorly directed force stresses the posterior cruciate ligament. In either case only one cruciate ligament is loaded while the other one remains unloaded. In addition, observations from knee joint specimens[33, 34] show that the rotational stiffness of the tibia about its longitudinal axis decreases if cruciates are missing (**Fig. 14.26**). As measured from specimens, the tensile strength of the anterior cruciate ligament ranges between 1000 N and 2000 N.[35] The tensile strength of the posterior cruciate ligament of healthy, physically active individuals is in the order

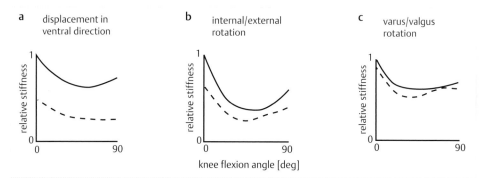

Fig. 14.26a–c Comparison of the stiffness of the knee after sectioning of the anterior cruciate ligament with the stiffness of the intact knee. Solid curves, intact knee; dashed curves, knee without anterior cruciate ligament. (Adapted from Crowninshield et al.[33])

a Ventral displacement of the tibia.

b Internal/external rotation of the tibia.

c Varus/valgus motion.

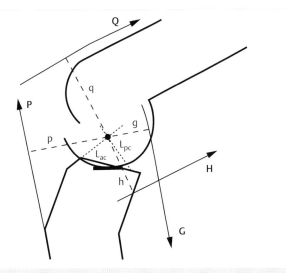

Fig. 14.27 Model of the knee joint. **G, H, P, Q**, forces of the gastrocnemius, hamstrings, patellar tendon, and quadriceps; g, h, p, q, appertaining moment arms related to the center of rotation of the joint; L_{ac} and L_{pc}, anterior and posterior cruciate ligaments. (Adapted, with permission, from O'Connor et al.[36])

of 4000 N. These observations support the conjecture that the cruciates are highly loaded in everyday life. (The argument is that a ligament exposed to only minor loading would adapt to its mechanical requirements and exhibit only a low tensile strength.)

Model calculations determining the loading of the cruciate ligaments have been published by several authors (see, for example, O'Connor et al[36] and Pandy and Shelburne[37]). The knee joint is spanned by the quadriceps and gastrocnemius muscles and the hamstrings. In addition, forces can be transmitted by the cruciate ligaments and the femorotibial joint. Due to the many unknowns, calculations cannot be performed without simplifications and/or additional assumptions. **Fig. 14.27** illustrates the model of O'Connor et al.[36] Input data are, at each flexion angle, the direction of the muscle forces and the moment arm derived from anatomical observations for quadriceps, gastrocnemius, and hamstrings, and the direction of the patellar and quadriceps tendons. The center of rotation is assumed to be located at the intersection of the cruciate ligaments. The model shown in **Fig. 14.27** can be used to help visualize the loading of the cruciate ligaments in specific postures. For example, if the quadriceps is activated with the knee extended, the anteriorly forward-oblique orientation of the patellar tendon gives rise to an anteriorly directed force exerted on the tibia and the anterior cruciate ligament comes under load. If, however, the knee is flexed 90°, the patellar tendon is aligned in the vertical direction. The tendon is under load, but because of its direction there is no generation of shear force with respect to the tibial plateau. Now the anterior cruciate ligament is not under load.

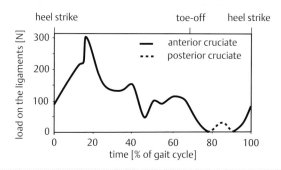

Fig. 14.28 Load on the cruciate ligaments during gait. (Adapted, with permission, from Shelburne et al.[38])

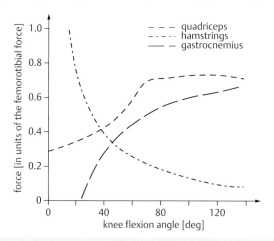

Fig. 14.29 Simultaneous activation of quadriceps, gastrocnemius, and hamstrings effecting mechanical equilibrium above 20° of knee flexion. Up to 20° of flexion, equilibrium of forces can be achieved merely by activation of the quadriceps and hamstrings. (Adapted, with permission, from O'Connor et al.[36])

Fig. 14.28 shows the results of a model calculation of the load on the cruciate ligaments during gait.[38] Here again the peak loading of the anterior cruciate ligament is seen after heel strike in the phase of knee extension and maximum activation of the quadriceps. (The combination of extended knee and activation of the quadriceps will be referred to again below in the discussion of potential causes of injury of the anterior cruciate ligament.)

There are some people who exhibit virtually normal gait despite an injury to the anterior cruciate ligament. In such cases the only documented abnormality is an increased bending angle of the knee at heel strike and prolonged activity of the hamstrings.[39] From **Fig. 14.27** it can be seen that the force of the hamstrings generates

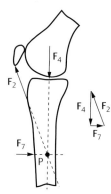

Fig. 14.30 Forces acting on the tibia during isometric activation of the quadriceps. If the lines of action of the three forces intersect at P, the sum of their moments equals zero. (Adapted from Zavatsky et al.[41])

a posteriorly directed shear force on the tibia. This force may (at least partially) compensate an anteriorly directed shear force on the tibia. O'Connor[40] showed that in the context of his model complete unloading of the anterior cruciate ligament by antagonistic activation of quadriceps and hamstrings is possible, but only at bending angles below 20°. At larger bending angles, antagonistic (angle-dependent) activation of the gastrocnemius is required in addition (**Fig. 14.29**). By what means persons with an injured anterior cruciate ligament control the angle-dependent activation of the three muscle groups to achieve normal gait remains unresolved.

Zavatsky et al[41] used the model of O'Connor and coworkers to analyze the loading of the cruciate ligaments during isometric activation of the quadriceps or the hamstrings, both commonly prescribed exercises during the rehabilitation of patients with cruciate ligament injuries. **Fig. 14.30** depicts the equilibrium of forces at the tibia during isometric activation of the quadriceps. The tibia is acted upon by the force of the patellar tendon F_2, the femorotibial force F_4, which is oriented perpendicular to the tibial plateau, and the external force F_7, which impedes rotational motion of the lower leg and thus a change in length of the quadriceps. If in this configuration the force F_7 is applied so that the lines of action of F_2, F_4, and F_7 intersect at a single point P, the sum of their moments equals zero: that is, there is equilibrium of moments. The magnitude of F_7 depends on the magnitudes of F_2 and F_4; in mechanical equilibrium the sum of these three forces must equal zero (**Fig. 14.30**, right-hand diagram). No additional forces are then required to maintain mechanical equilibrium. In other words, in this geometrical configuration the cruciate ligaments are not under load. If the bending angle of the knee is changed, the location of point P shifts due to the change in the direction of the patellar tendon. **Fig. 14.30** shows that, to keep the cruciate ligaments free from load, the point of application of force F_7 must be shifted distally when the bending angle of the knee is increased (**Fig. 14.31**). Analogous arguments hold for the isometric activation of the hamstrings.

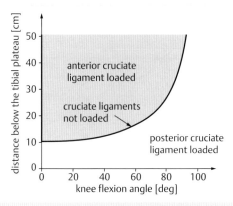

Fig. 14.31 Point of application of force on the tibia in relation to the flexion angle of the knee for the case that the cruciate ligaments remain unloaded during isometric activation of the quadriceps. If the point of force application moves from the point shown, the result will be a load on the anterior or posterior cruciate ligament. (Adapted from Zavatsky et al.[41])

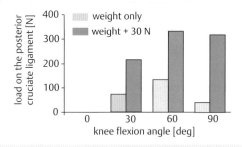

Fig. 14.32 Setup for loading the hamstrings against gravity or against an additional resistance acting at the ankle joint in an open-chain exercise. (Adapted, with permission, from Mesfar and Shirazi-Adl.[42])

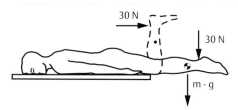

Fig. 14.33 Loading of the posterior cruciate ligament in the exercise illustrated in **Fig. 14.32**. During this exercise, the load on the anterior cruciate ligament was less than 6 N. (Adapted, with permission, from Mesfar Shirazi-Adl.[42])

Mesfar and Shirazi-Adl[42] calculated the load on the cruciate ligaments when the knee is flexed against gravity and against additional loads of 30 N acting at the ankle joint (**Fig. 14.32**). Depending on the flexion angle, this exercise resulted in a load on the anterior cruciate ligament of less than 6 N while the load on the posterior cruciate ligament rose as high as approximately 300 N (**Fig. 14.33**).

Toutoungi et al[43] recorded the motion of the knee joint during isokinetic and isometric exercises as well as during squats and calculated the load on the cruciate ligaments with the help of a model (**Table 14.2**). They point out that a load of 0.55 times body weight corresponds to approximately 25% of the tensile strength of the anterior cruciate ligament of a young person. A load of 4.6 times body weight corresponds to approximately 85% of the tensile strength of the posterior cruciate ligament of a young person. Even if the model calculation overestimated the load on the posterior cruciate ligament, it is the case that in the exercises investigated the load on the posterior cruciate ligament far exceeded the load on the anterior cruciate ligament. As an alternative to model calculations, the load on the anterior cruciate can be derived from measuring its length change during various exercises or postures.[44]

Types of sport like soccer, handball, basketball, and other ball games are linked with an increased risk of injury to the anterior cruciate ligament. In the majority of cases (> 70%) there was no physical contact with another player at the time of injury.[45] Video recordings of injury episodes demonstrate, however, that in many cases the intended motion had been disturbed before the accident happened, for example by a push from another player.[46] Injury typically occurs when a large ground reaction force is exerted on the extended leg; in addition, moments in the direction of valgus, varus, or internal rotation might act on the tibia.[47] Examples of such episodes are a sudden deceleration combined with a change in direction during running, or landing on the floor after a jump.

Posture and load status at the time of injury point to the force of the quadriceps as the cause of injury. With the knee close to full extension, the patellar tendon points obliquely in the anterior direction. Activation

Exercise	Anterior cruciate load [× body weight]	Posterior cruciate load [× body weight]
Extension, isokinetic, 120°/s	0.45	0.08
Flexion, isokinetic, 120°/s	–	3.3
Extension, isometric	0.55	–
Flexion, isometric	–	4.6
Squat, downward phase (heel off ground)	0.12	2.7
Squat, upward phase (heel off ground)	0.06	2.8

Table 14.2 Maximum values of the load on the cruciate ligaments, averaged over the cohort of eight persons investigated

Source: Data from Toutoungi et al.[43]

of the quadriceps generates an anteriorly directed component of the tendon force onto the tibia, and this force loads the anterior cruciate ligament. In principle, such an anteriorly directed shear force could be compensated by antagonistic activation of the hamstrings. Obviously, however, when injury happens this mechanism is ineffective; weakness or delayed activation of the hamstring muscles are regarded as risk factors.

A conspicuous phenomenon is the higher injury risk among women compared with men.[48] In the risky episodes with high ground reaction forces, females are observed to keep their legs generally less flexed than males. Other potential contributors under debate are anatomical differences in the shape of the condyles, differences in the mechanical properties of the cruciate ligaments, and hormonal influences affecting the tone of the ligaments.[49] To prevent injury when jumping, it is advisable not to keep the leg fully extended during take-off or landing. It is also advisable to load the forefoot when landing, leaning the trunk forwards, so as to decrease the moment arm of the ground reaction force in relation to the knee. However, the present state of knowledge about risk factors and injury mechanisms is still inadequate to serve as a basis for prevention programs.[50]

References

1. Frost HM. Orthopaedic Biomechanics. Springfield: Thomas; 1973

2. Maquet PGJ. Biomechanics of the Knee. Berlin: Springer; 1976

3. Seedholm BB, Takeda T, Tsubuku M, Wright V. Mechanical factors and patellofemoral osteoarthrosis. Ann Rheum Dis 1979;38(4):307–316

4. Charnley J. The lubrication of animal joints in relation to surgical reconstruction by arthroplasty. Ann Rheum Dis 1960;19:10–19

5. Linn FC. Lubrication of animal joints. II. The mechanism. J Biomech 1968;1(3):193–205

6. Menschik A. Mechanik des Kniegelenkes. 1. Z Orthop Ihre Grenzgeb 1974;112(3):481–495

7. Müller W. Das Knie. Form, Funktion und ligamentäre Wiederherstellungschirurgie. Berlin: Springer; 1982

8. van Dijk R, Huiskes R, Selvik G. Roentgen stereophotogrammetric methods for the evaluation of the three dimensional kinematic behaviour and cruciate ligament length patterns of the human knee joint. J Biomech 1979;12(9):727–731

9. Fuss FK. Anatomy of the cruciate ligaments and their function in extension and flexion of the human knee joint. Am J Anat 1989;184(2):165–176

10. Li G, DeFrate LE, Sun H, Gill TJ. In vivo elongation of the anterior cruciate ligament and posterior cruciate ligament during knee flexion. Am J Sports Med 2004;32(6):1415–1420

11. Freeman MA, Pinskerova V. The movement of the normal tibio-femoral joint. J Biomech 2005;38(2):197–208

12. Komistek RD, Dennis DA, Mahfouz M. In vivo fluoroscopic analysis of the normal human knee. Clin Orthop Relat Res 2003;410(410):69–81

13. Moro-oka TA, Hamai S, Miura H, et al. Dynamic activity dependence of in vivo normal knee kinematics. J Orthop Res 2008;26(4):428–434

14. Piazza SJ, Cavanagh PR. Measurement of the screw-home motion of the knee is sensitive to errors in axis alignment. J Biomech 2000;33(8):1029–1034

15. Blankevoort L, Huiskes R, de Lange A. Helical axes of passive knee joint motions. J Biomech 1990;23(12):1219–1229

16. Nietert M. Untersuchungen zur Kinematik des menschlichen Kniegelenks im Hinblick auf ihre Approximation in der Prothetik [dissertation]. Berlin: Technical University Berlin, 1975

17. Schipplein OD, Andriacchi TP. Interaction between active and passive knee stabilizers during level walking. J Orthop Res 1991;9(1):113–119

18. Zelle J, Barink M, De Waal Malefijt M, Verdonschot N. Thigh-calf contact: does it affect the loading of the knee in the high-flexion range? J Biomech 2009;42(5):587–593

19. Morrison JB. Bioengineering analysis of force actions transmitted by the knee joint. Biomed Eng 1968;3(4):164–170

20. Paul JP. Force actions transmitted by joints in the human body. Proc R Soc Lond B Biol Sci 1976;192(1107):163–172

21. Shelburne KB, Torry MR, Pandy MG. Muscle, ligament, and joint-contact forces at the knee during walking. Med Sci Sports Exerc 2005;37(11):1948–1956

22. Heinlein B, Kutzner I, Graichen F, et al. ESB Clinical Biomechanics Award 2008: Complete data of total knee replacement loading for level walking and stair climbing measured in vivo with a follow-up of 6-10 months. Clin Biomech (Bristol, Avon) 2009;24(4):315–326

23. Fukubayashi T, Kurosawa H. The contact area and pressure distribution pattern of the knee. A study of normal and osteoarthrotic knee joints. Acta Orthop Scand 1980;51(6):871–879

24. Wojtys EM, Chan DB. Meniscus structure and function. Instr Course Lect 2005;54:323–330

25. Lee SJ, Aadalen KJ, Malaviya P, et al. Tibiofemoral contact mechanics after serial medial meniscectomies in the human cadaveric knee. Am J Sports Med 2006;34(8):1334–1344

26. Rath E, Richmond JC. The menisci: basic science and advances in treatment. Br J Sports Med 2000;34(4):252–257

27. Reilly DT, Martens M. Experimental analysis of the quadriceps muscle force and patello-femoral joint reaction force for various activities. Acta Orthop Scand 1972;43(2):126–137

28. Cohen ZA, Roglic H, Grelsamer RP, et al. Patellofemoral stresses during open and closed kinetic chain exercises. An analysis using computer simulation. Am J Sports Med 2001;29(4):480–487

29. Huberti HH, Hayes WC. Patellofemoral contact pressures. The influence of q-angle and tendofemoral contact. J Bone Joint Surg Am 1984;66(5):715–724

30. Huberti HH, Hayes WC. Contact pressures in chondromalacia patellae and the effects of capsular reconstructive procedures. J Orthop Res 1988;6(4):499–508

31. Selfe J. The patellofemoral joint: a review of primary research. Crit Rev Phys Rehabil Med 2004;16(1):1–30

32. Brechter JH, Powers CM. Patellofemoral stress during walking in persons with and without patellofemoral pain. Med Sci Sports Exerc 2002;34(10):1582–1593

33. Crowninshield R, Pope MH, Johnson RJ. An analytical model of the knee. J Biomech 1976;9(6):397–405

34. Li G, Gill TJ, DeFrate LE, Zayontz S, Glatt V, Zarins B. Biomechanical consequences of PCL deficiency in the knee under simulated muscle loads—an in vitro experimental study. J Orthop Res 2002;20(4):887–892

35. Vieira AC, Guedes RM, Marques AT. Development of ligament tissue biodegradable devices: a review. J Biomech 2009;42(15):2421–2430

36. O'Connor J, Shercliff T, FitzPatrick D, Biden E, Goodfellow J. Mechanics of the knee. In: Daniel DM, Akeson WH, O'Connor JJ, eds. Knee Ligaments. Structure, Function, Injury and Repair. New York: Raven Press; 1990:201–238

37. Pandy MG, Shelburne KB. Dependence of cruciate-ligament loading on muscle forces and external load. J Biomech 1997;30(10):1015–1024

38. Shelburne KB, Pandy MG, Anderson FC, Torry MR. Pattern of anterior cruciate ligament force in normal walking. J Biomech 2004;37(6):797–805

39. Beard DJ, Soundarapandian RS, O'Connor JJ, Dodd CAF. Gait and electromyographic analysis of anterior cruciate ligament deficient subjects. Gait and Posture 1996;2:83–88

40. O'Connor JJ. Can muscle co-contraction protect knee ligaments after injury or repair? J Bone Joint Surg Br 1993;75(1):41–48

41. Zavatsky AB, Beard DJ, O'Connor JJ. Cruciate ligament loading during isometric muscle contractions. A theoretical basis for rehabilitation. Am J Sports Med 1994;22(3):418–423

42. Mesfar W, Shirazi-Adl A. Knee joint biomechanics in open-kinetic-chain flexion exercises. Clin Biomech (Bristol, Avon) 2008;23(4):477–482

43. Toutoungi DE, Lu TW, Leardini A, Catani F, O'Connor JJ. Cruciate ligament forces in the human knee during rehabilitation exercises. Clin Biomech (Bristol, Avon) 2000;15(3):176–187

44. Heijne A, Fleming BC, Renstrom PA, Peura GD, Beynnon BD, Werner S. Strain on the anterior cruciate ligament during closed kinetic chain exercises. Med Sci Sports Exerc 2004;36(6):935–941

45. Boden BP, Dean GS, Feagin JA Jr, Garrett WE Jr. Mechanisms of anterior cruciate ligament injury. Orthopedics 2000;23(6):573–578

46. Krosshaug T, Nakamae A, Boden BP, et al. Mechanisms of anterior cruciate ligament injury in basketball: video analysis of 39 cases. Am J Sports Med 2007;35(3):359–367

47. Shimokochi Y, Shultz SJ. Mechanisms of noncontact anterior cruciate ligament injury. J Athl Train 2008;43(4):396–408

48. Yu B, Garrett WE. Mechanisms of non-contact ACL injuries. Br J Sports Med 2007;41(Suppl 1):i47–i51

49. Alentorn-Geli E, Myer GD, Silvers HJ, et al. Prevention of non-contact anterior cruciate ligament injuries in soccer players. Part 1: Mechanisms of injury and underlying risk factors. Knee Surg Sports Traumatol Arthrosc 2009;17(7):705–729

50. McLean SG. The ACL injury enigma: we can't prevent what we don't understand. J Athl Train 2008;43(5):538–540

15   Mechanical Aspects of the Lumbar Spine

15.1   Load on the Lumbar Spine

15.1.1 Plane Model Calculation

The load on the lumbar spine when a mass is held in the hands can be estimated in a plane model calculation if some simplifying assumptions are made. In **Fig. 15.1** the gravitational force of the mass acts perpendicularly downwards. Its moment arm is the distance between the center of mass of the load and the
center of rotation, assumed to be in the center of the intervertebral disk. The force of the extensor muscles
is represented by a single muscle force **F**; its direction is approximately equal to the direction of the gravitational force. The moment arm of the muscle force **F** is to be estimated. Its minimum value is equal to the
distance from the center of the disk to the nearest muscle; its maximum value is equal to the distance from
the center of the disk to the surface of the skin. As a compromise we accept as moment arm the distance
between the center of the disk and the geometrical center of the cross-sectional area of the extensor muscles. This corresponds roughly to a distance of 5 cm. With a mass of 20 kg held in the hands (corresponding
to a weight of approximately 200 N) and a moment arm of the gravitational force of 25 cm, we obtain from
the equilibrium of moments (signs according to the sign convention for moments):

(15.1)
$$F \cdot 5 - 200 \cdot 25 = 0 \text{ Ncm}$$
$$F = 1000 \text{ N}$$

If we count the downward directed force components (muscle and gravitational force) as negative, we
obtain from the equilibrium condition of forces the component G of the joint load **G**.

(15.2)
$$G - 200 - F = 0 \text{ N}$$
$$G = 1200 \text{ N}$$

The positive sign of G indicates that the direction of **G** is opposite to the direction of the muscle and gravitational forces. The joint is loaded in compression.

If the total load on the lumbar spine is to be estimated in the posture shown in **Fig. 15.2**, the moment
of the body weight cranial to the segment in question has to be taken into consideration in addition to the
moment of the weight held in the hands. To simplify the model calculation and to allow easy adaptation to
different postures, the body is subdivided into the segments head, arms, and trunk (**Fig. 15.2**). The masses
and the locations of the centers of mass of the segments are approximately known (see Chapter 11). With
m_1 and L_1 as the mass and moment arm of the hand-held mass, m_2 to m_4 and L_2 to L_4 as the masses and
moment arms of the head, arms, and trunk segments, g as gravitational acceleration, and **F** and L_5 as the
force and moment arm of the extensors of the back, we obtain in equilibrium of moments:

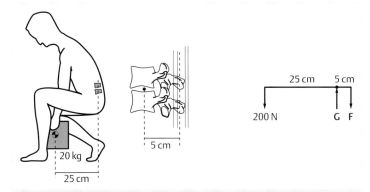

Fig. 15.1 Calculation of the increased load on the lumbar spine due to a mass held in the hands. In this example the directions of the gravitational force and of the force of the extensor muscles of the back are assumed to be parallel. The moment arm of the gravitational force is given by the perpendicular distance of the center of mass from the center of rotation, located at the center of the disk. This moment arm is assumed to amount to 25 cm. The moment arm of the extensor muscles of the back is given by the distance of the center of the cross-sectional area of these muscles from the center of the disk. This moment arm is estimated to amount to 5 cm.

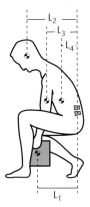

Fig. 15.2 Total load on segment L4/L5 when a mass is held in the hand. For the purpose of calculation, the body cranial to L4 is imagined to be divided into the segments of trunk, arms, and head, with masses m_2, m_3, and m_4. The segmented circles designate the centers of mass of these segments; L_2, L_3, and L_4 are the moment arms of the gravitational forces. The total load is obtained as the sum of four addends: one contribution from holding the mass (cf **Fig. 15.1**) and three contributions from the body segments.

(15.3) $$-L_1 \cdot m_1 \cdot g - L_2 \cdot m_2 \cdot g - L_3 \cdot m_3 \cdot g - L_4 \cdot m_4 \cdot g + L_5 \cdot F = 0$$

In equilibrium of forces G is calculated as

(15.4) $$G = m_1 \cdot g + m_2 \cdot g + m_3 \cdot g + m_4 \cdot g + F$$

It is concluded from this equation that, even without any external load (m_1 = zero), the lumbar spine is loaded by the body weight and in addition by the muscle force required to balance the moment of the weight of the head, arms, and trunk in the forward bent posture. This load increases with increased forward bending.

If an object is not only held or lifted very slowly but is noticeably accelerated in the lifting process, inertial forces have to be taken into account. When a mass is being lifted (**Fig. 15.3**) the accelerations of the mass and the body segments are directed upwards. Thus the inertial force $F_{in} = -m \cdot a$ is directed downwards and points in the same direction as the gravitational force. It follows that, when the object and the body segments are being accelerated (dynamic case), the extensor muscles of the back have to develop a higher force than during pure holding of the object (static case). Employing realistic data for the acceleration of objects being lifted, obtained by observation in industrial workplaces, Leskinen et al[1] calculated that the load on the L5/S1 segment during lifting of a mass of 15 kg using four different lifting techniques amounted to between 5800 and 6600 N. A static calculation (excluding inertial forces) showed loads between 3900 and 4600 N. This comparison demonstrates that inertial forces can contribute substantially to spinal loading.

As an extreme example of spinal loading, Granhed et al[2] calculated the load on the L3 vertebra of weight lifters. With masses of over 300 kg being lifted, a load of over 30 kN is predicted. A load of this magnitude

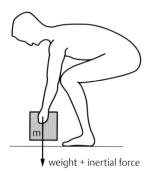

weight + inertial force

Fig. 15.3 When a mass is lifted, the acceleration **a** is directed upwards. The inertial force $F_{in} = -m \cdot a$ is directed downwards. During the lifting, the sum of the gravitational and inertial forces, $m \cdot g + m \cdot a$, acts on the hand. Consequently, the force on the hand is higher when the mass is being lifted upwards than during pure holding of a mass.

amounts to several times the normal compressive strength of L3 (see Section 15.2.1). To explain how it is possible to perform such exercises at all, the authors point to the unusually high bone density in the spine of these athletes. One has to assume that their vertebrae are composed almost entirely of compact bone.

15.1.2 Three-Dimensional Model Calculations

In the plane model described in the section above, muscle forces were represented by a single muscle force. Employing this model, loading configurations in the sagittal plane can be analyzed with adequate accuracy. An advantage of this procedure is that no additional assumptions have to be made to solve the equations. If, however, the load on the lumbar spine is to be estimated in any given posture or with any given directions of external forces, a model with only a single muscle is no longer applicable. To the contrary, all the muscles of the trunk need to be taken into account. For example, in a posture with the trunk bent forwards and rotated sideways, the calculation must take into account not only the muscle forces of the extensors, but also those of the obliques.

For the foundation of a three-dimensional model calculation, a detailed model of bones, muscles, and joints has to be compiled. The points (or areas) of insertion of muscles and tendons, the directions of their tensile forces, and their moment arms in relation to the joints have to be determined from anatomical observations. If more than a single muscle is taken into account, the equilibrium equations form an indeterminate system. However, the multitude of solutions can be reduced to a single solution by making additional assumptions. Various assumptions (objective functions) have been proposed. It can, for example, be postulated that the joint load, or the sum, or the sum of the squares of the muscle stresses has a minimum value. The choice of postulate is based on assumptions about the neuromuscular control strategy. Is it intended to limit joint loading? Are the muscles intended to be protected from overload or fatigue? The results of such model calculations do, of course, depend on the choice of assumptions, but the resulting uncertainty seems small compared with the uncertainties inherent in the anatomic models.

Schultz and Andersson[3] proposed a model incorporating ten muscle groups (**Fig. 15.4**). Minimization of the joint load was used as the objective function; in addition a maximum value of the muscle stress (muscle force divided by muscle cross section) was prescribed. This limiting value, known from muscle physiology (approx. 40 N/cm^2), ensures that individual muscles are not assigned unphysiologically high muscle forces in the calculation.[4] The model of Schultz and Andersson[3] has been applied for calculating the load on the lumbar spine in asymmetric body postures. Jäger[5] developed a model which represented the musculature of the back and the abdomen by eight muscles. The objective function employed by Jäger was the sum of the muscle forces. This model has been applied for determining loads on the lumbar spine in the workplace—for example, in one-handed brick laying, or when transporting waste containers.[6,7]

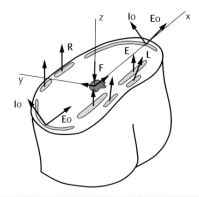

Fig. 15.4 Ten-muscle model to estimate the load on the lumbar spine. E, erector spinae; Eo, external oblique; Io, internal oblique; L, latissimus dorsi; R, rectus abdominis. (Adapted from Schultz and Andersson.[3])

In certain postures, antagonistic muscle activation is inevitable. If, for example, the trunk is bent forwards and simultaneously rotated to the right, the force of the oblique muscles must be compensated (due to their location anterior to the spine) by additional generation of force from the extensor muscles. A model calculation using objective functions allows correctly for this effect. However, any additional anticipated or involuntary, mechanically "unnecessary" activation of muscles cannot be taken into account without additional information or assumptions. As a simple example, the reader is referred to the calculation of the load on the elbow joint with activation of the biceps and triceps (see Chapter 12 and **Fig. 12.7**). If, in addition to the force of the biceps required for equilibrium, the triceps is activated voluntarily, there is no way to calculate the joint load. To find a solution for this, the magnitude of the additional muscle force has to be known.

To deal with the antagonistic muscle activation that occurs in certain postures and during certain activities, so-called electromyography (EMG)-based model calculations have been developed (see, for example, Granata and Marras[8]). These model calculations are likewise based on a model of the architecture of muscles and joints, but the muscle forces in the postures or during the activities under investigation are not calculated but are determined from EMG measurements. Insertion of these forces in the anatomical model then allows the joint loads to be calculated in a second step. To do this, the EMG signal must have been calibrated against the muscle force before the measurements are carried out. This is done in pilot experiments that determine the conversion factors between the maximum muscle force and the EMG signal amplitude. EMG signals are then recorded during the activity under investigation by means of electrodes placed on the skin, and correction factors are applied to account for the effect of length change and shortening velocity of the muscles. The study by Knapik and Marras[9] presents an example of an EMG-driven model calculation. A discussion of the foundations of the various model calculations is presented in the paper by Reeves et al.[10]

15.1.3 Intra-abdominal Pressure and the Load on the Lumbar Spine

Experience shows that many subjects spontaneously generate a pressure in the abdomen when they lift a heavy object. Why the intra-abdominal pressure is generated and what its effect is on the load of the lumbar spine is still a subject of debate. Some investigators hypothesize that the intra-abdominal pressure relieves the load on the lumbar spine. The reasoning is that a pressure in the abdominal cavity acts in all directions, resulting in a force F_1 on the diaphragm and a force F_2 on the floor of the pelvis (**Fig. 15.5**). These forces generate an extension moment in the opposite direction to and partially compensating the flexion moment generated by the load in the hands. In consequence, it is argued, the force of the extensor muscles and the load on the spine will decrease.

A closer look at the muscles generating the intra-abdominal pressure prompts some doubts about this argument. The pressure in the abdominal cavity is generated essentially by activation of the oblique and the transversus abdominis muscles. The forces of these muscles have components whose direction is parallel to the spine (**Fig. 15.5**), and these force components load the lumbar spine. In addition, the extensor muscles must develop higher forces to prevent forward bending of the trunk when the oblique muscles are activated. (This additional tensing of the extensors can easily be verified by palpating them while voluntarily generating intra-abdominal pressure.) In effect, the generation of muscle forces posterior and anterior to the spine results in an increase in spinal load. At best this increase can be partially compensated by the

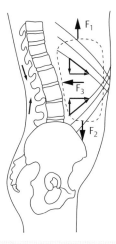

Fig. 15.5 Generation of intra-abdominal pressure by activation of the external and internal oblique muscles. Thin arrows represent muscle forces decomposed into components that are parallel and components that are perpendicular to the spine. F_1 and F_2, forces on the diaphragm and the pelvis; F_3, force on the lumbar spine.

extension moment generated by the intra-abdominal pressure. The conclusion that the generation of intra-abdominal pressure increases the load on the spine is in agreement with the observations of Nachemson et al.[11] These authors documented an increase in intradiskal pressure during voluntary generation of intra-abdominal pressure. This also agrees with observations in patients with spinal complaints: when they generate intra-abdominal pressure—for example, when they cough—their load-dependent symptoms increase.

Various conjectures have been put forward in answer to the question of why intra-abdominal pressure is generated (since it obviously does not unload the spine). It is possible that generation of intra-abdominal pressure is not intentional but merely a by-product of the contraction of the muscles of the trunk. Activation of these muscles serves to stabilize the upper with respect to the lower trunk. Marras et al[12] showed that, in rapid lifting exercises, peak values of the pressure are reached before peak values of the external moment are observed. This agrees with the observation that healthy subjects activate the transversus abdominis muscle before an anticipated activation of the deltoid muscle and subsequent movement of the arm is made.[13] In addition, the above hypothesis is supported by the observation that a high intra-abdominal pressure is usually generated during sit-up exercises. In these exercises the extension moment due to the pressure is directed in the opposite direction to the intended movement (that is, flexion) of the trunk.[14]

On the other hand, the pressure generated in the abdominal cavity is usually not very high; peak values of 100 mmHg (corresponding to 13.3 kPa) are exceeded only when lifting very heavy objects.[15,16] However, the pressure acts on a relatively large area and generates a posteriorly directed force on the lumbar spine (F_3 in **Fig. 15.5**). This posteriorly directed force may serve to prevent an excessive increase in the lordotic curvature if the spine is under high axial (longitudinally directed) load.[17] In any event, the intra-abdominal pressure permits the muscles of the trunk to contract while preventing a collapse of the abdominal cavity.

Despite the many unanswered questions, broad belts are available commercially that promise to reduce the load on the spine in physically demanding workplaces. Measurements have demonstrated, however, that wearing such belts neither increases the isometric force of the extensor muscles of the back, nor decreases the rate of injuries to the lumbar spine.[18-20] At most, belts limit the range of motion of the trunk with respect to flexion.[21,22]

15.1.4 Recommendations for Lifting and Carrying

Guidelines and recommendations for lifting and carrying at the workplace, in the household, and in leisure activities serve several goals[23]:

- They are intended to protect people against muscular exhaustion and cardiovascular overload. For this purpose, maximum values for the frequency of lifts performed are recommended, related to the mass lifted and the posture attained. The recommended limits are based on measurements of heart rate and energy turnover derived from respiratory gas analysis.

- They are intended to prevent accidents. For this purpose, risk factors such as slippery floors, missing handles, or obstruction of the view due to excessive size of the objects being handled have to be eliminated.

- They are intended to protect the lumbar spine against overload. Injuries due to a single episode of overloading or to repeated high loads are to be avoided by limiting the maximum mass of the objects handled and by avoiding certain postures when lifting and carrying. The recommended limits of the masses are based both on epidemiological studies and on a comparison of the results of biomechanical model calculations with the experimentally determined compressive strength of vertebral bodies and disks. Strictly speaking, it would be more correct to state limits for the moments exerted on the spine rather than limits for the masses handled, because spinal loading depends on the moments and not on the magnitude of the masses. However, specifying just the masses and the postures makes it easier to apply the recommendations.

The moment of a mass handled is proportional to its moment arm. For practical applications it follows that, for a given mass, the load on the lumbar spine will be smallest when the moment arm chosen is the smallest possible. For this reason it is recommended that objects being lifted or carried should be positioned as close as possible to the spine. If the object is carried anteriorly, the minimum magnitude of the moment arm is limited by the presence of the abdomen to approximately 20 cm (**Fig. 15.6**). Backward bending of the upper trunk, shifting the common center of mass of the body and the object closer to the spine, will bring about a reduction of spinal load in this posture.

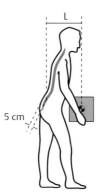

Fig. 15.6 Since the moment arm of the extensor muscles of the lumbar spine is virtually constant (approximate value 5 cm), the additional load on the lumbar spine in a given posture depends on the magnitude of the mass handled and on its moment arm L. The additional load on the lumbar spine is smallest when the moment arm L of the external load is selected to be as small as possible.

If the arms hang down and a weight is held in the hands (for example when carrying a suitcase or a stretcher, or when lifting a wheelbarrow), the moment arm in relation to the spine is small. If an object is carried posteriorly (for example when lifting a piece of furniture behind the back), the moment arm may well be less than 10 cm. At the same time, the moment arm of the abdominal muscles balancing the moment of the weight is substantially larger than that of the extensors of the back. It follows that lifting posteriorly may unload the spine in comparison with an anterior lift.

The components of the force loading the spine that are directed perpendicular to the vertebral end-plates and those that are directed parallel to them follow a characteristic pattern that depends on posture (**Fig. 15.7**). Ignoring for the time being the natural curvature of the spine, the moment arm L of a mass being carried in the erect posture is virtually constant. The moment of the gravitational force, the required muscle force, and the resulting force directed longitudinally along the spine are thus virtually identical in all segments of the lumbar spine. In this posture, the magnitude of shear forces acting in the plane of the disks is small. This is true even for the L5/S1 segment, which is tilted some 45° out of the horizontal. This is because by far the largest part of the spinal load stems from the force of the extensor muscles, and the direction of the muscles closely follows the direction of the spine.

By contrast, in the forward bent posture the moment arm of the weight increases in the craniocaudal direction and, consequently, so does the additional axial load (directed perpendicular to the endplates)

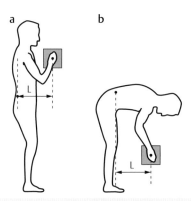

Fig. 15.7a, b Craniocaudal trend of the additional compressive load on the lumbar spine due to holding a mass in the hands.
a In the erect posture, the moment arm and thus the additional load are virtually equal for all segments (disregarding for the sake of simplicity the curvature of the spine in the sagittal plane).
b In the forward bent posture, the moment arm L and thus the compressive load increase in the craniocaudal direction. In this posture, loading by the shear force generated by the gravitational force of the mass and acting in the plane of the disks is approximately equal for all segments.

on the lumbar spine. To some extent the lumbar spine is adapted to increased loading in the craniocaudal direction, as the compressive strength of the vertebral bodies increases from T12 to L5. In the forward bent posture, the magnitude of the shear force acting in the plane of the disks (again ignoring the curvature of the spine) equals the weight of the mass handled in addition to the weight of the body mass located cranial to the segment under consideration. The shear force is largely resisted by the facet joints, and to a much lesser extent by the disks.

It is generally correct that, in any given posture, the load on the lumbar spine will be smallest when the moment arm of the object being lifted or carried is selected to be as small as possible. Further recommendations on specific postures to be assumed when lifting or carrying can, however, be problematic, for a number of reasons.

- **Fig. 15.8** compares lifting an object with the trunk bent forwards and lifting with the knees bent. It is assumed that the dimensions of the object are such that it cannot be lifted between the knees. In forward bending (**Fig. 15.8a**) the moment arm of the object related to the L5/S1 segment is smaller than it is in posture (b) where the knees are bent. The moment arm of the body weight, by contrast, is greater in the forward bending posture (**Fig. 15.8a**) than in the knees-bent posture (**Fig. 15.8b**). In the borderline case of a very heavy object and very lightweight lifter, therefore, posture **a** would result in minimal spinal loading and would thus be advantageous, whereas in the case of a heavy lifter and a lightweight

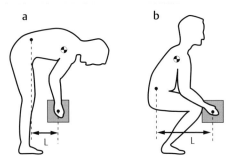

a   b

Fig. 15.8a, b Comparison of the load on the lumbar spine in lifting a mass with the trunk bent forward (**a**) or with the knees bent (**b**). Segmented circles show the center of mass of the body cranial to L5/S1. In posture **a** the moment arm L of the external load related to segment L5/S1 is smaller than it is in posture **b**. By contrast, the moment arm of the gravitational force of the body mass is greater in posture **a** than in posture **b**. Depending on the body mass and the mass being handled, the compressive load on the lumbar spine may be greater in either posture **a** or posture **b**. The loading of the knee joints is greatest in posture **b**.

object, posture **b** would be preferable. If the mass of the subject and the mass of the object are known, it is, of course, possible to decide which of the two postures results in the smaller axial load on the lumbar spine. If the masses are not known, no generally valid advice can be given. In other words: if only one posture were recommended for lifting and carrying, it might well be the wrong posture in a particular situation.[24]

- Even if a calculation in the individual case yielded the result that posture **b** loads the lumbar spine less than posture **a**, lifting with the knees bent cannot be recommended to all persons without reservation. This is because the load on the femorotibial and femoropatellar joints increases considerably as the bending angle of the knee increases. In elderly persons with incipient or advanced osteoporosis, a deep knee bend has the potential to damage the trabecular bone below the tibial plateau.

- In addition, it must be borne in mind that frequent lifting with the knees bent is energy-consuming and thus very tiring, because every straightening up from a knee bend requires lifting of the body's center of mass.

15.2 Strength of Lumbar Vertebrae

15.2.1 Compressive Strength

Strength is defined as the load that causes irreparable damage to a structure. In principle, bones can be loaded by compression, tension, shear, bending, torsion, or a combination of these. For vertebral bodies, the loading mode of interest is compression by a force directed perpendicular to the endplates. In both erect stance and forward bending, this force is transmitted to the vertebral bodies via the disks. Only at the limit of extension may a fraction of the load be transmitted by the facet joints and the vertebral arch, but the major part of the load is still exerted by axial compression. So far as fractures are concerned, tensile forces acting on the vertebral body via the ligaments or the disk are of importance only in situations of extreme load or in accidents. Forces acting in the plane of the disk and moments about the long axis of the spine are resisted by the facet joints. So long as the facet joints do not fracture (which almost never occurs except in accidents), shear forces and moments can be ignored when discussing the strength of vertebral bodies.

Fig. 15.9 shows the force–deformation curve of a lumbar vertebral body, determined in vitro. After an initial region under small load, deformation increases in line with force. Once a particular force value is reached, the curve deviates from a straight line: the deformation (compression) increases rapidly whereas the force hardly increases at all. This force value is called the *compressive strength* of the vertebra. If the force is now reduced to zero, the vertebra remains deformed. In almost all cases, the trabecular bone beneath the endplates fractures under overload, resulting in clefts and stepped or rounded impressions in the endplates, sometimes associated with intrusion of disk tissue into the trabecular bone. Wedge-type fractures or a decrease in the height of the entire vertebral body are less frequently seen. After a fracture,

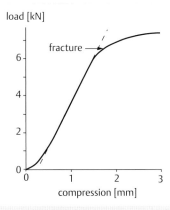

Fig. 15.9 Example of a force–deformation curve derived from in vitro strength testing of vertebral bodies. The point where the curve starts to deviate from a straight line designates a compression fracture. (Adapted, with permission, from Brinckmann et al.[25])

the vertebral body has a reduced load bearing capacity; in the example illustrated in **Fig. 15.9** this amounts to approximately 7 kN.

In addition to the compressive strength under one single loading cycle, the fatigue strength of lumbar vertebrae has been investigated.[26] The results show that the probability of a fatigue fracture undergoes a sharp increase if the amplitude of the cyclic load exceeds 50% of the load that results in vertebral fracture in one single loading cycle. The results of this experiment in vitro should, however, be regarded only as approximate values. In living persons the development of microdamage, eventually leading to fatigue fracture, competes with physiologic repair processes. In vitro experiments demonstrate that, unlike traumatic, multiple fractures, fatigue fractures rarely destroy a vertebral body completely. This suggests that the characteristic morphological alterations in vertebral shape seen in patients with advanced osteoporosis are in most cases due to fatigue fractures.

The results of in vitro strength tests of lumbar vertebrae allow elucidation of the parameters that determine compressive strength. As an example, **Fig. 15.10** shows the compressive strength of lumbar vertebrae measured in vitro in relation to the product of the bone density of the trabecular bone [mg/mL K_2HPO_4] and the area of one of the endplates [cm²].[25] The bone density in the central volume of the vertebrae and the endplate area were both determined by computed tomography (CT). To allow comparison of bone density measurements made on different scanners, the density is quoted not in milligrams per cubic centimeter [mg/cm³], but in units of the density of a potassium salt used as a reference substance for calibration [mg/mL K_2HPO_4]. The data from this experiment show that the compressive strength of vertebrae increases as the bone density and the dimensions of the vertebral body increase. The scatter of the data

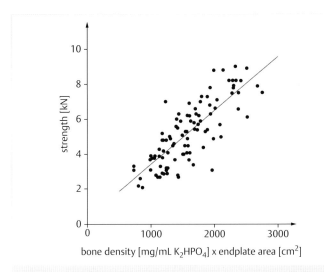

Fig. 15.10 Results of an in vitro study of the compressive strength of lumbar vertebrae T12 to L5. The regression line describing the statistical relation between the compressive strength and the product of density and endplate area is shown. (Adapted, with permission, from Brinckmann et al.[25])

about the regression line shown in **Fig. 15.10** indicates that compressive strength is influenced (though to a minor extent) by additional factors besides endplate area and bone density. The architecture and the material properties of the trabecular bone within the vertebral body may play a role here. If bone density and endplate area are measured in vivo by CT, the in vivo strength of vertebrae can be predicted from the data shown in **Fig. 15.10** within error limits of ± 1 kN. The study by Brinckmann et al[25] showed that in a given spine the bone densities of vertebrae T12 to L5 are virtually equal. The compressive strength of the vertebrae increases craniocaudally by approximately 300 N per segment; the increase is due to the increase in endplate area of the vertebrae.

Other investigators (see, for example, Eriksson et al[27]) correlated the in vitro strength of lumbar vertebrae with their bone mineral density as measured by dual photon or dual X-ray absorptiometry (DPA, DXA). For a discussion of the experiments and the results, see Ebbesen et al.[28] It turns out that the compressive strength of a vertebra can be predicted from the bone mineral density [g/cm] or from the product of the trabecular bone density [g/cm^3] and the endplate area [cm^2] with almost equal accuracy. This is because the dimensions of the bone are implicitly contained in the bone mineral density data: the product of volumetric density and area [g/cm^3 · cm^2 = g/cm] has the identical dimension to that of bone mineral density [g/cm]. The difference between the two measuring methods is due to the fact that volumetric bone density is determined only from the trabecular bone, whereas the measurement of bone mineral density also includes the cortical bone of the vertebral body. That both procedures still lead to approximately the same result is probably because there is a correlation between the densities of trabecular bone and cortical bone. It may be possible to achieve greater precision in the prediction of compressive strength if the model calculations into which the bone density measurements are fed take account of the individual architecture of the vertebra.[29]

15.2.2 Bone Density and Bone Mineral Density in Relation to Gender and Age

The trabecular bone density of lumbar vertebral bodies is age-dependent. Felsenberg et al[30] published normal values of bone density measured by CT in the age range between 20 and 89 years (**Fig. 15.11**). Bone density reaches its peak value between 20 and 30 years of age and then diminishes steadily with age. There is no significant gender-related difference. Regarding the influence of age and gender, the results of the measurement of the ash content of the L3 vertebra by Mosekilde[31] agree with the CT bone density results published by Felsenberg et al.[30] The ash content (**Fig. 15.12**) exhibits a steady drop with age; here too, there is no gender-related difference.

The U.S. reference standard for the bone mineral density of the lumbar spine shows a similar dependence on age (**Fig. 15.13**). In all age groups, however, bone mineral density is slightly higher in men than in women. This gender-related difference is probably caused by the fact that the mineral density of the cortical bone of the vertebral bodies and the posterior elements is included in the bone mineral density data. Because men are subjected to more physical stress on average than are women, their cortical bone may have developed greater thickness. Differences also exist between cohorts drawn from different countries. **Fig. 15.14** shows lumbar bone mineral density in a German cohort. Except in the two highest age groups, there is virtually no difference between males and females.

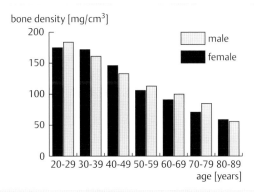

Fig. 15.11 Age dependence of trabecular bone density of lumbar vertebral bodies in a German cohort, measured by quantitative CT. (Data from Felsenberg et al.[30])

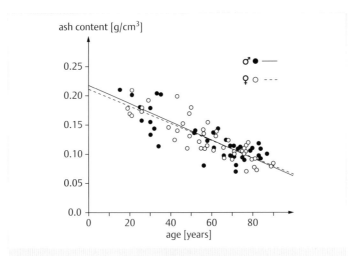

Fig. 15.12 Ash content of the trabecular bone from vertebra L3, by age and gender. (Adapted, with permission, from Mosekilde.[31])

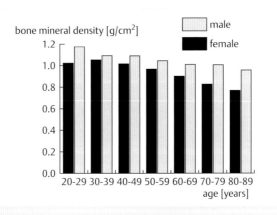

Fig. 15.13 Bone density of the lumbar spine by age and gender in a U.S. cohort, measured by dual X-ray absorptiometry (DXA). (Data courtesy of Thomas L. Kelly.[32])

Measuring bone density in the lumbar spine is costly and involves radiation exposure. For this reason, it was suggested in the past that bone density could instead be measured in the peripheral skeleton, preferably in the radius. Because of the correlation between the densities of the radius and the spine, data from the radius should allow conclusions to be drawn about vertebral bone density. **Fig. 15.15** shows that such a correlation between the volumetric bone densities does indeed exist. However, the scatter of the data about the regression line means that in the individual case it is impossible to draw conclusions about the bone density of the spine on the basis of the bone density of the radius. A similar correlation exists

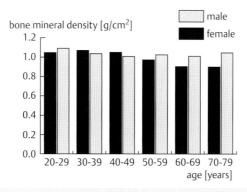

Fig. 15.14 Bone density of the lumbar spine in relation to age and gender in a German cohort, measured by DXA. (Data from Lehmann et al.[33])

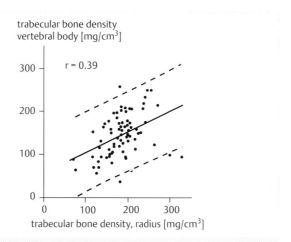

Fig. 15.15 Correlation of the trabecular bone density in the distal radius and the lumbar spine. Also shown are the regression line and two parallels (dashed lines) at a distance of twice the standard error. (Adapted from Grampp et al.[34] Reprinted with permission from the *American Journal of Roentgenology*.)

between bone mineral densities in the radius and the spine[35] but, again, the wide data scatter means that in the individual case no conclusions about the spine can be drawn from data about the radius.

Because of the age-related decrease of bone density or bone mineral density, we expect the compressive strength of lumbar vertebrae to reach its peak after skeletal maturation and then to drop steadily. Men and women undergo this loss of vertebral compressive strength equally. **Fig. 15.16** shows a compilation of compressive strength data of human lumbar vertebrae in vitro, in relation to age and gender. In addition,

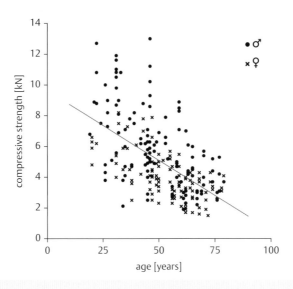

Fig. 15.16 Compressive strength of lumbar vertebrae (T12 to L5) in vitro in relation to gender and age. The regression line describing the statistical relation between strength and age is shown. On average, compressive strength decreases with age. However, the values for any given individual can deviate substantially from the statistical mean. (Adapted, with permission, from Biggemann and Brinckmann.[36])

the figure contains the regression line describing the overall statistical relation between strength and age. It can be clearly seen that (for the material investigated) strength decreases on average with age, but at any given age the strength data are scattered over a wide range. This is because of the variation in bone density and vertebral dimensions. Furthermore, it can be seen that women's vertebrae exhibit lower strength on average than men's vertebrae. This is because women's vertebrae are normally smaller than men's, not because of any gender-related differences in the material properties of bone. We hypothesize that the difference in strength due to the difference in size accounts for insufficiency fractures in osteoporosis being seen more frequently in women than in men, and at a younger age.

Insufficiency fractures of osteoporotic vertebrae are expected to occur in both men and women, but later in men because their vertebrae are, on average, larger. **Fig. 15.17** does indeed show that the incidence of fractures in the male cohort of 70–74 years of age is virtually the same as that the female cohort of 60–64 years of age, and the incidence in the male cohort of 75–79 years of age is virtually the same as that in the female cohort of 65–69 years of age. The study by Biggemann et al[38] gives an indication of the compressive strength required to withstand everyday in vivo loading. In a cohort of 75 persons, these authors determined the strength of the L3 vertebra by measuring bone density and the endplate area (**Fig. 15.18**).

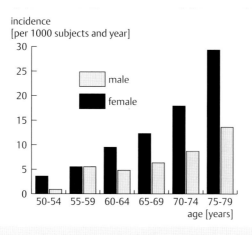

Fig. 15.17 Incidence of fractures in the lumbar spine in relation to age and gender. (Adapted, with permission, from Cummings et al.[37])

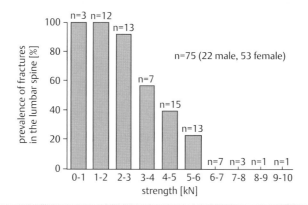

Fig. 15.18 Prevalence of fractures in the lumbar spine in relation to the strength of the L3 vertebra, predicted from trabecular bone density and endplate area. If the predicted strength of L3 falls below 3 kN, the prevalence of fractures approaches 100%. (Adapted, with permission, from Biggemann et al.[38])

It turned out that, in virtually all spines where the compressive strength of L3 was predicted to be lower than 3 kN, insufficiency fractures could be seen in the radiographs.

15.2.3 Fracture of the Vertebral Arch

A fracture of the vertebral arch in the pars interarticularis—that is, between the superior articular process and the inferior articular process—is not congenital but acquired. The fracture (spondylolysis) may lead to

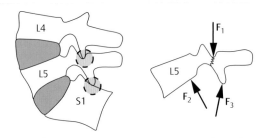

Fig. 15.19 Primary mechanical cause of fracture of the pars interarticularis of the vertebral arch. Bony contact between the inferior articular process and the lamina of the next vertebra down (dashed circles) can occur under simultaneous high axial loading and hyperextension. The vertebral arch is now subjected to three-point loading, with the maximum bending moment acting in the pars interarticularis. (Adapted from Suezawa and Jacob.[39])

anterior displacement of the vertebral body (spondylolisthesis) and to symptoms and disability requiring treatment. Suezawa and Jacob[39] explored the modes of loading that led to fracture of the vertebral arch and showed that a shear force directed parallel to the endplates can fracture the arch in the region of the pedicle but not in the pars interarticularis. They demonstrated that maximal extension in combination with high axial loading of the spine leads to a fracture in the pars interarticularis. In maximal extension (**Fig. 15.19**) bony contact can occur between the inferior articular process and the pars interarticularis of the next vertebra down. The center of rotation of the segment is then effectively shifted from the center of the disk to the point of bony contact. In the anterior longitudinal ligament and the anterior part of the disk, tensile stress is created; a compressive force acts at the point of bony contact. The arch is subjected to a bending moment and fracture may occur.

Epidemiological investigations demonstrate that the prevalence of fractures at the pars interarticularis is significantly higher in persons who engage in particular athletic disciplines such as gymnastics, high jump, and pole-vaulting than in the general population. It seems that the defect is acquired mainly at a young age. Whether the fracture is caused by a single overload episode or by fatigue due to repeated loadings cannot be determined in retrospect.

15.3 Segmental Motion

15.3.1 Description as Pure Rotation

In principle, the relative motion of two adjoining vertebrae can be described as pure rotation. For geometrical reasons, the center of rotation is expected to be located close to the center of the disk. If this were not the case, the height of the disk space would be subject to large variation during rotational motion, which is anatomically impossible. Penning et al[40] and Pearcy and Bogduk[41] reconstructed the location of the center of rotation of segments L2/L3 to L5/S1 by superimposing lateral radiographs of the lumbar spine in flexion and extension (**Fig. 15.20**). The location of the centers of rotation show as small regions of scatter that are shifted caudally and posteriorly relative to the centers of the disks. The caudal shift means that rotational motion of a vertebra is always associated with anterior or posterior displacement (translation). If, for example, the L3 vertebra is flexed in relation to the L4 vertebra, the whole of the L3 vertebra moves anteriorly, because of the position of the L3/L4 center of rotation.

The scatter of the measurements of the centers of rotation are due to biological variation and measurement error. The range of rotational motion of lumbar motion segments is normally in the order of 10°; in persons with back problems the range of motion can be reduced to between 2° and 5°. Errors in determining a center of rotation increase as the range of angular motion decreases (see Chapter 6). Locating centers of rotation is further complicated by the fact that it is not possible to provide precise definitions of distinctive points (landmarks) that are visible on radiographs. Past attempts to derive the location of centers of rotation from sagittal plane radiographs of individual patients, and to draw from them conclusions about pathological changes present in those patients, failed due to the large measurement errors encountered.

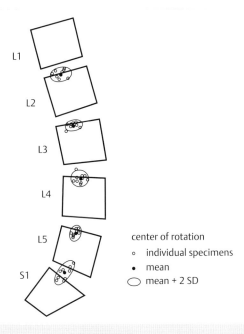

Fig. 15.20 Centers of rotation of the segments of the lumbar spine, determined from lateral radiographs in flexion and extension. (Adapted, with permission, from Pearcy and Bogduk.[41])

15.3.2 Description as Combination of Rotation and Translation

The conceptual difficulties involved in determining a center of rotation can be avoided if the relative motion of adjoining vertebrae is described as a combination of rotation and translation. In principle, it is always possible to describe a plane motion as a combination of rotation and translation; the angle of rotation is identical to the angle when the motion is described as a pure rotation (see Chapter 6). **Fig. 15.21** illustrates the proposal of Frobin et al.[42] The midpoints between the anterior and posterior corners of a vertebra define a straight line (the *midplane*). The change in the angle between the midplanes of adjoining vertebrae, measured from lateral radiographs taken in extension and flexion, defines the rotational motion. From the centers of the vertebrae (geometrical centers of corners 1–4), perpendiculars to the bisector of the angle between the midplanes are constructed. The distance between the intersections of these perpendiculars with the bisector is equal to the posteroanterior displacement of the vertebrae; the change in this displacement defines the translational motion. Both rotation and the translation can be measured with high precision on lateral radiographs of the lumbar spine. The study by Frobin et al[42] showed that the translational motion is in proportion to the rotational motion. In the individual patient, the measured rotation and translation values can be compared with reference values in healthy persons to see whether the segmental motion determined in the patient differs from normal motion.

Relative motion of vertebrae can be measured to a very high accuracy in vivo if metallic markers are implanted in the spine and stereoradiographs are taken and assessed.[43] Stereoradiography assesses translational motion with a precision (99% confidence limits) of about 0.5 mm and rotational motion with a precision of about 1°. As an invasive procedure, however, this investigation is restricted to postoperative studies.

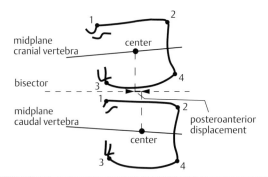

Fig. 15.21 Definition of rotational and posteroanterior translational motion in segments of the lumbar spine. (Adapted, with permission, from Frobin et al.[42])

15.4 Mechanical Function of Lumbar Disks

The component of the spinal load directed longitudinally along the spine is transmitted from vertebra to vertebra almost entirely by the intervertebral disks. As the surfaces of the lumbar facet joints face almost perpendicular to the transverse plane, they cannot normally transmit any of the axial load. Load transmission via the facet joints occurs only when bony contact is made between the caudal facet and the lamina of the lower vertebra, which means when segments are in maximum extension or have a very low disk height.[44] The component of the spinal load directed parallel to the endplates—the shear component—is transmitted almost entirely by the facet joints; the disks and the ligaments of the vertebral joint, because they are less stiff than bone, transmit only a small fraction of this load. If the vertebral arch is fractured, the only resistance to shear forces is provided by the disk and the ligaments. In such cases, anterior displacement of the cranial vertebra, often progressive, is frequently observed.

Fig. 15.22 illustrates the mechanical function of the disk:

- Because of the incongruency of the endplates of adjoining vertebrae, the disk has the task of ensuring a uniform pressure distribution.
- The mobility of the segments requires the disk tissue, which is virtually incompressible, to be capable of deforming and shifting within the intervertebral space.
- The vertebral body and intervertebral disk deform under load. The vertebral endplates bulge inwards; the disk also bulges outwards radially, and the height of the motion segment decreases.

Under a load close to the limit of the compressive strength, the inward bulge of the vertebral endplates is in the order of 0.5 mm and the radial bulge of the disk in the order of 1 mm compared with the unloaded state.[45,46] If the inward bulge of the endplates continues to grow, the maximum compressive strain of the trabecular bone in the interior of the vertebra is exceeded and the bone fractures. Disk tissue can then intrude into the vertebral body and the disk undergoes an irreversible loss of height.

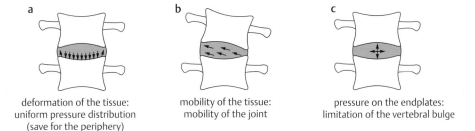

a deformation of the tissue: uniform pressure distribution (save for the periphery)

b mobility of the tissue: mobility of the joint

c pressure on the endplates: limitation of the vertebral bulge

Fig. 15.22a–c Mechanical function of the disk: it generates uniform distribution of the pressure over the endplates (**a**), enables motion between adjacent vertebral bodies (**b**), and (through the intradiskal pressure) restricts radial bulging of the disk (see Section 15.4.2) (**c**).

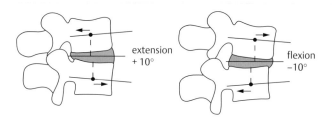

Fig. 15.23 Ventral and dorsal radial bulge of a lumbar disk in extension and flexion.

In flexion and extension the disk space becomes wedge-shaped (**Fig. 15.23**). The radial bulge of the disk is at its smallest on the side where the wedge opens, that is, posteriorly in flexion and anteriorly in extension. The bulging is limited by the tensile stress of the fibers of the anulus fibrosus, which is directed longitudinally along the spine.

15.4.1 Pressure Distribution at the Interface between the Intervertebral Disk and the Vertebral Body

Under load, the distribution of compressive stress (pressure) over the endplates of the vertebrae is almost uniform (**Fig. 15.24**). Tensile stress exists only in a zone about 1 to 2 mm wide along the periphery of the

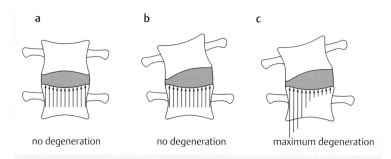

no degeneration   no degeneration   maximum degeneration

Fig. 15.24a–c Pressure distribution at the interface of the disk and the vertebral body. (Adapted from Horst et al.[47])
a In nondegenerated or moderately degenerated disks there is uniform pressure over the entire vertebral endplate save for a 1- to 2-mm-wide zone along the periphery, where the outer layer of the anulus fibrosus is under tensile stress.
b The uniformity of the pressure distribution is not changed under flexion or side bending.
c In highly degenerated disks the pressure is greater in those regions where the endplates approach each other under flexion or side bending.

intervertebral disk, where the outermost fiber layers of the anulus fibrosus insert.[47] The uniformity of the pressure distribution is preserved when the endplates of the adjoining vertebrae are no longer parallel but tilted against each other. Only in maximally degenerated disks and at the limit of the range of motion did Horst et al observe increased pressure at the location where the endplates approach each other in side bending, flexion, or extension.[47] Recent measurements performed with a miniature pressure probe showed additional details of the pressure distribution (**Fig. 15.25**).[48] While the pressure in disks with grade I degeneration (no degeneration) was virtually uniform, disks with grade II–IV degeneration (moderate to marked degeneration) regularly exhibited pressure maxima in the region of the posterior anulus. The maximum values increased when the segment was moved in extension.

The underlying cause of the occurrence of these differences in the uniformity of pressure distribution can be understood qualitatively if the mechanical properties of disk tissue are considered to lie somewhere between the properties of an ideal fluid and a solid. In contrast to the properties of a solid, no force is required to deform a fluid. Nondegenerated or only slightly degenerated disk tissue can be deformed easily and is able to move (within certain limits) within the disk space. For this reason such disks effect a virtually uniform pressure distribution over the vertebral endplates, irrespective of the geometry of the disk space. The mechanical properties of highly degenerated tissue, on the other hand, or those of tissue dehydrated by long-term loading, increasingly resemble those of a solid. The tissue is more resistant to deformation

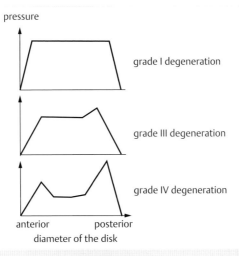

Fig. 15.25 Distribution of the vertical component of the compressive stress over the diameter of the intervertebral disk. In disks with grade I degeneration (no degeneration) the pressure is almost uniformly distributed. Disks with grade II–IV degeneration (noticeable or marked degeneration) exhibit pressure maxima in the peripheral region of the anulus. (Adapted, with permission, from Adams et al.[48])

and less mobile within the disk space. If the disk space becomes wedge-shaped, peak values of compressive stress are observed at locations where the endplates approach each other and the tissue cannot "slip aside." A similar result is obtained where disk height is very low. Without sufficient available disk tissue, it is not possible to equalize the pressure in a wedge-shaped disk space.

15.4.2 Relation between Intradiskal Pressure and Radial Bulge

Nachemson[49] showed in his pioneering study that the relation between load F and pressure p at the center of the disk is described by

(15.5)
$$p = 1.5 \cdot F / A$$

where F denotes the compressive force directed perpendicular to the plane of the disk and A the cross-sectional area of the disk. The numerical value of the experimentally determined factor of proportionality between pressure and the quotient of force and area indicates that the disk cannot simply be regarded as an elastically deformable, intermediate layer between the endplates. If it were, a factor of proportionality equal to 1.0 instead of 1.5 would be expected.

In the following the origin and function of the intradiskal pressure are discussed qualitatively using the model shown in **Fig. 15.26**; for the appertaining formulae see Brinckmann et al.[50] The disk tissue contains

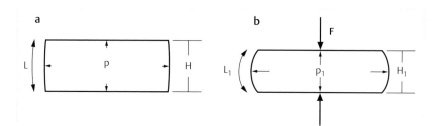

Fig. 15.26a, b Model of an intervertebral disk used to derive the relation between intradiskal pressure and radial disk bulge: incompressible material enclosed between rigid endplates and an outer membrane of high tensile strength (the outer layer of the anulus fibrosus). (Adapted, with permission, from Brinckmann et al.[50])

a Unloaded state. H, L, and p designate the height of the disk, the length along the enclosing membrane, and the intradiskal pressure.

b State under external load. The disk bulges outwards and the height decreases to the value H_1. The length of the membrane increases from L to L_1. Consequently, the tensile stress of the membrane increases. To fulfill the equilibrium condition of forces, the intradiskal pressure increases and assumes the value p_1. This pressure generates a radially directed force on the anulus and a perpendicularly directed force on the adjoining endplates.

compounds that have the ability to bind water via an electrochemical process. This ability to bind water is greatest under low pressure and decreases as pressure increases. In the state of low loading (at night, for example) there is a net water uptake by the disk, by diffusion from the surrounding body fluid. The height of the disk increases. The height increase tightens the fibers of the anulus fibrosus in the longitudinal direction of the spine; the radial bulge of the disk is small (**Fig. 15.26a**). When the fluid-saturated disk is loaded, intradiskal pressure is generated. The pressure acts uniformly in all directions, on both opposing endplates as well as (radially) on the anulus fibrosus (**Fig. 15.26b**). The anulus bulges outwards and, because part of the disk tissue shifts into the anular bulge, the disk height decreases. The outermost fiber layers of the anulus are stretched, generating tensile stress which acts on the opposing endplates. As a consequence, the pressure within the disk must increase to balance (in addition to the load F) the resulting tensile force acting at the periphery of the endplates. Due to this mechanism the intradiskal pressure actually rises above the magnitude of the mean pressure F/A.

The intradiskal pressure acts uniformly in all directions, on the endplates of the adjoining vertebrae as well as radially on the anulus fibrosus. The intradiskal pressure causes the radial bulge of the disk. However, since the circumferential area of the anulus (disk circumference times disk height) is smaller than the area of the endplates, the force (pressure times area) on the endplates limits the radial bulge, in effect maintaining the disk height. As an analogy, consider the mechanical system of an automobile or bicycle tire, which is very similar to that of a disk. Inside the tire is pressure; the wall of the tire is under tensile stress. When the tire pressure is increased by pumping air into it, its height increases and its radial bulge decreases. If air is let out of it, its height decreases and its radial bulge increases. The tire model predicts that any loss of disk tissue, whether caused by disk extrusion, endplate fracture, or surgical intervention, results in decreased disk height, decreased intradiskal pressure, and an increased radial bulge. These predictions agree with in vitro observations on human lumbar spine specimens and with in vivo follow-up studies after chemonucleolysis (therapeutic enzymatic digestion of disk tissue).[51] **Fig. 15.27** shows the change in disk height, intradiskal pressure, and radial disk bulge in relation to the amount of tissue excised from the interior of a lumbar disk.[50]

The method of in vivo measurement of intradiskal pressure was employed by Nachemson and Elfström[52] to determine load on the lumbar spine. The advantage of this protocol is that the measured pressure data can be used directly, without further model assumptions, to quantify the spinal loading. If different postures or activities are compared (standing and sitting, for example), it must be taken into account that the intradiskal pressure depends not only on the load on a segment but also on the relative angular orientation of the vertebrae. Under constant load the intradiskal pressure changes in relation to the angle, because the tensile strain and thus the tensile stress in the outer layers of the anulus change as the angle changes.

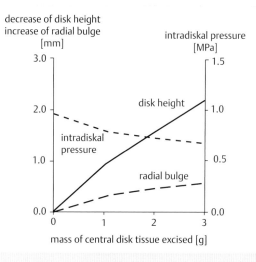

Fig. 15.27 Example of disk height, intradiskal pressure, and radial disk bulge, measured in vitro during incremental excision of central disk tissue (nucleotomy); constant load of 1 kN. (Adapted, with permission, from Brinckmann et al.[51])

The change in height of the intervertebral disks due to the inflow or outflow of fluid results in a measurable change in stature. Since the study by DePuky,[53] it has been known that body height is at its maximum in the morning and decreases during the course of the day by about 1 to 2 cm. The rate at which body height decreases is highest in the morning and slows down over the day.[54] Eklund and Corlett[55] proposed utilizing the observed change in stature to determine spinal loading. Using a refined measurement protocol, Althoff et al[56] employed stadiometry to determine spinal loading in standing relative to sitting as well as under additional shoulder loads and during exposure to whole-body vibration.

15.5 Disk Prolapse

A lumbar disk prolapse occurs when a separate tissue fragment extrudes or sequestrates through a complete tear of the anulus. The high axial compressive loading of lumbar disks, often in combination with side bending or rotation of the trunk, as well as case reports from patients, seem to suggest that lumbar disk prolapse has a primary mechanical cause. The designation "primary" is chosen to make it clear that we are discussing the causal event(s) at the very outset of the process ending in a disk prolapse. This is in contrast to a "secondary" mechanical contribution leading to prolapse of a disk already impaired by other, nonmechanical factors.

15.5.1 Hypotheses Relating to Mechanical Causes of Disk Prolapse

Several in vitro studies have been performed to explore whether high axial loading of motion segments of the lumbar spine may lead to disk prolapse. Under axial overload of a motion segment, however, vertebral body fracture invariably occurs first.[25,57,58] Injury of the anulus fibrosus or a prolapse of disk tissue was not observed. This holds for single overload episodes as well as for fatigue fractures.[26]

The role of tears (fissures) of the anulus fibrosus in triggering disk prolapse has been investigated in specimens of motion segments. The disks were experimentally incised, with the incision starting from the center of the disk and extending right through the entire anulus save for an outer layer about 1–2 mm thick.[59] Under overload these "injured" segments exhibited only vertebral fractures; disk prolapse was not observed. However, when fissures extending up to 2 mm short of the periphery were created in the posterior region and the tissue in the region of the nucleus pulposus was dissected in small fragments, prolapse of the fragments was observed at the location of the fissure.[60] In specimens in which the anulus fibrosus was completely cut through, Simunic et al[61] observed disk prolapse in flexion under high axial load. These observations suggest that prolapse must be preceded by fissures and fragmentation.

If lumbar motion segments are loaded in hyperflexion (that is, flexion beyond the physiological limit), the posterior anulus may rupture or tear from the vertebral endplate. With this loading mode, Adams and Hutton[62] produced a prolapse in a number of the specimens investigated. The mechanism simulated by Adams and Hutton may account for prolapses seen as the result of accidents, sometimes in combination with a fracture of the posterior rim of the vertebral body. In the majority of symptomatic cases, a disk prolapse does not seem to be associated with injury to the dorsal ligaments.

The influence of axial rotation in the etiology of disk prolapse has been investigated both experimentally and by means of biomechanical model calculations.[63,64] These studies concluded that, without facet damage, axial rotation (approximately 2° in the lumbar spine) is insufficient to cause disk injury leading to prolapse.

The conjecture that a forward bent posture of the trunk encourages the development of disk prolapse has not so far been substantiated. In contrast to previously held opinion, the dorsal radial bulge of the disk decreases in flexion (see **Fig. 15.23**). This is true of nondegenerated as well as degenerated disks. The higher incidence of disk prolapse in the L4/L5 and L5/S1 segments as compared with the segments of the upper lumbar spine seems at first sight to point to a mechanical etiology. It is, however, unclear whether these segments exhibit the largest incidence of prolapse or the largest incidence of prolapse in need of treatment. In addition, it has to be considered that during lifting and carrying in the erect posture all segments of the lumbar spine are exposed to approximately the identical load. Because the disks in the proximal region of the lumbar spine are smaller, the mechanical stress caused by the external load is larger in the proximal part of the lumbar spine than in the distal part.

Disk tissue obtained during disk surgery has been studied histologically to obtain a clue to whether the fragments originated from the nucleus pulposus or the anulus fibrosus.[65-67] Virtually all the fragments contained central disk tissue, combined in a high percentage of cases with fragments of endplate cartilage. No convincing hypothesis has been put forward to explain what mechanical process could cause fragmentation of the central disk tissue and its detachment from the bony endplates. The tissue at the center of the disk is under minimal tensile strain during flexion, extension, side bending, and axial rotation. If tensile strain of the tissue were to play a role, therefore, one would expect fragmentation of the disk to be initiated at its periphery.

As diagnostic methods become more refined, an increasing prevalence of pathological but asymptomatic alterations of lumbar disks is being observed.[68-70] Protrusions (local increases in radial disk bulge) seem to be frequent, but extrusions (tissue fragments almost or completely separated from the rest of the disk) seem to be rare. So far, it has not proved possible to document the time course of the development of disk protrusions. In a longitudinal study of 48 persons with asymptomatic disk prolapse in the thoracic spine, Wood et al[70,71] observed virtually no alterations in the existing protrusions. Boos et al[72] confirmed in a longitudinal study of 46 symptom-free individuals that pathological findings can be frequently observed in lumbar disks. Over the 5-year observation period, the protrusions did not change, and only one person developed a disk prolapse.

It must be pointed out that present knowledge derived from experiments in vitro and model calculations is severely limited. Due to enzymatic decomposition of the tissue it is not yet possible to preserve disk specimens for long periods (essentially, for longer than 1 day) in a state suitable for biomechanical experimentation. Thus, we see at present no possibility of investigating the effects of long-term static or cyclic loading in the laboratory. To simulate highly recurrent loading, the specimens have to be subjected to a large number of load cycles within a short time (see, for example, Callaghan and McGill[73]). In addition it must be kept in mind that long-term processes are always in competition with physiologic tissue repair. At present such repair (if it exists for disk tissue) cannot be reliably simulated either in experiments or in model calculations.

15.5.2 Epidemiological Studies

The relationship between long-term heavy physical work and the risk of symptomatic disk prolapse has been investigated in epidemiological studies. The case–control studies of Braun,[74] Kelsey et al,[75,76] and Heliövaara[77] compared cohorts whose work exposed them to long-term heavy physical work with age- and gender-adjusted controls. According to Braun,[74] men with highly loaded spines have a significantly increased risk of symptomatic disk prolapse, against which the risk in women with heavily loaded spines is surprisingly small. Braun suggests that the explanation may lie in unknown confounding factors in his study that shifted the probability of receiving treatment in hospital for symptomatic disk prolapse (the only way for cases to be captured in the statistics), but not the rate of actual incidence, to higher values in men than in women.

In the studies by Kelsey and coworkers,[75,76] too, lifting and carrying of heavy loads entails a higher risk of disk prolapse. These studies, however, have methodological shortcomings. For example, to classify spinal loading, data collection comprised only the weight of the objects handled but not the moment (product of weight and distance) exerted in relation to the lumbar spine. With respect to sitting as a risk factor, the results reported by Kelsey and coworkers in their 1975 and 1984 studies[75,76] were contradictory.

According to Heliövaara,[77] the risk of being hospitalized due to disk prolapse is significantly increased for men performing physically demanding work, whereas (in conformity with Braun[74]) highly loaded women exhibit only a slight increase in this risk. Agricultural workers exhibit a moderately increased risk, while persons in sedentary occupations exhibit no increased risk. In the light of these findings, Heliövaara[77] urges that the results of his study be interpreted with caution. The risk factors established might be confounded by differences in opportunity and willingness to undergo conservative or surgical treatment. According to the author, the results of the study should not be interpreted as proof of a relationship between spinal loading and the development of disk prolapse.

Heliövaara[77] proposed that prospective studies (intervention studies) should be conducted to clarify the issue. The performance of prospective studies is, however, complicated by the fact that symptomatic lumbar disk prolapse is a rare disease. The number of new cases requiring treatment (incidence) ranges from about 6 to 8 · 10^{-4} per year and person.[78] The follow-up of such a rare disease in a prospective study would, if it were to produce statistically significant results, require large cohorts and long follow-up times with spinal loading conditions remaining essentially unchanged. To illustrate the problem, here is an example using actual numbers. We assume that (1) the incidence of lumbar disk prolapse is 10^{-3} per year and person (rounded value to facilitate calculation) and (2) heavy spinal loading by physically demanding work doubles the incidence of prolapse (a drastic effect). Under these assumptions, with cohorts of 200 persons and observation times of 10 years we would expect two cases of prolapse in the control cohort (10^{-3} per year and person · 10 years · 200 persons) and four cases in the heavily loaded cohort (**Table 15.1**). The statistical significance of this result would be low. The χ^2 test tells us that, with a probability of over 40%, this numerical result might have been obtained by chance, with no relation existing in reality between heavy

	Disk prolapse	No disk prolapse	n
Heavy spinal loading	4	196	200
No heavy spinal loading	2	198	200

Table 15.1 The 2 × 2 contingency table for a study of the relationship between heavy spinal loading and the incidence of lumbar disk prolapse, with two groups of 200 persons each

	Disk prolapse	No disk prolapse	n
Heavy spinal loading	20	980	1000
No heavy spinal loading	10	990	1000

Table 15.2 The 2×2 contingency table for a study of the relationship between heavy spinal loading and the incidence of lumbar disk prolapse, with two groups of 1000 persons each

spinal loading and disk prolapse. To increase the statistical significance, either the size of the cohorts or the follow-up period would have to be increased. In a study surveying a total of 2000 subjects over 10 years we would expect, under the above assumptions, 10 cases of prolapse in the control cohort and 20 cases in the heavily loaded cohort (**Table 15.2**). The probability of obtaining such a result by chance would still range between 5% and 10% (χ^2 test).

At present, the issue of the relation between heavy spinal loading and incidence of lumbar disk prolapse remains unresolved. Up to now, experiments in vitro have failed to identify a primary mechanical cause of prolapse. The exceptions are traumatic episodes with simultaneous hyperflexion and high axial loading of the spine. Epidemiological studies indicate that persons in certain types of workplace have an increased probability of being hospitalized for lumbar disk prolapse. The differences seen between exposed men and women and between industrial and agricultural workers have yet to be clarified. The results of the epidemiological studies and of the experiments in vitro are consistent with the conjecture that mechanical influences can trigger prolapse of a disk that already has pre-existing damage from another (unknown) cause. Whether or not there is a relationship between degeneration of lumbar disks (as indicated by height loss, fluid loss, and tissue alteration) and the incidence of disk prolapse remains unclear. It is evident that genetic elements play a role in the development of disk degeneration.[79] Whether the same holds for disk prolapse cannot be determined because of the low case numbers.

References

1. Leskinen TP, Stålhammar HR, Kuorinka IA, Troup JD. A dynamic analysis of spinal compression with different lifting techniques. Ergonomics 1983;26(6):595–604

2. Granhed H, Jonson R, Hansson T. The loads on the lumbar spine during extreme weight lifting. Spine 1987;12(2):146–149

3. Schultz AB, Andersson GB. Analysis of loads on the lumbar spine. Spine 1981;6(1):76–82

4. Bean JC, Chaffin DB, Schultz AB. Biomechanical model calculation of muscle contraction forces: a double linear programming method. J Biomech 1988;21(1):59–66

5. Jäger M. Biomechanisches Modell des Menschen zur Analyse und Beurteilung der Belastung der Wirbelsäule bei der Handhabung von Lasten. Düsseldorf: VDI Verlag; 1987. Fortschritt-Berichte 17/33

6. Jäger M, Luttmann A, Laurig W. Biomechanisches Modell des Transports von Müllgroßbehältern über Bordsteinkanten. Zbl Arbeitsmedizin 1983;33:251–259

7. Jäger M, Luttmann A, Laurig W. Lumbar load during one-handed bricklaying. Int J Ind Ergon 1991;8:261–277

8. Granata KP, Marras WS. An EMG-assisted model of trunk loading during free-dynamic lifting. J Biomech 1995;28(11):1309–1317

9. Knapik GG, Marras WS. Spine loading at different lumbar levels during pushing and pulling. Ergonomics 2009;52(1):60–70

10. Reeves NP, Cholewicki J. Modeling the human lumbar spine for assessing spinal loads, stability, and risk of injury. Crit Rev Biomed Eng 2003;31(1-2):73–139

11. Nachemson AL, Andersson BJ, Schultz AB. Valsalva maneuver biomechanics. Effects on lumbar trunk loads of elevated intraabdominal pressures. Spine 1986;11(5):476–479

12. Marras WS, Joynt RL, King AI. The force-velocity relation and intra-abdominal pressure during lifting activities. Ergonomics 1985;28(3):603–613

13. Hodges PW, Richardson CA. Inefficient muscular stabilization of the lumbar spine associated with low back pain. A motor control evaluation of transversus abdominis. Spine 1996;21(22):2640–2650

14. McGill SM. The mechanics of torso flexion: situps and standing dynamic flexion manoeuvres. Clin Biomech (Bristol, Avon) 1995;10(4):184–192

15. Davis PR, Troup JDG. Pressures in the trunk cavities when pulling, pushing and lifting. Ergonomics 1964;7:465–474

16. Stubbs DA. Human constraints on manual working capacity: effects of age on intratruncal pressure. Ergonomics 1985;28(1):107–114

17. Cholewicki J, Juluru K, McGill SM. Intra-abdominal pressure mechanism for stabilizing the lumbar spine. J Biomech 1999;32(1):13–17

18. McGill SM. Abdominal belts in industry: a position paper on their assets, liabilities and use. Am Ind Hyg Assoc J 1993;54(12):752–754

19. Reyna JR Jr, Leggett SH, Kenney K, Holmes B, Mooney V. The effect of lumbar belts on isolated lumbar muscle. Strength and dynamic capacity. Spine 1995;20(1):68–73

20. Miyamoto K, Iinuma N, Maeda M, Wada E, Shimizu K. Effects of abdominal belts on intra-abdominal pressure, intra-muscular pressure in the erector spinae muscles and myoelectrical activities of trunk muscles. Clin Biomech (Bristol, Avon) 1999;14(2):79–87

21. Lüssenhop S, Deuretzbacher G, Steuber KU, Rehder U. Zur mechanischen Wirksamkeit von Präventivmiedern (Back Supports) - erste Ergebnisse einer biomechanischen Untersuchung. Orthop Praxis 1996;32:409–412

22. McGorry RW, Hsiang SM. The effect of industrial back belts and breathing technique on trunk and pelvic coordination during a lifting task. Spine 1999;24(11):1124–1130

23. Waters TR, Putz-Anderson V, Garg A, Fine LJ. Revised NIOSH equation for the design and evaluation of manual lifting tasks. Ergonomics 1993;36(7):749–776

24. Park KS, Chaffin DB. A biomechanical evaluation of two methods of manual lifting. AIIE Trans 1974;6:105–113

25. Brinckmann P, Biggemann M, Hilweg D. Prediction of the compressive strength of human lumbar vertebrae. Clin Biomech (Bristol, Avon) 1989;4(Suppl 2):1–27

26. Brinckmann P, Biggemann M, Hilweg D. Fatigue fracture of human lumbar vertebrae. Clin Biomech (Bristol, Avon) 1988;3(Suppl 1):i–S23

27. Eriksson SA, Isberg BO, Lindgren JU. Prediction of vertebral strength by dual photon absorptiometry and quantitative computed tomography. Calcif Tissue Int 1989;44(4):243–250

28. Ebbesen EN, Thomsen JS, Beck-Nielsen H, Nepper-Rasmussen HJ, Mosekilde L. Lumbar vertebral body compressive strength evaluated by dual-energy X-ray absorptiometry, quantitative computed tomography, and ashing. Bone 1999;25(6):713–724

29. Crawford RP, Cann CE, Keaveny TM. Finite element models predict in vitro vertebral body compressive strength better than quantitative computed tomography. Bone 2003;33(4):744–750

30. Felsenberg D, Kalender WA, Banzer D, et al. Quantitative computertomographische Knochenmineralgehaltsbestimmung. Fortschr Röntgenstr 1988;148(4):431–436

31. Mosekilde L. Sex differences in age-related loss of vertebral trabecular bone mass and structure—biomechanical consequences. Bone 1989;10(6):425–432

32. Kelly TL. Developing DXA reference databases [collection of reference data]. Bedford, MA: Hologic; 1996

33. Lehmann R, Wapniarz M, Randerath O, et al. Dual-energy X-ray absorptiometry at the lumbar spine in German men and women: a cross-sectional study. Calcif Tissue Int 1995;56(5):350–354

34. Grampp S, Jergas M, Lang P, et al. Quantitative CT assessment of the lumbar spine and radius in patients with osteoporosis. AJR Am J Roentgenol 1996;167(1):133–140

35. Mazess RB, Barden HS, Ettinger M. Radial and spinal bone mineral density in a patient population. Arthritis Rheum 1988;31(7):891–897

36. Biggemann M, Brinckmann P. Biomechanics of osteoporotic vertebral fractures. In: Genant HK, Jergas M, van Kuijk C, eds. Vertebral Fracture in Osteoporosis. San Francisco: Radiology Research and Education Foundation; 1995:21–34

37. Cummings SR, Melton LJ. Epidemiology and outcomes of osteoporotic fractures. Lancet 2002; 359(9319):1761–1767

38. Biggemann M, Hilweg D, Seidel S, Horst M, Brinckmann P. Risk of vertebral insufficiency fractures in relation to compressive strength predicted by quantitative computed tomography. Eur J Radiol 1991;13(1):6–10

39. Suezawa Y, Jacob HAC. Zur Aetiologie der Spondylolisthesis. Stuttgart: Hippokrates; 1981. Die Wirbelsäule in Forschung und Praxis; Band 94

40. Penning L, Wilmink JT, van Woerden HH. Inability to prove instability. A critical appraisal of clinical-radiological flexion-extension studies in lumbar disc degeneration. Diagn Imaging Clin Med 1984;53(4):186–192

41. Pearcy MJ, Bogduk N. Instantaneous axes of rotation of the lumbar intervertebral joints. Spine 1988;13(9):1033–1041

42. Frobin W, Brinckmann P, Leivseth G, Biggemann M, Reikerås O. Precision measurement of segmental motion from flexion-extension radiographs of the lumbar spine. Clin Biomech (Bristol, Avon) 1996;11(8):457–465

43. Axelsson P, Johnsson R, Strömqvist B. Radiostereometry in lumbar spine research. Acta Orthop Suppl 2006;77(323):1–42

44. el-Bohy AA, Yang KH, King AI. Experimental verification of facet load transmission by direct measurement of facet lamina contact pressure. J Biomech 1989;22(8-9):931–941

45. Brinckmann P, Frobin W, Hierholzer E, Horst M. Deformation of the vertebral end-plate under axial loading of the spine. Spine 1983;8(8):851–856

46. Brinckmann P, Horst M. The influence of vertebral body fracture, intradiscal injection, and partial discectomy on the radial bulge and height of human lumbar discs. Spine 1985;10(2):138–145

47. Horst M, Brinckmann P. Measurement of the distribution of axial stress on the endplate of the vertebral body. Spine 1981; 6(3):217–232

48. Adams MA, Dolan P, McNally DS. The internal mechanical functioning of intervertebral discs and articular cartilage, and its relevance to matrix biology. Matrix Biol 2009;28(7):384–389

49. Nachemson A. Lumbar intradiscal pressure. In: Jayson MIV, ed. The Lumbar Spine and Back Pain. 2nd ed. London: Pitman; 1985:341–358

50. Brinckmann P, Grootenboer H. Change of disc height, radial disc bulge, and intradiscal pressure from discectomy. An in vitro investigation on human lumbar discs. Spine 1991;16(6):641–646

51. Leivseth G, Salvesen R, Hemminghytt S, Brinckmann P, Frobin W. Do human lumbar discs reconstitute after chemonucleolysis? A 7-year follow-up study. Spine 1999;24(4):342–347, discussion 348

52. Nachemson A, Elfström G. Intravital dynamic pressure measurements in lumbar discs. A study of common movements, maneuvers and exercises. Scand J Rehabil Med Suppl 1970;1:1–40

53. DePuky P. The physiological oscillation of the length of the body. Acta Orthop Scand 1935;6:338–347

54. Reilly T, Tyrrell A, Troup JDG. Circadian variation in human stature. Chronobiol Int 1984; 1(2):121–126

55. Eklund JA, Corlett EN. Shrinkage as a measure of the effect of load on the spine. Spine 1984; 9(2):189–194

56. Althoff I, Brinckmann P, Frobin W, Sandover J, Burton K. An improved method of stature measurement for quantitative determination of spinal loading. Application to sitting postures and whole body vibration. Spine 1992;17(6):682–693

57. Perey O. Fracture of the vertebral end-plate in the lumbar spine; an experimental biochemical investigation. Acta Orthop Scand Suppl 1957;25:1–101

58. Hutton WC, Cyron BM, Stott JR. The compressive strength of lumbar vertebrae. J Anat 1979;129(Pt 4): 753–758

59. Brinckmann P. Injury of the annulus fibrosus and disc protrusions. An in vitro investigation on human lumbar discs. Spine 1986;11(2):149–153

60. Brinckmann P, Porter RW. A laboratory model of lumbar disc protrusion. Fissure and fragment. Spine 1994;19(2):228–235

61. Simunic DI, Broom ND, Robertson PA. Biomechanical factors influencing nuclear disruption of the intervertebral disc. Spine 2001;26(11):1223–1230

62. Adams MA, Hutton WC. Prolapsed intervertebral disc. A hyperflexion injury. Spine 1982;7(3):184–191

63. Ahmed AM, Duncan NA, Burke DL. The effect of facet geometry on the axial torque-rotation response of lumbar motion segments. Spine 1990;15(5):391–401

64. Duncan NA, Ahmed AM. The role of axial rotation in the etiology of unilateral disc prolapse. An experimental and finite-element analysis. Spine 1991;16(9):1089–1098

65. Reimers C. Untersuchungen zur Entstehung der lumbalen Bandscheibenhernie. Wirbelsäule in Forschung und Praxis 1961;25:89–106

66. Brock M, Patt S, Mayer HM. The form and structure of the extruded disc. Spine 1992;17(12):1457–1461

67. Moore RJ, Vernon-Roberts B, Fraser RD, Osti OL, Schembri M. The origin and fate of herniated lumbar intervertebral disc tissue. Spine 1996;21(18):2149–2155

68. McRae DL. Asymptomatic intervertebral disc protrusions. Acta Radiol 1956;46(1-2):9–27

69. Jensen MC, Brant-Zawadzki MN, Obuchowski N, Modic MT, Malkasian D, Ross JS. Magnetic resonance imaging of the lumbar spine in people without back pain. N Engl J Med 1994;331(2):69–73

70. Wood KB, Garvey TA, Gundry C, Heithoff KB. Magnetic resonance imaging of the thoracic spine. Evaluation of asymptomatic individuals. J Bone Joint Surg Am 1995;77(11):1631–1638

71. Wood KB, Blair JM, Aepple DM, et al. The natural history of asymptomatic thoracic disc herniations. Spine 1997;22(5):525–529, discussion 529–530

72. Boos N, Semmer N, Elfering A, et al. Natural history of individuals with asymptomatic disc abnormalities in magnetic resonance imaging: predictors of low back pain-related medical consultation and work incapacity. Spine 2000;25(12):1484–1492

73. Callaghan JP, McGill SM. Intervertebral disc herniation: studies on a porcine model exposed to highly repetitive flexion/extension motion with compressive force. Clin Biomech (Bristol, Avon) 2001;16(1):28–37

74. Braun W. Ursachen des lumbalen Bandscheibenvorfalls. Stuttgart: Hippokrates; 1969. Wirbelsäule in Forschung und Praxis; Band 43

75. Kelsey JL. An epidemiological study of the relationship between occupations and acute herniated lumbar intervertebral discs. Int J Epidemiol 1975;4(3):197–205

76. Kelsey JL, Githens PB, White AA III, et al. An epidemiologic study of lifting and twisting on the job and risk for acute prolapsed lumbar intervertebral disc. J Orthop Res 1984;2(1):61–66

77. Heliövaara M. Occupation and risk of herniated lumbar intervertebral disc or sciatica leading to hospitalization. J Chronic Dis 1987;40(3):259–264

78. Berney J, Jeanprêtre M, Kostli A. Epidemiological factors of lumbar disk herniation [in French]. Neurochirurgie 1990;36(6):354–365

79. Battié MC, Videman T, Kaprio J, et al. The Twin Spine Study: contributions to a changing view of disc degeneration. Spine J 2009;9(1):47–59

16   Mechanical Aspects of the Shoulder

The upper extremity is designed to fulfill a large variety of tasks. The "link chain" of upper arm, lower arm, and hand permits motion in a large volume of space. The hand can reach almost any point within a sphere centered at the center of the humeral head and a with radius equal to the length of the arm. The almost unrestricted mobility of the hand enables objects to be gripped and manipulated under visual control as well as in regions out of sight (behind the back, for example). Upper arm, lower arm, and hand can execute quick and forceful as well as fine, very accurately guided movements. Forces and moments can be oriented in virtually any direction. The maximum values of such forces and moments depend on the location and orientation of the hand relative to the trunk. Knowledge of this dependence on position and orientation is of practical importance in the design of workplaces or orthopedic aids and appliances. Further information on this topic is presented in textbooks of ergonomics.

16.1   Link Chain of the Upper Extremity

In humans, as in all other vertebrates, the limbs are fixed to the trunk by means of "girdles," whose architecture is adapted to the mechanical function of the limbs. The pelvic girdle consists of the iliac bones and the sacrum, joined together by the symphysis and the iliosacral joints. Both these joints are characterized by being very stiff and having a small range of motion. The joint between the sacrum and the fifth lumbar vertebra forms the junction with the trunk. The pelvic girdle is adapted to the function of the legs, which is to support the body weight and locomotion.

Fig. 16.1 shows an overview of the architecture of the shoulder girdle and the arm. The shoulder girdle consists of the clavicle and scapula, connected by the acromioclavicular joint. The scapula glides on the posterior thoracic wall; it is fixed to the trunk by muscles alone. It can translate about 10 cm upwards, downwards, or laterally, and can rotate about an axis perpendicular to its own (imagined) plane. To a small extent, it can also be tilted with respect to the thorax. The clavicle is connected laterally to the acromion (acromioclavicular joint) and medially to the sternum (sternoclavicular joint). These two joints at either end of the clavicle can be described in mechanical terms as ball-and-socket joints which allow the clavicle to rotate in addition about its long axis. The range of motion of these joints is strongly restricted by their ligamentous connections. In point of fact, the shoulder girdle articulates with the rest of the skeleton only via the clavicle. The link between the scapula and the thorax is sometimes called the "scapulothoracic joint," but it is not a joint in the anatomical sense. Due to its deformability and its loose attachment to the trunk, the shoulder girdle is superbly adapted to upper-extremity functions such as touching, grasping, manipulating, and climbing.

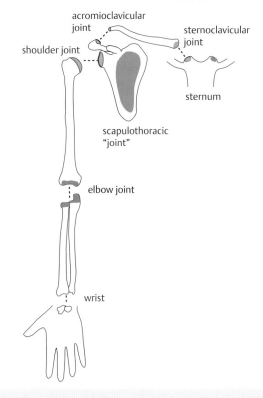

Fig. 16.1 Joints of the shoulder girdle and "link chain" of the upper extremity. Right shoulder, anterior view.

The shoulder joint (glenohumeral joint) links the upper arm to the shoulder girdle. It is a ball-and-socket joint with a large range of motion. The joint surface of the humeral head is spherical; it articulates with the shallow socket of the glenoid cavity of the scapula. The surface area of the glenoid cavity (which is about 6 cm^2) is much smaller than the surface area of the humeral head (which is about 24 cm^2).[1] Whether there is a precise fit between the head and the socket or whether the radius of the socket is slightly larger than that of the head is a matter of some debate. Radiographic views can simulate an incongruency between head and socket, as the cartilage is thicker at the periphery of the socket than at its center. According to Graichen et al,[2] in addition to rotational motion, translational motions in the order of a few millimeters are possible in the shoulder joint due to the incongruency of head and socket.

The elbow joint, the link between upper and lower arm, moves very much like a hinge joint. The wrist, the link between lower arm and hand, also moves like a hinge joint, and motion is also possible in the plane of the palm of the hand, in the direction of the thumb or the little finger (radial or ulnar deviation). The multiplicity of possible hand motions is further augmented by the rotation of ulna and radius (**Fig. 16.2**).

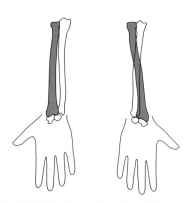

Fig. 16.2 Rotation of radius and ulna as the hand turns over (supination/pronation). (Adapted from Tillmann et al.[3])

The relative change in position of these bones permits supination and pronation (rotation about the long axis of the hand) even when the elbow joint is held firm.

The upper arm and shoulder girdle, like the femur and the pelvic girdle, are linked by ball-and-socket joints. Compared with a hinge joint, a ball-and-socket joint has a larger range of motion. To increase the range of motion of the upper extremity as much as possible, the socket (glenoid cavity) is not fixed rigidly but follows the motion of the upper arm. When the upper arm is raised, the scapula undergoes displacement and rotation relative to the thorax (**Fig. 16.3**). This is made possible by the joints between the scapula

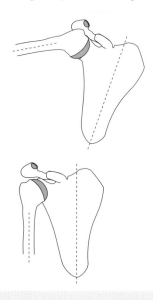

Fig. 16.3 Movement of the scapula accompanying the elevation of the upper arm (scapulohumeral rhythm). Right shoulder viewed from anterior in a plane fitted to the scapula.

and the thorax (as we have said, not "a joint" in the anatomical sense) and between the scapula and the clavicle, which have no counterparts in the pelvic girdle.

Viewed in a plane fitted to the scapula, the ratio of the rotational motion of the upper arm to that of the scapula for arm elevation angles above 30° ranges between 5:4 and 3:1.[4,5] This interplay between the motions of upper arm and scapula is called the *scapulohumeral rhythm*. In the individual case the scapulohumeral rhythm is well reproducible and in the case of small loads is virtually independent of the load on the shoulder.[6] With increasing age the concomitant motion of the scapula decreases.[7] The concomitant motion of humeral head and glenoid cavity stabilizes the shoulder joint (see Section 16.4). It also ensures that the humerus does not impinge on the acromion when the arm is elevated above 90°.

16.2 Muscles of the Shoulder Region

The large number of muscles in the shoulder region accords with the wide variety and range of motion of the shoulder. The muscles can be categorized according to their areas of insertion (**Table 16.1**).

Origin and insertion	Muscles
Trunk and upper arm	Pectoralis major, latissimus dorsi
Trunk and scapula	Levator scapulae, rhomboid, trapezius, serratus anterior, pectoralis minor
Trunk and clavicle	Trapezius, subclavius
Scapula and upper arm	Subscapularis, supraspinatus, infraspinatus, teres minor, teres major, deltoid
Origin in the shoulder region, crossing the elbow joint	Biceps, triceps

Table 16.1 Muscles of the shoulder region, by origin and insertion areas

Fig. 16.4 provides an overview of the muscles that move the upper arm forwards, backwards, or to the side, or rotate it about its long axis. Since even simple motions usually involve the activation of several muscles, it is easy to see from the figure that biomechanical models of the shoulder must necessarily be complex. The muscle group consisting of teres minor, infraspinatus, supraspinatus, and subscapularis is called the *rotator cuff* (**Figs. 16.5** and **16.6**). Activation of these muscles generates a force that presses the humeral head into the glenoid cavity, thus preventing instability of the shoulder joint. If these muscle forces are absent or a tendon is ruptured, instability of the joint may ensue. Except at the end of the range of motion, the shoulder joint capsule is slack and cannot provide stability.

16.3 Stability of the Shoulder Joint

In mechanical terms, a configuration is referred to as stable if it returns to its initial state after a small external perturbation. A configuration is called unstable if a small perturbation suffices to change it completely (see Section 1.7). In reference to joints of the body, the terms *stable* and *unstable* are sometimes

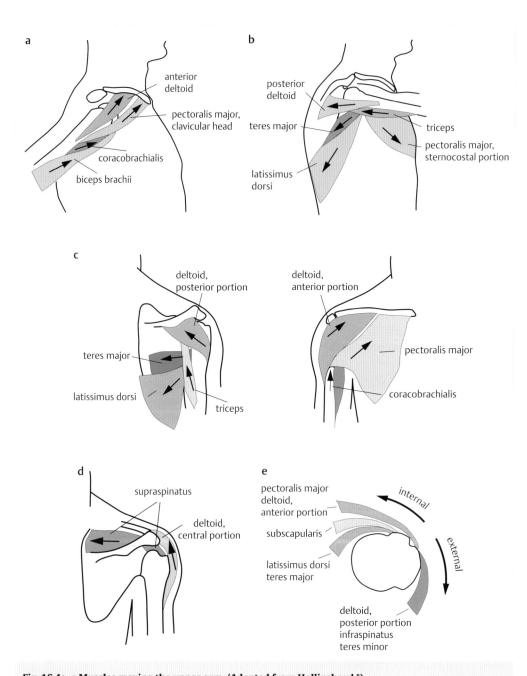

Fig. 16.4a–e Muscles moving the upper arm. (Adapted from Hollinshead.[8])

a Anteflexion.

b Retroflexion (extension).

c Adduction (left: posterior view, right: anterior view).

d Abduction.

e Internal and external rotation (seen from above).

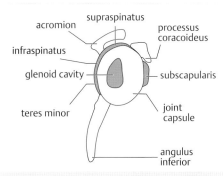

Fig. 16.5 Rotator cuff. Lateral view of the right shoulder, seen from the right side. (Adapted, with permission, from van der Helm.[9])

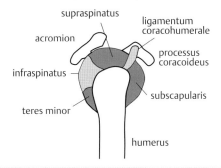

Fig. 16.6 View of the rotator cuff. Right shoulder, seen from the right. (Adapted from Tillmann et al.[3])

used imprecisely. The term *instability* is sometimes used when merely an increased range of motion is observed. For example, an increased range of motion of adjoining lumbar vertebrae compared to the norm in healthy persons is called *segmental instability* of the spine. Correctly, it should be called *hypermobility*, because the articulating bones can always return to their initial position. In the mechanical sense, a joint is unstable only when the articulating bones cannot return to their initial positions after being acted on by an external force or after performing a particular movement.

Instability of the shoulder joint exists if the humeral head dislocates from the glenoid cavity because of low muscle tone or under the influence of an externally applied force. Dislocation may occur during small, everyday movements such as putting on a coat or turning over in bed. This event is analogous to the luxation of the hip seen in patients with a dysplastic acetabulum. Displacement of the shoulder joint is termed *caudal*, *anterior* (the most common), or *posterior*, depending on the direction in which the humeral head dislocates. Athletes in disciplines requiring forceful overhead movements of the arm (javelin throwing, for example) are at increased risk of dislocations of the shoulder joint.[10]

The predisposition of the shoulder joint to instability is the price paid for the large range of motion of this joint. To facilitate a large range of motion, the shoulder joint is designed as ball-and-socket joint. This type of joint permits angular motion in a large range and simultaneous rotation about the long axis of the bone (**Fig. 16.7**). To prevent the ball, or sphere, of the loaded joint from being pushed out of the socket, the socket must enclose a part of the sphere. The more the sphere is enclosed, the smaller the risk of its being pushed out. At the same time, however, the more the sphere is enclosed, the smaller the joint's range of motion. The range of motion of ball-and-socket joints in the human body is end-stopped by contact between the articulating bone and the rim of the socket. In the example shown in **Fig. 16.7** the socket encloses the sphere by 180°. The range of motion α is, however, much less than 180°. If the diameter of the long bone where it transitions into the sphere were smaller, this would increase the range of motion—but the diameter of the bone cannot be reduced too much without excessively compromising its strength.

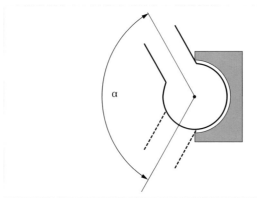

Fig. 16.7 The range of motion of a ball-and socket joint is end-stopped by contact between the articulating bone and the rim of the socket. If the ball, or sphere, is enclosed 180° by the socket, the range of motion α is much less than 180°.

Alternatively the range of motion can be increased by reducing the extent to which the sphere is enclosed by the socket. Nature chose this design in the shoulder joint, combining the spherical head of the humerus with a shallow socket (**Fig. 16.8**). However, when the socket encloses only a small portion of the sphere, the risk of instability increases. In a friction-free ball-and-socket joint the vector of the joint load is perpendicular to the joint surface; it intersects the center of the sphere. In the absence of additional safety measures, the sphere will always be pushed out of the socket when the line of action of the joint load **F** does not intersect the socket. In the example shown in **Fig. 16.8**, the force **F** generates a moment in relation to the lower rim of the socket

(16.1) $$M = -L \cdot F$$

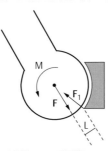

Fig. 16.8 Increasing the range of motion by having a shallower socket. If the load vector **F** does not point at the socket, the moment $| M | = L \cdot F$ tends to lever the sphere out of the socket and the joint is unstable. The reaction force $\mathbf{F}_1$ cannot stabilize the joint.

which tends to lever the sphere out of the socket (the minus sign results from the sign convention for moments). In this situation, a reaction force $\mathbf{F}_1$ acting from the socket on the sphere cannot alone—that is, without additional muscle or tendon forces—establish mechanical equilibrium.

The shoulder joint is protected against instability in three ways. First, in the scapulohumeral rhythm the socket follows the motion of the arm. This increases the likelihood that the line of action of the load vector, which always points approximately along the direction of the upper arm, will intersect the socket. Secondly, the muscles of the rotator cuff can exert an additional force on the humeral head, pressing the head into the socket. As an example, **Fig. 16.9** shows a joint load vector **F** which initially does not point into the socket. However, if, in addition to the force **F**, a muscle force $\mathbf{F}_m$ is exerted, the vector sum $\mathbf{F}_r$ of the two forces points into the socket and provides joint stability. Thirdly, the shoulder joint is stabilized by the joint capsule and the ligamentous connections between humerus and scapula (coracohumeral and glenohumeral ligaments). Slack in the middle of the range of motion, these structures become tight at the end of the range, where they assist in stabilizing the joint.[11]

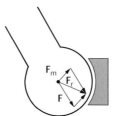

Fig. 16.9 If, in addition to the force **F**, a muscle force $\mathbf{F}_m$ is exerted, the resulting force $\mathbf{F}_r$ points to the socket and the joint is stable.

16.4 Loading of the Shoulder Joint

In contrast to the hip joint, where interest is focused on repetitive loading during walking, the shoulder joint is subject to widely varying modes of loading. The studies discussed below relate to specific problems, such as the load on certain muscles or tendons or the load on the shoulder joint resulting from forces acting on the arm or the hand. Forces act on the hand, for example, when objects are held and lifted, or a ball is thrown, or a wheelchair is being propelled. Apart from their academic interest, the aim of these studies is the identification of risks due to overloading or the provision of basic data for the construction of artificial joint replacement.

Model calculations of the loading of the shoulder joint are complicated by the fact that in virtually all postures and movements several muscles have to be taken into account. As for all model calculations, assumptions have to be made about the activation pattern of these muscles. Furthermore, because of the spatial architecture of the muscles, activation of a muscle to generate a moment to equilibrate the moment of an external force may simultaneously generate "unwanted" moments about other axes, which then have to be equilibrated by the activation of further muscles. For example, the pectoralis major generates a moment that lowers the forward-raised arm. Due to the insertion of this muscle at the clavicle, the arm is simultaneously pulled medially and rotated (Veeger et al[12]; see also **Fig. 16.4b**). If a purely downward movement is intended, additional muscles have to be activated—in this case the supraspinatus and infraspinatus. Moreover, since the muscles move along with the arm, their lever arms with respect to the shoulder joint may change during the course of the movement. In some situations muscles change their mechanical function, as when, in the course of a movement, the line of action of the muscle force shifts to the other side of the center of rotation.

The following sections discuss different approaches to determining shoulder joint load. The results of the calculations give an impression of the order of magnitude of the load. The results can be compared with recent measurements of shoulder joint load obtained by means of an instrumented artificial joint replacement.

16.4.1 Static Plane Model Calculations

Fig. 16.10 shows a simplified model for calculating the load on the shoulder joint when the straight arm is held horizontally abducted.[13] The gravitational force $\mathbf{F}_1$ of the arm acts at the center of mass (close to the elbow joint). It is assumed that the equilibrium of moments is fulfilled exclusively by the force $\mathbf{F}_2$ of the deltoid (see **Fig. 16.4d**). In equilibrium it holds that

(16.2)
$$L_2 \cdot F_2 - L_1 \cdot F_1 = 0$$

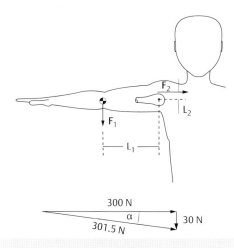

Fig. 16.10 Estimating the load on the shoulder joint with the arm horizontally abducted. (Adapted from Poppen and Walker.[13])

By inserting estimated values of 30 cm for L_1, 3 cm for L_2, and 30 N for the weight of the arm (corresponding to 5% of the body weight of a person of 60 kg mass), we obtain for the magnitude of the force $\mathbf{F}_2$ of the
deltoid muscle

(16.3)
$$F_2 = F_1 \cdot L_1 / L_2$$
$$F_2 = 300 \text{ N}$$

The joint load $\mathbf{G}$ is opposite and equal to the vector sum of muscle and gravitational force. Since the angle
between the muscle and the gravitational force amounts to 90°, the magnitude of the joint load is calculated as

(16.4)
$$G = \sqrt{300^2 + 30^2} = 301.5 \text{ N}$$

This force is transmitted to the trunk via the scapulothoracic and the sternoclavicular joints. The vector of
the joint load forms an angle α

(16.5)
$$\alpha = \operatorname{atan}(30 \text{ N} / 300 \text{ N}) = 5.7°$$

with the horizontal. Whether or not the line of action of this vector intersects the socket—and thus whether
or not activation of the deltoid alone will keep the joint stable—depends on the orientation of the socket.

If, keeping the same posture, mass held in the hand is added, increased force from the deltoid is required
to maintain equilibrium. Inserting estimated values of 10 N additional load (corresponding to an additional
mass of approximately 1.0 kg) and a moment arm of the additional load of approx. $2 \cdot L_1$, we obtain for the
additional force F_3 of the deltoid

(16.6)
$$F_3 = 10 \cdot 2 \cdot 30 / 3 = 200 \text{ N}$$

and for the joint load G, as the sum of the muscular and gravitational forces,

(16.7) $$G = \sqrt{(300+200)^2 + (30+10)^2} = 501.6 \text{ N}$$

To estimate the load on the shoulder joint when the upper arm is raised in the plane of the scapula, Poppen and Walker[13] developed another model that took a number of muscles into account. Electromyography (EMG) measurements were used to determine which muscles were activated during this movement: supraspinatus, deltoid, subscapularis, infraspinatus, and latissimus dorsi. The moment arms of these muscles in relation to the center of rotation of the joint were determined from specimens. The muscle forces were assumed to be proportional to the cross-sectional area of the muscles multiplied by the integral of the EMG signal. Under these assumptions the load on the shoulder joint amounted to 0.05 times body weight when the arm was hanging at the side. When the arm was raised to 90° anteflexion the load increased to 0.8 times body weight, and when the arm was raised to 150° anteflexion the load fell to 0.4 times body weight.

16.4.2 Static Three-Dimensional Model Calculations

Van der Helm[9] presented a detailed model of the shoulder region consisting of the bony elements thorax, sternum, clavicle, scapula, and humerus, and 20 muscles, including those muscles which run from the shoulder region to the lower arm. The geometry of the skeleton, the areas of insertion, and cross-sectional areas of the muscles were obtained from anatomical studies. The scapulohumeral rhythm was taken into account. In order to enforce an unequivocal solution for the mechanically indeterminate system, the sum of the squares of the tensile stress generated by muscles was postulated to assume a minimum. The maximum tensile stress generated by muscles was assumed to amount to 37 N/cm². The calculation yielded muscle forces and joint loads were obtained (not just the load on the shoulder joint, but also those on the sternoclavicular and acromioclavicular joints and the force between scapula and thorax). The direction of the vector of the load on the shoulder joint in relation to the socket provides information on the stability of the joint.

According to van der Helm[9], with the elbow extended, the load on the shoulder joint, on the sternoclavicular and acromioclavicular joints, and on the contact area between the scapula and the thorax depends on the angle of anteflexion of the arm. Maximum values are observed at angles close to 90°. At this angle the load on the shoulder joint amounts to approximately 340 N. If an additional force of 75 N acts on the hand, the load rises to approximately 550 N. In this posture and without additional load in the hand the acromioclavicular joint is loaded by approximately 150 N; a load of 75 N on the hand increases this load to about 270 N.

Hughes and An[14] determined the force of the muscles of the rotator cuff (teres minor, infraspinatus, supraspinatus, subscapularis) by means of a model calculation. The model included 10 muscles in the shoulder region. Their cross sections and moment arms in relation to the center of rotation of the shoulder joint were determined from specimens. In a cohort of healthy subjects, the maximum moments exerted in vivo in the direction of internal and external rotation with the upper arm in different postures were measured (**Fig. 16.11**). The results of the calculation showed that generating maximum moments requires particularly high forces of the muscles of the rotator cuff, especially the subscapularis and infraspinatus. By comparison, the muscle forces that occur when the arm is lifted against gravity or against an additional external resistance are smaller. When evaluating exposure to physical exertions in the workplace, or when giving advice to patients with shoulder complaints, it has to be borne in mind that in the posture with abducted upper arm and flexed elbow (**Fig. 16.12**) a gravitational force **F** on the hand generates an adduction moment and at the same time an internal rotation moment acting on the upper arm.

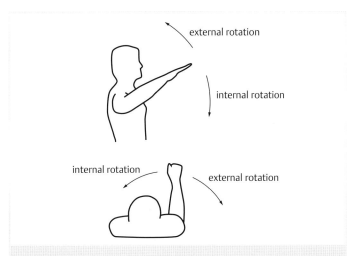

Fig. 16.11 Postures of the arm during determination of maximum internal and external rotation moments. (Adapted from Hughes and An.[14])

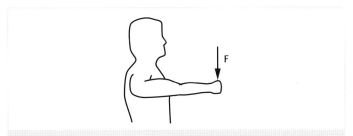

Fig. 16.12 In the posture shown (upper arm 90° abduction, elbow 90° flexion), a gravitational force **F** exerts adduction as well as internal rotation moments on the upper arm. The internal rotation moment exerts load on the muscles of the rotator cuff. (Adapted form Hughes and An.[14])

Anglin et al[15] determined the load on the shoulder joint for five activities: rising from a chair with the help of the arms, sitting down with the help of the arms, walking with a cane, lifting a 5-kg box from floor to shoulder height, and lifting a 10-kg suitcase. The authors regarded these loads as typical of everyday loading episodes in elderly subjects and in patients with artificial shoulder replacement. Six persons aged above 50 years were studied. The motion of the right arm and the trunk was traced by optical methods. The model calculation took the bones of the shoulder girdle and arm as well as 22 muscles into account. The calculation was quasi-static as the accelerations of the body segments, the box, and the suitcase were small enough to ignore. **Fig. 16.13** shows an overview of the results; the graph cites the mean values of the maximum shoulder load observed during five repetitions of the exercises. The calculated load varied considerably between repetitions. The authors hypothesize that this is due to slight modifications to the arm postures and to the objective function employed (minimization of the sum of the squares of the muscular tensile stresses together with a limiting value for the muscular tensile stress). In all activities investigated the load vector intersected the glenoid cavity (the socket) in its anterior, upper quadrant. This last-mentioned result is of importance for the development of artificial joint replacements, especially in terms of fixation of the socket.

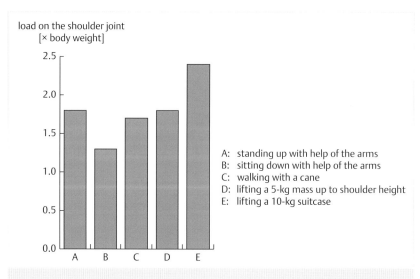

Fig. 16.13 Loads on the shoulder joint caused by five everyday activities. (Adapted from Anglin et al.[15])

16.4.3 Dynamic Three-Dimensional Model Calculations

If, in addition to the effects of external static forces and moments, the influence of inertial forces and moments is to be determined, the arm is subdivided into the segments hand, lower arm, and upper arm. If the masses, locations of the centers of mass, moments of inertia, linear and angular accelerations, and external forces are known, the technique of inverse dynamics can be used to calculate the force and moment transmitted from the upper arm to the trunk. To obtain the load on the shoulder joint, in a second step a model of the joint has to be developed: based on anatomical observations, it must specify which muscles actually generate the moment transmitted from the upper arm to the trunk (similar to the calculation of hip joint load using gait analysis, see Chapter 13).

If, however, the intention is merely to compare the loads on the shoulder joint in different activities, it may in certain cases suffice to compare the net moments exerted on the shoulder joint. This is so because, in identical postures of the joint—that is, with given moment arms and directions of the muscle forces—the joint load is virtually equal to the vector sum of the muscle forces and thus proportional to the moment transmitted. (If the postures are different, this is strictly no longer true, because moment arms, directions of muscle forces, and activation patterns of the muscles may change depending on the posture.) We will now consider two examples of the determination of dynamic shoulder load. An overview of other relevant literature, especially in the field of rehabilitation, will be found in Slavens and Harris.[16]

Veeger et al[17] determined the motion sequence of the arm in propelling a wheelchair as well as the force and the moment acting on the hand. Employing models of the muscles of the shoulder region[8] and of the arm,[18] the force of 17 muscles of the shoulder region and the load on the shoulder joint were obtained. At a wheelchair velocity of 3 km/h and a power level of 20 W, the load on the shoulder joint in the propulsion phase amounted on average to 700 N; in the phase where the arm was retracted the load amounted to approximately 300 N. In the propulsion phase the subscapularis was the most highly stressed muscle (approximately 200 N); in the retraction phase the deltoid was the most highly loaded (approximately 200 N). In general the forces of the muscles of the rotator cuff (subscapularis, infraspinatus, and supraspinatus) were comparable in magnitude to the forces of the deltoid, biceps, and triceps. The authors point out that the muscle forces determined are not particularly high, but overload damage may still occur due to the high repetition rate in wheelchair propulsion.

In a cohort of wheelchair users that included both paraplegic and tetraplegic patients and able-bodied persons, van Drongelen et al[19] determined the moments acting on the elbow and shoulder during the following activities: propulsion on a level floor and a slope of 3%, lifting the body to take the weight off the seat, grasping an object, and negotiating a curb 10 cm high. The force and moment acting on the hand were measured and the motion of the segments of the arm (hand, lower arm, upper arm) was documented. Transmitted moments were calculated applying the technique of inverse dynamics. **Fig. 16.14** shows the maximum values of the moments transmitted by the shoulder in the subgroup of paraplegic individuals. Negotiating a curb and lifting the body off the seat by exerting force with the arms on the pushrims result in high shoulder loads. By comparison, the load when propelling the wheelchair is quite small. For three of the above-mentioned activities, a model of the muscles of the shoulder region was employed to calculate

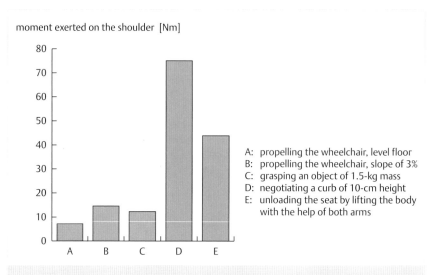

moment exerted on the shoulder [Nm]

A: propelling the wheelchair, level floor
B: propelling the wheelchair, slope of 3%
C: grasping an object of 1.5-kg mass
D: negotiating a curb of 10-cm height
E: unloading the seat by lifting the body
   with the help of both arms

Fig. 16.14 Moments exerted on the shoulder during wheelchair propulsion (paraplegic subjects). (Adapted, with permission, from van Drongelen et al.[19])

the load on the shoulder joint.[20] Among the paraplegic patients, the peak shoulder load for propulsion on a plane was approximately 300 N, that for grasping an object approximately 600 N, and for lifting the body off the seat approximately 1300 N. The authors remark that when estimating the risk of overload damage in wheelchair users, it has to be kept in mind that the repetition rate of the activities investigated varies widely.

16.4.4 Measurement of Shoulder Load by Means of an Instrumented Joint Prosthesis

Westerhoff et al[21] carried out measurements of the load on the shoulder joint in vivo. For this purpose, the shafts of shoulder joint prostheses were fitted with strain gauges enabling measurement of the deformation of the shafts under the influence of forces and moments. The electric circuits received their power supply from an induction coil and the data were transmitted telemetrically to an external receiver. Prior to implantation the instrumented artificial joint was calibrated in the laboratory by applying known forces and moments to the head of the prosthesis and measuring the resulting deformations. After implantation it was possible, therefore, to compute the three-dimensional forces and moments at work from the measured deformation values. Direct measurement of the joint load has the advantage that the result depends neither on assumptions about the numbers, directions, moment arms, or activation patterns of the muscles involved, nor on the choice of objective functions. However, due to the considerable technical and medical costs of measuring joint loading in vivo, it can only be done in a small number of people. In addition, there are only certain tasks and exercises that patients with an artificial joint can be asked to perform.

Westerhoff et al[21] report the loads on the shoulder joint measured in four patients while they were performing everyday activities: holding a mass, combing their hair, turning a steering wheel, and hammering in a nail at eye height. Lifting a coffee pot (1.5 kg) with the arm stretched forwards exerted a load amounting to an average of 1.1 times body weight. As the coffee pot was put down, a higher load of 1.2 times body weight was measured, probably due to the activation of additional muscles in order to avoid "banging" the pot down. Maximum load values were observed when the arm was raised anteriorly or abducted 90° with additional weight in the hand. Placing a 2-kg mass onto a shelf at eye height loaded the joint by approximately 1.3 times body weight. Holding a 10-kg mass laterally at hip height (with a small moment arm in relation to the shoulder joint) loaded the shoulder joint by 0.12 times body weight. When the mass was slowly lifted from this position, the load on the shoulder joint increased to about 0.9 times body weight. The direction of the vector of the joint load showed only minor deviations from the direction of the upper arm. This is easy to understand, as the muscles move with the upper arm. On the other hand, it also means that the direction of the load on the glenoid cavity varies considerably in the course of the motion of the upper arm. In addition to the forces, Westerhoff et al[21] observed the moment acting on the head of the prosthesis. This moment originates from friction between the joint surfaces and from the deformation of the loaded joint (analogous to rolling friction).

The measured data can be compared with results from previous model calculations. Van der Helm[9] determined the load on the shoulder joint with the arm horizontally extended to be 340 N, and with an additional load of 75 N on the hand it was 550 N. Assuming a linear relation between additional hand load and additional shoulder load, one extrapolates a shoulder load of approximately 380 N for a hand load of 15 N (as employed by Westerhoff et al[21]). This is lower than the value of 1.1 times body weight actually measured by Westerhoff et al. With 86 kg as the mean body mass in the cohort investigated, 1.1 times body weight corresponds to $1.1 \cdot 86 \text{ kg} \cdot g = 928 \text{ N}$. Thus, the model calculation cited underestimated the load on the shoulder joint.

Nikooyan et al[22] compared the load on the shoulder joint measured with an instrumented prosthesis with the load determined from model calculations based on the Delft shoulder and elbow model[18] (a further development of the model of van der Helm[9]). When the arm is moved in anteflexion or abduction there is overall satisfactory agreement between the measured and the calculated load. However, some systematic differences exist; **Fig. 16.15** shows an example. The calculations were performed using two different objective functions (muscle tensile stress and energy consumption) and with the model adjusted for the height and weight of the individuals being studied. In the region between 0° and 90° elevation, **Fig. 16.15** shows good agreement between the measured and the calculated load. It seems that the choice of objective functions plays only a minor role in the context of the model calculation; compared with this, the adjustment of the model parameters to the individual case has a greater influence on the results. With

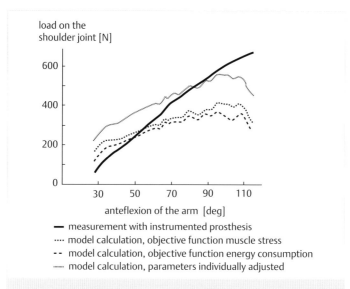

measurement with instrumented prosthesis
···· model calculation, objective function muscle stress
-- model calculation, objective function energy consumption
······ model calculation, parameters individually adjusted

Fig. 16.15 Load on the shoulder joint when the arm is raised in the frontal plane. In vivo measurement with an instrumented prosthesis, model calculations using different objective functions, and model calculation adjusted for segmental masses, body weight, and body height in the individual case. (Adapted, with permission, from Nikooyan et al.[22])

elevation above 90°, the measured load shows a further increase whereas the calculated load decreases. A fall in the calculated shoulder load above 90° elevation might be expected even on the basis of simple model calculations, because the moment arm of the gravitational force of the arm is greatest at 90° and decreases at angles greater than 90°. Nikooyan et al[22] speculate that the load increase above 90° is caused by antagonistic muscle activation. In theory this could be verified by EMG measurements, but in practice this is difficult because several muscles in the shoulder region are not accessible to measurement by EMG.

References

1. Putz R. Biomechanik des Schultergürtels. Manuelle Medizin 1986;24:1–7

2. Graichen H, Hinterwimmer S, von Eisenhart-Rothe R, Vogl T, Englmeier KH, Eckstein F. Effect of abducting and adducting muscle activity on glenohumeral translation, scapular kinematics and subacromial space width in vivo. J Biomech 2005;38(4):755–760

3. Tillmann B, Töndury G, eds. Bewegungsapparat. 2nd ed. Stuttgart: Thieme; 1998. Leonhardt H, Tillmann B, Töndury G, Zilles K, eds. Rauber/Kopsch: Anatomie des Menschen; Band 1

4. Poppen NK, Walker PS. Normal and abnormal motion of the shoulder. J Bone Joint Surg Am 1976;58(2):195–201

5. Högfors C, Sigholm G, Herberts P. Biomechanical model of the human shoulder—I. Elements. J Biomech 1987;20(2):157–166

6. Högfors C, Peterson B, Sigholm G, Herberts P. Biomechanical model of the human shoulder joint—II. The shoulder rhythm. J Biomech 1991;24(8):699–709

7. Endo K, Yukata K, Yasui N. Influence of age on scapulo-thoracic orientation. Clin Biomech (Bristol, Avon) 2004;19(10):1009–1013

8. Hollinshead WH. The Back and Limbs. Philadelphia: Harper & Row; 1982. Anatomy for Surgeons; vol 3

9. van der Helm FC. Analysis of the kinematic and dynamic behavior of the shoulder mechanism. J Biomech 1994;27(5):527–550

10. Blevins FT. Rotator cuff pathology in athletes. Sports Med 1997;24(3):205–220

11. Itoi E, Hsu HC, An KN. Biomechanical investigation of the glenohumeral joint. J Shoulder Elbow Surg 1996;5(5):407–424

12. Veeger HE, van der Helm FC. Shoulder function: the perfect compromise between mobility and stability. J Biomech 2007;40(10):2119–2129

13. Poppen NK, Walker PS. Forces at the glenohumeral joint in abduction. Clin Orthop Relat Res 1978; (135):165–170

14. Hughes RE, An KN. Force analysis of rotator cuff muscles. Clin Orthop Relat Res 1996;(330):75–83

15. Anglin C, Wyss UP, Pichora DR. Glenohumeral contact forces. Proc Inst Mech Eng H 2000;214(6):637–644

16. Slavens BA, Harris GF. The biomechanics of upper extremity kinematic and kinetic modeling: applications to rehabilitation engineering. Crit Rev Biomed Eng 2008;36(2-3):93–125

17. Veeger HE, Rozendaal LA, van der Helm FC. Load on the shoulder in low intensity wheelchair propulsion. Clin Biomech (Bristol, Avon) 2002;17(3):211–218

18. Veeger HE, Yu B, An KN, Rozendal RH. Parameters for modeling the upper extremity. J Biomech 1997;30(6):647–652

19. van Drongelen S, Van der Woude LH, Janssen TW, Angenot EL, Chadwick EK, Veeger DH. Mechanical load on the upper extremity during wheelchair activities. Arch Phys Med Rehabil 2005;86(6):1214–1220

20. van Drongelen S, van der Woude LH, Janssen TW, Angenot EL, Chadwick EK, Veeger DH. Glenohumeral contact forces and muscle forces evaluated in wheelchair-related activities of daily living in able-bodied subjects versus subjects with paraplegia and tetraplegia. Arch Phys Med Rehabil 2005;86(7):1434–1440

21. Westerhoff P, Graichen F, Bender A, et al. In vivo measurement of shoulder joint loads during activities of daily living. J Biomech 2009;42(12):1840–1849

22. Nikooyan AA, Veeger HE, Westerhoff P, Graichen F, Bergmann G, van der Helm FC. Validation of the Delft Shoulder and Elbow Model using in-vivo glenohumeral joint contact forces. J Biomech 2010;43(15):3007–3014

17   Biomechanics of the Foot

The foot has static, kinematic, and dynamic functions. It carries the weight of the body, which is distributed roughly equally to both feet in stance. The foot is also capable of carrying the entire body weight for a short time. Along with static stability, this also requires an ability to regulate dynamic balance. When standing, and even more when walking and running, the foot must be able to adapt to the conditions of the ground beneath it. Extensive and secure contact with the ground is necessary in the stance phase, even when the ground is sloping or uneven. On the other hand, sufficient ground clearance must be ensured during the swing phase. This requires that the effective length of the leg is shortened by flexing the knee and ankle. The foot transmits forces that not only control balance but also provide locomotion. In the push-off phase of the gait cycle the foot forms a rigid moment arm that transmits a propulsive force generated by the extension moment in the knee and ankle joint. The opposing braking force is transmitted by the contralateral leg on heel strike.

To meet these diverse requirements the foot has a complex structure (**Fig. 17.1**). The foot skeleton consists of 26 bones. Some of them articulate with several neighboring bones. The foot is held together by muscles and ligaments. These allow the foot to adjust its position, its shape, and its rigidity as necessary.

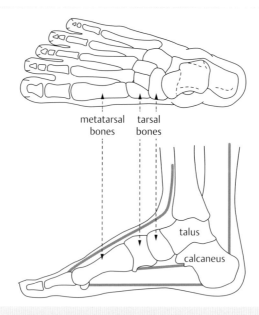

Fig. 17.1 Upper: Outline and skeleton of the right foot, proximal view. Lower: Medial view of the right foot. The bones of the second to fifth rays are not shown. The Achilles tendon, the fascia containing the plantar aponeurosis, the long plantar ligament, and the tendons of the toe extensors are depicted in gray.

The bones of the foot are grouped functionally and anatomically into the hindfoot, the midfoot, and the forefoot.

In the ankle or talocrural joint the distal ends of the tibia and fibula articulate with the trochlear surface of the talus. This is shaped roughly like a cylinder. It is flanked by the articular facets of the tibial and fibular malleoli. The talus has two further joint surfaces on its plantar aspect, which articulate posteriorly with the calcaneus and anteriorly with the calcaneus and the navicular. A bony canal, the tarsal sinus, runs between the anterior and posterior joint compartments. The joint complex comprising the talocalcaneal joint and the talonavicular joint is called the talocalcaneonavicular joint[1] or subtalar joint.

All the bones of the foot below the talus comprise the subtalar footplate.[2,3] The hindfoot consists of the talus and calcaneus. It is bounded by the Chopart joint, which articulates with the cuboid and navicular bones. Together with the three cuneiform bones, the talus, calcaneus, cuboid, and navicular comprise the tarsal bones, which are separated from the metatarsal bones by the Lisfranc joint. The tarsal and metatarsal bones constitute the midfoot,[4] though they are sometimes assigned to the forefoot,[5] which also includes the 14 phalanges of the toes. The metatarsals and phalanges are grouped into five rays. The first ray comprises the metatarsal and phalanges of the great toe, and the fifth ray accordingly those of the little toe.

The arrangement of the bones of the foot forms a characteristic longitudinal arch. It extends from the calcaneus to the metatarsal heads. The transverse arch is less obvious and its actual existence is sometimes disputed; it may be identified most readily at the level of the cuneiform bones. Only the lateral part of this arch is in contact with the ground. The arches are sustained by the plantar fascia and ligaments as well as by muscular action. The most important fasciae are the plantar aponeurosis and the long plantar ligament.

17.1   The Kinematic Chain of the Foot

Drawing on general mechanical terminology, the foot and hand are also referred to as "branched open kinematic chains." What this means is that they each consist of a series of different, distinct joints linked together from proximal to distal. The term is intended to suggest how a distal limb carries out a movement that is composed of the individual movements of the more proximal joints along the same branch.

Abduction and adduction of the foot, leading to external and internal rotation, originate in the hip and knee. The ankle, comprising the talocrural joint and the subtalar joint, allows movements around two different anatomical axes (**Fig. 17.2**) and composite movements involving both axes. More distally, in the Chopart and Lisfranc joints the foot may perform small movements mainly to adapt to the conditions of the ground beneath it, though these movements are limited by the tension of the fasciae.

The kinematic properties of the foot are mainly due to the talocrural joint (sometimes also termed the ankle proper) and the subtalar joint. From various points of view the two joints can be regarded as a functional unit. This is due to the fact that the talus is involved in and connects the two joints. A particular

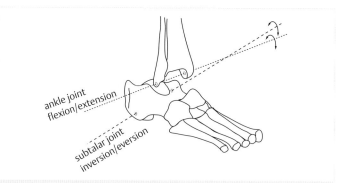

Fig. 17.2 Location and orientation of the axes of the talocrural and subtalar joints between the malleoli above and the calcaneus below. For simplicity, the talus has been omitted. The axis of the talocrural joint is nearly transverse, and the subtalar joint axis runs obliquely from posterior and inferolateral to anterior and superomedial. (Adapted from Debrunner and Jacob.[6])

feature of the talus is that no muscles are attached to it, and instead it is fixed by ligaments only. This means that it cannot be kept in position or moved specifically by muscular action. All the muscles involved in foot movements cross the talus, the ankle, and subtalar joint. Consequently, the forces from the forefoot, hindfoot, and tibia that act on the talus must compensate each other and no moment can be transmitted. In addition, the axes of the two joints differ in orientation but they intersect near the tarsal sinus, that is, in the region of the talus.[5] It remains unclear whether the two axes do actually intersect or merely pass close to one another.

The relative positions of the axes of the talocrural and subtalar joints suggest comparison with a technical joint, for example a universal or Cardan joint. However, in contrast to an engineered universal joint, the two axes of the ankle joint are not orthogonal. The axis of the talocrural joint runs roughly transversely and it allows dorsiflexion and plantar flexion of the whole foot in the sagittal plane. The axis of the subtalar joint runs obliquely from the medial dorsal aspect of the navicular bone to the lateral plantar aspect. Rotatory movements about this axis lead to a coupled movement, in which an outward or inward movement of the tip of the foot occurs simultaneously with lowering and elevation of the medial border of the foot.

Unfortunately the nomenclature for these movements is not uniform. Only the movement about the axis of the talocrural joint is consistently named: *plantar flexion* and *dorsiflexion*. Kummer[5] describes the movement around the subtalar joint axis as "pronation/supination," while Mann[7] describes it as "inversion/eversion" (see **Fig. 17.2**). The International Society of Biomechanics[8] recommends the terms "inversion" and "eversion" to describe the composite rotation around the longitudinal axis of the foot, in contrast to the American Academy of Orthopaedic Surgeons (AAOS)[9] and various textbooks,[10] where "inversion/eversion" describes the movement around the axis of the subtalar joint and "supination/pronation" means movement around the longitudinal axis of the foot. A detailed discussion may be found in Debrunner and Jacob.[6]

The basic studies to measure the joint axes in the ankle joint complex were conducted by Isman and Inman[11] and Inman.[12] They performed measurements in cadaver specimens and determined the means and standard deviations for the position and orientation of the axes. The orientation of the talocrural axis is defined by reference to the axis of the shank and the longitudinal axis of the foot, which is itself defined by Inman as the line connecting the center of the heel to the gap between the second and third toes. The axis of the talocrural joint is nearly perpendicular to the plane spanned by these two axes. In the frontal plane it inclines approximately 10°, with the lateral end lower than the medial end. In the transverse plane the axis is inclined by approximately 6°, with the lateral end lying further back than the medial end. The lateral end of the axis of the subtalar joint lies behind and below the medial end. In the proximal view the axis forms an angle of $23 \pm 11°$ with the longitudinal axis of the foot, and in the lateral view it forms an angle of $41 \pm 9°$ with the horizontal. The strikingly large standard deviations are due to the fact that interindividual variation is so great.

Measurements of the location and orientation of the axes of the ankle and subtalar joints are subject not only to individual variations but also to technical inaccuracies if measurements are not based on specimens or performed using imaging techniques or with intracortical bone pins.[13] As the talus is not directly accessible from outside, its position cannot be indicated by markers. Furthermore, the value of such measurements is limited by the fact that the position and orientation especially of the axis of the subtalar joint depend on the direction of movement (flexion or extension) and loading of the joint.[14] For clinical studies, individual modeling and description of the kinematics are necessary. Using X-ray stereophotogrammetry, Lundberg et al[15] confirmed the earlier results of Hicks,[16] who found that the orientation of the talocrural axis in the frontal plane changes depending on dorsiflexion and plantar flexion, but in the horizontal plane it remains stable; that is, it continues to pass through the malleoli.

17.2 Statics of the Foot

Because of its longitudinal arch, the loading of the foot during standing occurs mainly in two anatomical regions: the heel region, with the calcaneus as one bony support, and the ball of the foot, with the metatarsal heads as the other bony support. The fifth ray contributes a minor degree of lateral support in the midfoot region, but this can be ignored for the purpose of calculations. To ensure a secure stance, the line of gravity—the line of action of the gravitational force **W**—must pass through the foot at a point between the supports in the forefoot and hindfoot. In doing so, it gives rise to two moment arms, one of the forefoot and one of the hindfoot, denoted by d_f and d_h respectively. The ground reaction forces acting on the forefoot and the hindfoot are denoted by $\mathbf{R}_f$ and $\mathbf{R}_h$ respectively. In equilibrium of moments (**Fig. 17.3**)

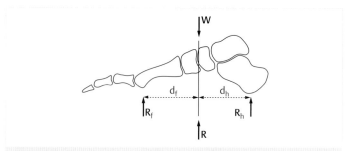

Fig. 17.3 Diagram of the foot with a cross section through the second ray showing the moment arms of the forefoot and hindfoot for transmission of the ground reaction force **R**. d_f is the moment arm of the forefoot and d_h that of the hindfoot.

$$d_f \cdot R_f = d_h \cdot R_h$$
(17.1)
$$d_f / d_h = R_h / R_f$$

The sum of $\mathbf{R_f}$ and $\mathbf{R_h}$ is equal to the ground reaction force $\mathbf{R}$. $\mathbf{R}$ is opposite and equal to the gravitational force $\mathbf{W}$.

In relaxed stance the line of gravity runs through the foot near the Lisfranc joint and the distances d_f and d_h are in an approximate ratio of 2 : 3, so $\mathbf{R_f}$ and $\mathbf{R_h}$ amount to approximately 60% and 40% of the body weight respectively. The position of the line of gravity is variable, however, changing relative to the foot during the phases of gait and on changes in posture. The further forward it is, the greater the proportion of the reaction force acting below the forefoot. When the line of gravity runs through the ball of the foot, the magnitude of the reaction force R_f equals the body weight. In this position, compensatory movements to ensure stable stance are no longer possible without involving the toes.

17.2.1 Loading of the Ankle

In normal stance the left and right ankle each support half of the weight of the body less the weight of the respective foot, which amounts to 1.5% of body weight. However, loading of the ankle is increased if the line of gravity does not pass midway between the two ankles but is shifted forwards. The load on one foot— generated by half the body weight—can be estimated by a model calculation similar to the one used for the hip in Chapter 13, though, in this case, the model is set up in the sagittal plane. The gravitational force $\mathbf{W}$ acts vertically, parallel to the y-coordinate, and is denoted below by $\mathbf{W_y}$ (**Fig. 17.4**). The moment around the ankle joint produced by the gravitational force is compensated by the force $\mathbf{A}$ in the Achilles tendon. For simplicity, only the y-component will be considered and will be denoted as $\mathbf{A_y}$. The resulting force $\mathbf{R_y}$ acts on the ankle. Its line of action must intersect the axis of the ankle joint, as otherwise it would produce

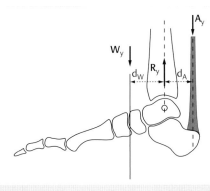

Fig. 17.4 Equilibrium above the ankle joint. The Achilles tendon is depicted in gray. The center of rotation in the talus is indicated by a circle. Besides the gravitational force $\mathbf{W}_y$, the diagram shows only the vertical components of force $\mathbf{A}_y$ of the Achilles tendon and the reaction force $\mathbf{R}_y$ on the talus. The variables d_W and d_A indicate the moment arms of W_y and A_y.

a moment around the ankle in contradiction of the conditions of equilibrium. Limiting the discussion to these three forces means that antagonists such as the dorsal flexor muscles of the foot and toes are ignored, although their action is necessary for a stable stance and they further increase the actual load on the ankle.

The plantar flexion moment exerted by the triceps surae muscle through the Achilles tendon is

(17.2)
$$M_A = A_y \cdot d_A$$

The opposing moment due to the gravitational force is

(17.3)
$$M_W = -W_y \cdot d_W$$

Because of their different directions of rotation, the two moments have opposite signs. In static equilibrium

(17.4)
$$M_A + M_W = 0$$

Therefore the magnitude of force $\mathbf{A}_y$ in the Achilles tendon can be obtained from

(17.5)
$$A_y = (d_W / d_A) \cdot W_y$$

According to the equilibrium condition, the three forces must add up to 0, that is,

(17.6)
$$A_y + W_y + R_y = 0$$

After substitution the magnitude of the reaction force $\mathbf{R}_y$ acting on the subtalar joint is obtained:

(17.7)
$$R_y = -(d_W + d_A) / d_A \cdot W_y$$

The distances d_W and d_A are about the same and therefore $\mathbf{R}_y$ has about twice the magnitude of the gravitational force $\mathbf{W}$. Quantitatively the distance d_A amounts to approximately 5 cm.[17] Therefore, for a person of 75 kg mass and standing on both feet the plantar flexion moment according to Eq. 17.2 is

(17.8) $$M_A = 0.05 \cdot 37.5 \cdot 9.81 = 18.39 \ [\text{Nm}]$$

Measurements by Smith[18] yielded moments between 8.3 Nm and 25 Nm, thus confirming the order of magnitude of this estimate. One reason for the large variability of the results is postural sway, which is accompanied by swaying of the line of gravity and hence by variations in the moment arm d_W. If the line of gravity intersects the ball of the foot, d_W exceeds d_A by a factor of approximately 3. The load on the ankle then amounts to four times the body weight. This model can be extended to one-legged stance as well, so long as it is confined to the sagittal plane. In this case the whole body weight is supported by one foot alone, so the load is doubled.

If this calculation is used to model joint loading during the push-off phase of gait, account must be taken of dynamic forces that increase the ground reaction force during toe-off in normal walking to 120% of body weight. Moments are then generated in excess of 100 Nm.[19] However, this model reaches its limits when detailed analyses are required, and more complex models become necessary, involving dynamic analysis, the action of agonists and antagonists in different phases of gait, and the changes in the moment arms during the stance phase.[20]

17.2.2 Internal Forces in the Arch

The vertical reaction force $\mathbf{R}_y$ exerted by the talus on the tibia is generated by the supporting forces under the forefoot and under the heel and by the tension in the Achilles tendon. The vertical forces acting on the calcaneus produce a moment which is compensated by horizontal forces generated by the tension of the fasciae. The same is true for the forefoot, where the vertical force which supports the forefoot and toes produces an oppositely directed moment, which in turn is compensated by the moment generated by the fasciae. For simplicity the following assumptions are made: it is assumed that, in contrast to the plantar aponeurosis, the force exerted by the long plantar ligament on the calcaneus and forefoot can be neglected because of its weaker structure and less efficient moment arm. It is also assumed that the plantar aponeurosis runs approximately horizontally.

The vertical forces acting on the forefoot and hindfoot produce a moment of the same magnitude but in opposite directions. The same is true of the horizontal components. Therefore, in equilibrium it is sufficient to consider either the forefoot or the hindfoot alone to determine the force $\mathbf{P}$ in the plantar aponeurosis. The moment arms of the hindfoot can be taken from the center of the ankle joint (**Fig. 17.5**). In equilibrium of moments

(17.9) $$-d_h \cdot R_h - d_A \cdot A_y + d_P \cdot P = 0$$

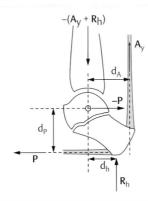

Fig. 17.5 Tensile force **P** in the plantar aponeurosis. The ground reaction force **R**$_h$ under the heel and the force **A**$_y$ of the Achilles tendon apply a moment to the fulcrum of the talocalcaneal joint, which counteracts the moment of the plantar aponeurosis. The respective moment arms are d$_p$, d$_h$, and d$_A$. The load of the tibia on the talus amounts to (**A**$_y$ + **R**$_h$). Mobility between the talus and calcaneus is neglected.

Therefore the plantar aponeurosis stabilizes the calcaneus with force **P**, whose magnitude is given by

(17.10) $$P = (d_h \cdot R_h + d_A \cdot A_y) / d_p$$

As the plantar aponeurosis is countersupported by the metatarsal heads, the horizontal component of the force in the forefoot is equal to −**P**. The magnitude of **P** depends implicitly on the location of the line of gravity. If the foot is supported only under the hindfoot, the Achilles tendon relaxes and in the term

(17.11) $$d_h \cdot R_h + d_A \cdot A_y$$

A$_y$ becomes zero, thus minimizing the force in the plantar aponeurosis, which then can be written

(17.12) $$P_h = d_h \cdot W / d_p$$

with the index h indicating loading of the hindfoot. W is the magnitude of the gravitational force. As d$_h$ and d$_p$ are roughly equal, P$_h$ is roughly equivalent to the body weight. If, on the other hand, the foot is supported only under the forefoot, the ground reaction force R$_h$ under the heel vanishes. Instead, the Achilles tendon is activated. As described above, on forefoot loading the force of the Achilles tendon is approximately three times the weight of the body and its moment arm d$_A$ is roughly the same size as d$_p$. The resulting magnitude of tension **P**$_f$ in the plantar aponeurosis is therefore

(17.13) $$P_f = d_A \cdot 3W / d_p$$

387

where the index f indicates forefoot support. P_f amounts to about three times the gravitational force—in agreement with corresponding measurements[21] and finite element calculations.[22]

The variation of tension in the fascia of the plantar aponeurosis therefore depends on the location of the line of gravity, with important consequences for the behavior of the foot during the stance phase. When the heel comes into contact with the ground, the tension in the Achilles tendon and in the plantar fascia is relatively low. Thus the ability of the foot to deform due to the irregular joint surfaces of the Lisfranc and Chopart joint is not inhibited and the foot can adjust to the form of the ground. However, as the line of gravity moves forwards, the tension in the plantar aponeurosis increases and mobility reduces as the joint surfaces become wedged together. In this way the foot becomes stiff and acts as a rigid lever for push-off.

The windlass mechanism as described by Hicks[23] acts to reinforce this effect. Because the plantar aponeurosis inserts into the joint capsules of the metatarsophalangeal joints and extends functionally beyond them, the aponeurosis can be tensed by lifting the toes. The same happens during roll-off over the toes, which flexes the metatarsophalangeal joints and thus further tenses the aponeurosis (**Fig. 17.6**).

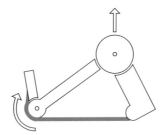

Fig. 17.6 Windlass mechanism. When the toes are lifted, tension in the plantar aponeurosis increases through a windlass mechanism and the foot becomes more arched.

A further important aspect is the height d_p of the ankle above the ground. Eq. 17.10 shows that P is inversely proportional to this height, that is, P increases when d_p decreases. Under normal conditions, brief vertical loading of the ankle causes the arch to give elastically and then recover. The descent of the talus is limited by the increase of tension in the fascia. A finite element calculation quantifies this effect.[24] However, severe overloading with increased descent of the talus increases the tension in the bones so greatly that microfractures and partial destruction of the trabecular structure may lead to shortening of the bones involved, with consequent irreversible reduction of the height of the arch. This in turn increases the tension in the plantar aponeurosis, risking bone damage. This risk is especially raised where bone strength is compromised, for instance, as a result of metabolic disorders such as diabetes. This may lead to accelerated repetition of the overload injuries and eventually to collapse of the longitudinal arch and fragmentation of the involved bones as in Charcot arthropathy.[25]

17.2.3 Internal Forces in the Forefoot

The internal forces in the forefoot between the talus and the metatarsophalangeal joints are determined primarily by the tension of the plantar aponeurosis, which inserts in the metatarsophalangeal joint capsules. However, the anterior ground reaction force $\mathbf{R}_f$ beneath the forefoot can be displaced forwards beyond the ball of the foot by using the toes. This affects the internal forces in the forefoot and hindfoot: involvement of the toes transmits forces to the ankle and lower leg through the forefoot, while the lengthened forefoot lever requires an increased compensating force in the Achilles tendon.

The most important contributor to the forces in the toes is the first ray. Cadaver measurements by Jacob[26] reveal the ratio of moment arms L_1 and L_2 (**Fig. 17.7**) to be

(17.14)
$$L_1 / L_2 = 2.2$$

so that

(17.15)
$$L_1 \cdot F - L_2 \cdot F_{hl} = 0$$

gives the magnitude of the force $\mathbf{F}_{hl}$ acting along the tendon of the flexor hallucis longus:

(17.16)
$$F_{hl} = 2.2 \cdot F$$

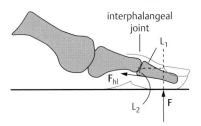

Fig. 17.7 Section through the first ray to determine the load on the interphalangeal joint. $\mathbf{F}$ is the ground reaction force, $\mathbf{F}_{hl}$ the force of the flexor hallucis longus, and L_1 and L_2 are the moment arms of the ground reaction force and flexor hallucis longus respectively. (Adapted, with permission, from Jacob.[26])

The magnitude of force $\mathbf{F}_{hl}$ therefore is 2.2 times the magnitude of ground reaction force $\mathbf{F}$. From the vector sum of the two forces (taking into account an inclination of the flexor hallucis tendon of 15° to the horizontal), the magnitude of the resultant force across the joint can be calculated as 2.6 times the ground reaction force. The force $\mathbf{F}$, by which the toe pushes off from the ground, cannot be estimated on the basis of a model but has to be measured. Plantar pressure distribution measurement during push-off shows the magnitude of $\mathbf{F}$ to be approximately 25% of body weight.[27] As the loading of the joint is 2.6 times the ground reaction force, the resultant joint loading is 65% of body weight. Similar calculations for the more proximal metatar-sophalangeal joint reveal higher loading because the moment arm of the ground reaction force is longer. The loads on the toes of the other rays are smaller and are calculated in the same way, with anatomic and geometric parameters modified as appropriate.

17.2.4 Deformation of the Foot

Elastic deformations in the foot are normally small. Anthropometric investigations by Xiong et al[28] in young adults compared the descent of the malleoli under minimal foot loading and when loaded by the entire body weight. They found that the medial malleolus descent was approximately 1 mm (1.3 mm in men, 0.7 mm in women). On the basis of in vivo radiographic measurements, Carlsöö and Wetzenstein[29] attributed the height loss primarily to soft tissue deformation and found no evidence of changes in the foot skeleton. Gefen[24] quantified the height loss due to weight bearing as 0.15 mm, likewise using radiographic methods. Finite element calculations predict significantly greater loss of height if the plantar aponeurosis is lengthened surgically or its elastic properties are changed with corresponding effect.

17.3   Posturography

In normal stance on both legs the body's center of mass is located a few centimeters anterior to the lumbar spine at about the level of the fourth lumbar vertebra. It is not possible to give a generalized, anatomically precise localization, since the body's center of mass depends on the positions of the centers of mass of the different body segments, which in turn vary according to the segments' distribution of mass and their position. To ensure stable stance and prevent falling, the base of support (the area beneath and between the feet) must be below the center of mass. As this condition must also be met during changes of loading, a complex regulatory (sensing and controlling) mechanism is needed to keep the center of mass over the base of support and allow dynamic balance. Measuring this postural control by measuring the ground reaction forces is termed *posturography*.

In biomechanics the dynamics of balance is commonly described by reference to the model of the inverted pendulum. A simple example of this is balancing a stick on the fingertip and keeping it vertical. If the center of mass of the stick is not kept exactly above its base, the stick starts to lean over to one side or the other and it falls over. To avoid this, the finger must follow the stick, moving the point of application of the reaction force. This model cannot be applied directly to the analysis of posture as the supporting base cannot be moved, but the point of application of the ground reaction force can be shifted by changing the load distribution in the feet.

Fig. 17.8 is a schematic lateral diagram of the foot based on Winter[30] with the aim of describing the fundamental mechanisms involved in maintaining dynamic balance. The x-coordinate axis, with its origin

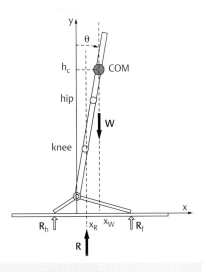

Fig. 17.8 Posturography. The origin of the xy-coordinate system is located in the support plane beneath the ankle joint. The gravitational force **W** acts at the center of mass. Its line of action does not coincide with that of the ground reaction force **R**, thus producing a moment, leading to an increase in the angle of inclination θ in the situation illustrated here. COM, center of mass.

below the ankle, runs in the support plane. The foot is supported in the forefoot and hindfoot regions where the reaction forces R_f and R_h act. For reasons of simplicity only the vertical components are considered below. The line of action of the ground reaction force **R** crosses the base line at x_R. The center of mass of the body is located at height h_c above the ankle joints. The trunk is inclined by the angle θ so that the center of mass and consequently the line of action of the gravitational force **W** are displaced by x_W with reference to the ankle joint.

(17.17)
$$x_W = h_c \cdot \tan\theta$$

As θ is very small, a good approximation is

(17.18)
$$x_W = h_c \cdot \theta$$

The two forces **R** and **W** acting in opposite directions exert a moment that rotates the trunk around the ankle joint. The angular acceleration $\ddot{\theta}$ is derived from the angular momentum equation

(17.19)
$$-x_R \cdot R + x_W \cdot W = I \cdot \ddot{\theta}$$

where I denotes the moment of inertia of the trunk relative to the axis of the ankle. To simplify the calculation, the difference between the magnitudes of the gravitational force **W** and ground reaction force **R** is ignored by setting

(17.20)
$$|R| = |W|$$

Furthermore, by using Eq. 17.18 the angular acceleration $\ddot{\theta}$ can be replaced so that the acceleration in x-direction $\ddot{x}_W$ of the center of mass can be written

(17.21)
$$(-x_R + x_W) \cdot W = \ddot{x}_W \cdot I / h_c$$
$$\ddot{x}_W = (x_W - x_R) \cdot h \cdot W / I$$

This means that the distance $(x_W - x_R)$ between the two lines of action of the gravitational force and the ground reaction force is decisive for the tilting movement. Whether this pair of forces acts more posteriorly or more anteriorly is unimportant, but they must act within the support area. This is evident for the ground reaction force, as it can be generated only inside the support area. This means that the line of gravity must be restricted to this area. If it moves beyond these limits, the ground reaction force can no longer follow, and falling can be avoided only by either moving the center of mass (for instance, by moving the arms or trunk) or by expanding the area of support (for instance by a step forwards or backwards).

In **Fig. 17.8** x_W is greater than x_R, so that $\ddot{x}_W$ is positive, meaning that the center of mass is accelerating its forward tilting movement. This means that the application point of the ground reaction force (coordinate x_R) has to be moved forward beyond the line of gravity (coordinate x_W) by activation of the plantar flexors— the triceps surae, for example—so that the sign of angular acceleration is reversed and the center of mass starts moving backward. This produces the opposing reaction, namely to move the ground reaction force backward by relaxing the triceps surae and activating foot extensors such as the tibialis anterior muscle. These actions alternate, producing dynamic balance control.

Fig. 17.9 presents a typical time course of the two coordinates x_W and x_R. They are usually labeled COM (center of mass) and COP (center of pressure). The COP is equivalent to the point of force application in the

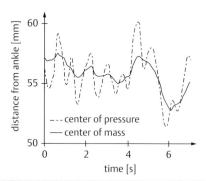

Fig. 17.9 Typical time course of the x-coordinate of the center of mass and of the ground reaction force in quiet standing. (Adapted, with permission, from Winter.[30])

support surface. The center of mass is a point in three-dimensional space, but here "COM" indicates the two-dimensional projection of the center of mass in the base of support. The COP is by definition bound to this plane. It can be seen that the two coordinates oscillate around a state of equilibrium approximately 55 mm in front of the ankle joint, the COP at a higher frequency and with a wider range than the COM. The higher frequency is required to ensure rapid regulatory reaction, while the larger amplitude is necessary to enable the COP to "capture" the COM. The amplitude of the COP is limited by the length of the foot; of necessity, that of the COM must be somewhat smaller.

Regulation of balance by shifting the COM by flexion and extension of the ankle is called *ankle strategy*. Another technique known as *hip strategy* can also be used; in this, the hip flexors and extensors move the COM relative to the COP. At the same time, other body segments may also be accelerated and their reaction forces may aid stabilization. This is most evident if the arms are also involved in balancing. However, the hip strategy is not often employed by healthy people.[31]

In the frontal plane, the situation is different. Dynamic balance must be established here as well, and the projection of the center of mass must fall within the base of support. During standing on both feet the hip strategy is employed, essentially consisting of elevation or lowering of the pelvis on one side. The resulting redistribution of load from one side to the other causes displacement of the COP along the z-axis. The ankle strategy plays only a small part in this, by rotating one foot inward about its longitudinal axis and the other foot outward so that the COP shifts medially in the one case and laterally in the other. However, because the foot is narrow, this strategy is of minor importance for balance.

This complexity means that a great variety of regulatory mechanisms are involved in successfully keeping the center of mass above the base of support. These include vision, the sense of balance, proprioception regarding the position of the ankles, perception of the loading of the feet, together with neuromuscular control of posture. Impairments of one or more of these sensory systems interfere with the regulatory mechanisms. As a consequence, the amplitude of oscillations may increase or their frequency may decrease. This has led to a wealth of different posturographic measurement and analysis techniques used to quantify disturbances of balance and of its regulation.

As the above considerations show, the movements of both COP and COM provide important information about the mechanisms of balance regulation, so measuring both of them is desirable. Measuring COP is comparatively simple. A force measurement platform (forceplate) working with a frequency of at least 50 Hz can deliver worthwhile results. For better temporal resolution, a sampling rate of 100 Hz or more should be used. **Fig. 17.10** shows two different images of a typical measurement of the COP oscillation in a healthy person. Measuring COM is a more elaborate undertaking. Direct measurement is not possible; instead all body segments must be recorded separately and the location of the COM is calculated from these. This can be done using optical techniques. An alternative is to measure the oscillations of the trunk alone, if the

393

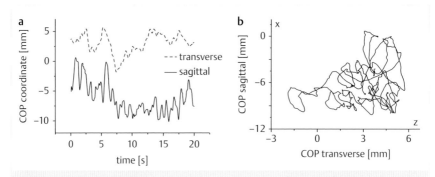

Fig. 17.10a, b Typical time course of the center of pressure (COP) in a healthy person measured for 20 seconds, presented in two ways: coordinate–time diagram (**a**) and x–z diagram showing the path of the COP in the support plane (**b**). The sagittal and transverse curves both exhibit small fluctuations and rapid balancing motions. The standard deviation of the sagittal component (x-component in **b**) is somewhat smaller than that of the transverse component (z-component in **b**). The sagittal (anteroposterior) component has higher frequencies than the transverse component.

arms do not move against the trunk, so that only the movements of the trunk need to be captured. This can be achieved using accelerometric techniques allowing the COM to be determined according to Eq. 17.21, if the COP is measured simultaneously.

In clinical practice two measurements taken under different conditions are often compared, such as "eyes open" and "eyes closed." For example, in patients with a diabetic foot, where sensory impairment due to neuropathy can be assumed, measurements taken with the eyes open and then closed are compared to discover how dependent the patient's balance regulation is on visual feedback. These investigations can be extended by integrating deliberate or random disturbances, such as changes in the slope of the support.[32] Characterization and quantitative analysis of COP oscillations are based on statistical methods.[33] The most important parameters record the length of the trajectory recorded in a given time, the mean frequency and frequency distribution, and the direction of the largest and smallest oscillations. The posturographic method is limited to analysis of the location and movement of the COP; it does not provide a detailed investigation of the plantar supporting forces. That is provided by plantar pressure distribution measurement.

17.4 Plantar Pressure Distribution

The calculation of forces in the joints of the forefoot as described in Section 17.2.3 ("Internal Forces in the Forefoot") shows that knowledge of the point of force application (the COP) and of the force acting there does not suffice for a detailed analysis of internal loads. For example, to calculate the internal forces in the forefoot, the force exerted by the ground on the great toe during push-off must be measured to obtain a numerical estimate of the joint forces. The more detailed the knowledge of the contributing forces—especially their point of application, direction, and magnitude—the more precise the information regarding loading of the individual bones, joints, or regions of the foot. Pedography, also known as pedobarography, is an important and widely employed method of measuring the plantar pressure distribution, although commercially available systems do not record the direction of the applied forces. Systems based on capacitive sensors measure only the normal component, while in other systems the signal depends on the magnitude of the force without specifying the direction. Separate and locally resolved measurement of shear force in sagittal or lateral directions is not possible with conventional systems but requires special custom-made sensor systems that can measure all three components of force simultaneously.[34,35]

17.4.1 Pressure Measurement: Requirements and General Solutions

Methods of measuring pressure distribution record the location and time course of forces acting on the sole of the foot. A variety of systems has been developed for this purpose. A good overview of the different methods of measuring normal and shear stress is given by Urry.[36]

The following description is limited to commercially available systems for measuring the pressure on the surface. Two different types are in common use: stationary platforms designed to measure the interface between the ground and the bare foot, and mobile measuring insoles designed to be worn at the interface between foot and shoe or between foot and shoe insert. The following discussion refers to insoles but also applies for the platforms. Measurement data from the two systems cannot be directly compared because of the interactions between the shod foot and its shoe, especially the walls and the toe box, which do not arise in the case of the unshod foot.

The systems for plantar pressure measurement feature a regular arrangement ("matrix") of force sensors of known area. When they are subjected to a compressive force they are deformed, thus altering their electrical properties. Sensors used for biomechanical measurements must meet several requirements:

- The sensor area must be as small as possible.
- The matrix of force sensors must completely cover the measurement area.
- The electronic readout from the individual sensors must be fast.
- They must provide low hysteresis and high reproducibility of measurements.
- For insoles: the substrate for the sensors must be flexible without interfering with accuracy even when it adjusts to the shape of the foot or the shoe insert.
- Repeated disinfection should be possible.

Commercial systems meeting these requirements most commonly use capacitive or FSR ("force-sensitive resistor") sensors. They measure the change in capacitance or resistance between two conducting surfaces caused by pressure. The sensors deliver the mean value of the force exerted on the entire sensor area. Therefore, the pressure p generated by a force of magnitude F acting on a sensor with area A is calculated as

(17.22) $p = F / A$

From this it is apparent that the area of the individual sensors is an important characteristic of the measurement system. Sensors with a large area deliver signals with a comparatively low level of noise and errors. On the other hand, large sensor areas deform readily on local loading, leading to nonlinearity of the characteristic curve. Moreover, misleading results may be obtained when the size of the structure under examination roughly matches the size of the sensor. Random displacements between the object and the sensor may then produce artifacts (**Fig. 17.11**).

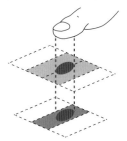

Fig. 17.11 Effect of pressure sensor positioning under the foot when small structures are being measured. If the toe covers two sensors instead of one, the loaded area is doubled and hence the pressure value halved.

Similar considerations apply to the arrangement of the sensors. They should cover the surface of the measuring device as completely as possible to avoid incomplete coverage of the contact area of the foot. If coverage is incomplete, the sum of forces from all the sensors will be less than the total reaction force as measured simultaneously with a force measuring platform. In systems where this effect cannot be ignored, calibration of the device to the patient is essential and must also take the patient's body weight into account. Fast readout from sensor elements is required to obtain a high measurement frequency. A typical frequency is 50 Hz; higher frequencies are usual in sports applications.

Various factors may interfere with the reproducibility of measurements. These include intraindividual deviations, for instance due to slight changes of the gait pattern in repeated measurements, as well as errors due to the measurement system. Positioning errors as discussed above may arise from different positioning of the foot relative to the sensors. **Fig. 17.12** shows typical results of repeated plantar pressure measurements together with the standard deviations. An example of the standard deviation of pressure data from a single sensor in repeated measurements is given in **Fig. 17.13**. The mean values for relative standard deviations

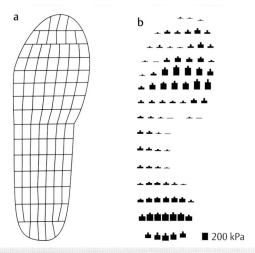

Fig. 17.12a, b Measuring plantar pressure.

a Arrangement of the 99 pressure sensors in a Pedar measurement insole (Novel GmbH, Munich, Germany) to determine plantar pressure in the foot.

b Typical pressure distribution (peak pressures) of a healthy person. Error bars show the standard deviation of repeated measurements on consecutive days. The relative standard deviation is 22% when averaged over all sensors but 16% when averaged only over sensors loaded with more than 100 kPa. The bar at the lower right indicates the scale.

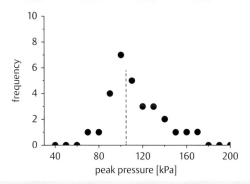

Fig. 17.13 Typical frequency distribution of pressure measurements from a sensor in the lateral heel region, with 29 measurements on 10 consecutive days. The mean peak pressure is 112 kPa (dashed line), and the values range between 70 and 170 kPa. The pressure values are rounded to the nearest ten.

of 16% and 22% can be regarded as typical. In similar investigations Putti et al[37] and Gurney et al[38] obtained similar results, although their studies bundled together multiple sensors in individual areas of the foot.

In clinical use the measurement system must be suitable for repeated use. It is therefore necessary that these systems are capable of being repeatedly disinfected without damage. Some manufacturers provide advice, but systematic investigations are lacking.

17.4.2 Pressure Measurement: Interpretation of Data

Each sensor defines a plantar measurement site and the system delivers a force–time curve for that site. **Fig. 17.14** shows two typical curves from different sites. Force–time measurements can be converted into pressure–time measurements by dividing the force values by the area of the sensor. As these curves are generated for each sensor, a large volume of data is produced which needs to undergo data reduction and analysis before it can be interpreted further. The first step consists of averaging over several gait cycles, if the investigator can ensure that the gait pattern did not change during the measurement. This reduces the effect of intraindividual variations between steps. Biomechanical analysis looks first at the shape of the whole footprint and then the local and temporal differences in the pressure distribution. The local analysis provides information on which regions are subject to greater loading and where there is an increased risk of tissue damage. The temporal analysis provides information on the gait pattern and the duration of loading. Various methods are available for the evaluation and analysis of the data, which may be used alone or in combination.

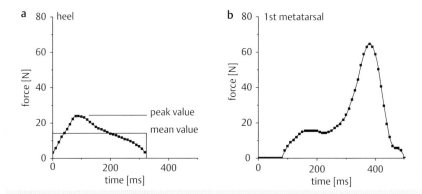

Fig. 17.14a, b Two synchronous force–time curves from two widely separated sensors using a Pedar measurement insole in a healthy subject. In both curves the time scale starts with the heel strike. The characteristic peak value and mean are used to describe the magnitude of loading. The area of the rectangle formed by the mean and the duration of loading is equal to the force–time integral.

a Heel.

b Metatarsal head of the first ray.

Local Analysis

Characteristic values are calculated to describe each particular force–time curve and pressure–time curve. These include the *peak pressure*, the *force–time integral* and *pressure–time integral*, and the *temporal mean value*. The peak pressure (see **Fig. 17.14**) represents the highest pressure measured by the respective sensor. Peak pressure is a parameter of great clinical importance as it is frequently employed to quantify the risk of soft tissue damage, although the biomechanical basis for this interpretation has not been confirmed. The force–time integral is the area under the force–time curve and is calculated by integration of this curve over time (although this is not done explicitly by the software provided by some manufacturers).[39] In mechanical terms, this integral describes the change in the momentum of the body effected by the force in the given time interval. Similar considerations apply for the pressure–time integral, which may also be termed the *pressure dose*.[40] The temporal mean is calculated as the ratio of the force–time integral or pressure–time integral and the duration of loading. The duration of loading may be defined in various ways: (1) as the individual loading time of each sensor; (2) as the ground contact time, that is, the time the foot (whether heel or toes) is in contact with the ground; or (3) as the cycle time, that is, the duration of either a single step or a stride (a left and a right step, or a right and a left). These parameters are usually presented graphically in the form of contour-like pressure distributions, with the measurement value of each sensor displayed either graphically or numerically (see **Fig. 17.12b**). Combined representation of the different parameters instead of separate representations is also possible,[40] for example by combining peak pressure, mean pressure, loading duration, and force–time integral in a single graphic.

Regional Analysis

Regional analysis is often used for investigations and comparisons in cohort studies. It is based on summation of the curves of neighboring sensors covering certain regions of the foot. A simple division distinguishes the hindfoot, midfoot, ball, and toes.[41] The development of smaller sensors allows more sophisticated analyses. They may be needed to calculate forces and loads in a small and precisely demarcated region, such as a single ray, as described in Section 17.2.3 ("Internal Forces in the Forefoot"). The graphical representation is the same as for local analysis, but the measurement results are assigned not to individual sensors but to regions of the foot. A special case—at least with capacitive sensors—arises if the sensors covering the whole foot are summed. The resulting force–time curve then corresponds to the curve of the normal component of the ground reaction force as measured by a force platform. Hence, in standing on one leg or when both feet are recorded together, the temporal mean value of the force–time curve is equal to the body weight.

Analysis of the Point of Force Application

When the entire sole of the foot is covered by pressure sensors, it is possible to calculate the instantaneous COP at each instant of ground contact. In a similar way to the calculation of the center of mass (see Eq. 11.2), the COP is calculated as a sum of coordinates weighted by the product of pressure times sensor area for each sensor. Results are shown graphically by the gait line that connects the COPs, which are calculated at regular time intervals. If the individual COP points are shown as well, a highly informative illustration of the roll-off movement of the foot is provided. In particular, the regions subject to particularly prolonged loading are visible as the COP points are clustered closely together there. The gait line is generally integrated into a representation of the pressure distribution. An alternative representation is obtained when the instantaneous ground reaction force is shown along with the movement of the point of force application along the x-axis.[42] **Fig. 17.15** is an example, with the ground reaction forces displayed as bars in the y-axis, their lengths indicating the magnitude of the force. For simplicity, the pressure distribution is omitted from this illustration.

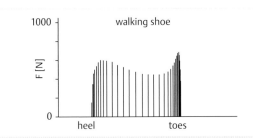

Fig. 17.15 Bar diagram representing the progression of the center of pressure (COP) from heel to toes during a typical gait cycle in a healthy person wearing a normal (walking) shoe. The x-coordinates of the COP and the corresponding ground reaction force F are obtained at regular intervals of 20 milliseconds from the normal component of the plantar forces. The dense sequences in the ball and toe region show the longer duration of loading.

Analysis of the Pressure Gradient

In this method the pressure distribution is analyzed according to differences between adjacent sites.[43] Sites with a large pressure difference over a given distance (pressure gradient) are of particular interest. This is because, biomechanically, high internal tissue stresses can be expected at sites with a steep gradient,[44] thus increasing the risk of tissue damage.

17.4.3 Ground Reaction Force and Plantar Pressure

In stance the ground reaction force is constant and is equal and opposite to the gravitational force. This force, when it acts on the sole of the foot, produces the plantar pressure. To estimate the order of magnitude of the expected pressures, a very simple assumption may be made, that the pressure distribution is uniform over the entire plantar area of the foot. A typical value for this area is 150 cm². Assuming that the ground reaction force of a person standing on two legs is 750 N distributed equally to both feet, the plantar pressure is

$$(17.23) \qquad 750 \text{ N} / 300 \text{ cm}^2 = 2.5 \text{ N/cm}^2 = 25 \text{ kPa}$$

Accordingly, the pressure doubles when the person stands on one foot, and if he or she stands on the ball of the foot alone, reducing the supporting area to about one-third, the pressure is three times as high, approximately 150 kPa. In reality, however, the pressure distribution under the sole is not uniform; the foot supports itself less in the midfoot region and more in the region of toes, ball, and heel, and laterally along the fifth ray, where higher pressures can be expected. The systolic pressure in the blood vessels of the foot is approximately 30 kPa. Perfusion there is interrupted when the plantar pressure exceeds this value. This occurs during prolonged motionless standing on a reduced plantar supporting area; however, it is counteracted by natural body sway, which suffices to limit the duration of lack of blood flow and so avoid ischemic injury.

Walking increases the loading of some regions of the foot in comparison with standing. There are various reasons for this:

- Except during the double stance phases in the course of a gait cycle, the entire body weight rests on only one foot at a time.
- The roll-off process reduces the ground contact area. This is especially true in phases of increased ground reaction forces, namely in deceleration during heel strike and in acceleration during push-off.
- Dynamic effects such as raising or lowering the body's center of mass modulate the ground reaction forces, thus producing the typical M-shaped curve (**Fig. 17.16**). In normal gait the two peak loads are approximately 1.2 times the body weight.
- Shear forces may occur in addition to the normal forces, mainly during the heel strike and push-off phases. These constitute only a fraction (typically one-quarter) of the normal forces.

17.4.4 Factors Influencing Plantar Pressure Distribution

Several longitudinal studies of barefoot walking have been performed to investigate functional and structural parameters that determine the distribution of plantar pressure.[46–48] From these very detailed investigations it is evident that, even with knowledge of the foot's architecture, joint mobility, plantar thickness, muscle status, and the patient's age and weight, peak pressures in the individual regions of the foot can be predicted with only 50% certainty. Therefore, when possible, clinical practice mainly relies on

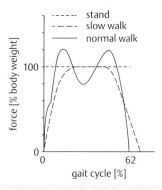

Fig. 17.16 Vertical component of the ground reaction force under different conditions. In standing and during the one-legged stance phase during slow walking, it equals 100% of the body weight. At a normal walking speed, dynamic forces are added and the characteristic M-shaped curve is produced. The contribution of the contralateral leg is not shown. (Adapted from Perry.[45])

intraindividual measurements, varying only one condition at a time while keeping the other potential influencing factors constant. This can be demonstrated for the influence of walking speed and step or stride length on peak pressure (see below).

Influence of Weight

Common sense would suggest that the patient's weight plays a decisive role. This is correct in the case of the force–time integral of the entire foot. The mean value over a complete gait cycle equals the exact weight, thus providing a good opportunity to test the calibration of the pressure measurement system. However, as soon as we come to the pressure–time integral, additional factors gain influence. For example, if a person both weighs more and has bigger feet, the result may be only a slight increase or even a decrease in the pressure–time integral, despite the increased weight. In the case of peak pressure, assumptions based on general principles are even more problematic. According to Morag and Cavanagh,[46] only for the midfoot region can it be concluded that peak pressure increases with weight; this conclusion cannot be made for the other regions. Similar results are reported by Bosch et al,[49] who state—again on the basis of barefoot measurements—that weight can be expected to influence peak pressure only in extreme cases of overweight.

Results obtained using measuring insoles with a simulated increase or decrease of body weight show a different picture. In these short-term longitudinal studies a clear linear relation was shown between weight reduction or additional loading on the one hand and peak pressure on the other.[50] Wearing a 20-kg weight vest increases the mean peak pressures in the heel and the ball of the foot by 26 and 60 kPa respectively. Conversely, if body mass is reduced by 20 kg by using a movable suspension, peak pressures fall by the same amount. These results showing a considerable effect of weight appear contradictory to the results described above, but the contradiction can be explained by considering long-term adaptation mechanisms, which might counteract the effects of weight gain on the loading pattern and peak pressures. Such adaptation processes might be enlargement of the sole area and/or fat deposition in the sole, a change of gait pattern, or change of walking speed.

Influence of Walking Speed and Step Length

Dynamic factors such as speed, cadence (number of steps per minute), and gait pattern have quite a large influence on the results of pressure distribution measurement. This means that in the clinical setting these conditions have to be very precisely controlled during assessment of functional deficits or when comparing findings before and after treatment. **Fig. 17.16** shows that the ground reaction force is increased by dynamic contributions when walking speed goes up from slow to normal. At a slow walking speed the ground reaction force is virtually equal to the body weight. At a customary speed the curve oscillates and exhibits two peaks with a trough between. The first peak is due to the "loading response" at the beginning of the ground contact phase when mainly the heel is loaded. The second peak occurs during the "terminal stance phase," which is characterized by the push-off phase. The effect of higher speed on peak pressure is shown in **Fig. 17.17**, where the peak signal in a single insole sensor is plotted against walking speed in a total of seven runs, with the subject walking slowly twice, at normal speed three times, and fast twice. The speed varied between 0.9 m/s and 1.5 m/s. The diagram shows that the peak pressures increase significantly as speed increases ($P \leq 5\%$). A significant linear correlation was found for the ball, the toes, and the heel,[40,51] though with varying slope.[52] In other regions, the slope is less pronounced or the peak pressures are so small that statistical measurement errors are predominant.

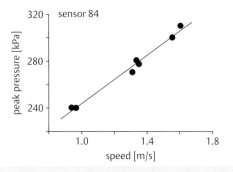

Fig. 17.17 Typical peak pressure values in a sensor under the first metatarsal head (sensor 84) of a healthy person during slow, normal, and fast walking.

In the example in **Fig. 17.17** the speed was increased without cadence or step length being monitored. In physiological walking, speed is increased by increasing the cadence and also, in proportion to the cadence, the step length.[53] These three parameters are linked by the formula

(17.24) $\qquad$ walking speed = step length $\times$ cadence / 60

The speed is measured in meters per second and step length in meters. As the cadence measures the frequency in steps per minute, it is converted by the factor 1/60 to meters per second.

The effect of speed and step length on plantar pressure distribution can be studied by changing step length while keeping the cadence constant. What this means in practice (**Fig. 17.18**) is that the cadence as measured during normal walking is kept constant but the step length is halved, so the speed is halved as well. The expectation is that the ground reaction forces and hence the peak pressures will also drop. This is due to two effects, both acting in the same direction. First, lower speed produces smaller dynamic forces, lowering pressures and peak pressures. Second, the shortened step length leads to shallower angles between the foot and the ground, resulting in a larger contact area with the ground, which also reduces pressures and peak pressures. **Fig. 17.19** shows a comparison of peak pressures measured in 20 healthy persons.[54] The peak pressure is particularly reduced in areas with great dynamic loading, most markedly in the toe region, where the reduction in the roll-off angle is most apparent. There is no obvious reduction in the midfoot region.

Further reduction of peak pressure can be accomplished by a shuffling gait,[55] as this largely avoids the one-legged stance phase. At the same time, flexion–extension movement in the ankle joint is reduced to minimize dynamic effects by smoothing the dynamic height excursions of the center of body mass. This

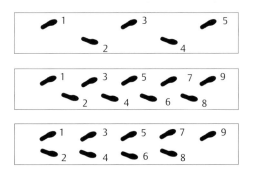

Fig. 17.18a–c Diagram of footprints illustrating three different gait patterns. Patterns **b** and **c** maintain the cadence of **a**.

a Normal gait.

b Step-over-step gait with half the step length of normal gait.

c Step-to gait, with the left foot leading with the same step length as in normal gait, while the right foot "trails" behind and is moved up level with the left foot. The left foot then starts a new cycle.

peak pressure (N = 20)

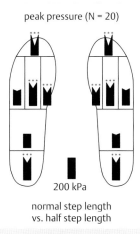

200 kPa

normal step length
vs. half step length

Fig. 17.19 Comparison of peak pressures in normal gait and with step length and speed halved. The height of the symbols (outer sides) shows the peak pressure during normal gait and the notching shows the reduction when step length is halved. A significant difference (P < 1%) is indicated by ***.

type of gait is referred to as the *hip strategy*, in contrast to the *ankle strategy*, where propulsion is generated by flexion and extension in the ankle joint.

Another gait pattern, one which has ceased to be symmetrical, is based on the "step-to" gait, which achieves a substantial reduction of peak pressure in one forefoot.[56] One foot (the "leading" foot) is brought forward and the other (the "trailing" foot) is then brought up to the level of the leading foot (**Fig. 17.18c**). If the length of the step taken by the leading foot is the same as that in normal gait and the cadence remains the same, again the walking speed is halved. Compared with the gait pattern in which step length is halved, the loading pattern of heel and forefoot is quite different and is asymmetrical. The leading foot covers the same distance as in normal gait so the ground reaction force and pressure distribution in the heel region should correspond to normal gait. The same is true for the trailing foot during push-off, where normal values can be expected in the forefoot region. However, there is no push-off in the leading foot and no heel strike and loading response in the trailing foot, so the associated loading is diminished.

From the step-to gait pattern illustrated in **Fig. 17.18** it can be expected that the heel of the leading left foot is normally loaded whereas the peak pressures in the forefoot are lowered. The opposite occurs in the trailing right foot, where a normal pressure distribution is expected in the forefoot and reduced pressures in the hindfoot. **Fig. 17.20** shows actual results. They agree with expectations (the comparison refers to a gait pattern with halved step length, so the speed is the same in both cases). A significant reduction of load is observed in the ball and toes of the leading foot, with increased loading on those of the trailing foot. The reverse occurs in the heel region, though this is less pronounced. The leading foot is subject to greater

peak pressure (N = 20)

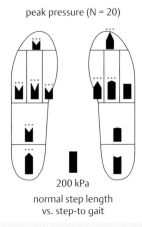

200 kPa

normal step length
vs. step-to gait

Fig. 17.20 Comparison of peak pressures in a gait with step length halved (outer sides) and in step-to gait (notching). Details as in **Fig. 17.19**.

loading, with a slight reduction in loading of the trailing foot. Similar results are observed for the regional force–time and pressure–time integrals.[54]

17.5 Particular Features of the Diabetic Foot

Chronic polyneuropathy is a frequent late complication of diabetes mellitus. The symptoms include lack of pain sensation and impaired balance regulation, which is characterized on posturography by slow excursions of the COP oscillation with increased amplitude (**Fig. 17.21**).

Patients suffering from diabetic neuropathy are at risk of major foot lesions. These include neuropathic osteoarthropathy (also known as Charcot foot), which causes progressive degeneration of the joints and

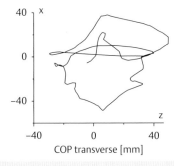

COP transverse [mm]

Fig. 17.21 Trajectory of the center of pressure of a diabetic patient with chronic neuropathy. As in the healthy person in **Fig. 17.10**, the measurement time was 20 seconds. The excursions are nearly 10 times larger and show considerably fewer high-frequency balancing motions.

bones that form the arch, followed by collapse of the arch. A more common complication is "diabetic foot" with its characteristic ulceration. These two conditions may occur in combination. In both the onset is often insidious, but in the early stages there is often a biomechanical component,[57] which is involved in the development of the Charcot or diabetic foot (see Wrobel and Najafi,[58] which also includes an overview of the literature). The main structures involved are:

- *Bones.* Their overall strength diminishes, although bone mineral density can sometimes even increase.
- *Skin.* Diabetes alone has little effect on the properties of skin. However, if neuropathy supervenes, the skin becomes more vulnerable and its elasticity diminishes. As a result, its protective cushioning effect is lost, and sharply localized pressure peaks may develop.
- *Muscles.* Diabetes causes a change in the muscle fibers, and neural muscle activation is affected by neuropathy. Overall, the muscles become weaker.
- *Joint mobility.* Microfractures lead to swelling of joint capsules, thus reducing their range of motion. At the same time, tendon elasticity is reduced. If diabetes and neuropathy are present together, the range of motion of the ankle and metatarsophalangeal joints is halved.
- *Tendons and plantar aponeurosis.* Elasticity is reduced while thickness increases, contributing to the reduction in joint mobility and limiting of the windlass mechanism.
- *Fat pads.* These act as shock absorbers, for example beneath the heel and the ball of the foot. Their effect becomes weakened in various ways over the course of diabetes and polyneuropathy: they atrophy, they become stiffer, and they respond to loading by migrating to less stressed neighboring regions.

Taken together, these alterations have major effects on gait.[59] The impact of heel strike is no longer damped sufficiently because the fat pad is missing. The additional damping mechanism via plantar flexion of the foot is also impeded, by the diminished mobility in the ankle joint. In the one-legged stance phase unsteady gait and increased oscillations of the center of mass lead to increased lateral shear forces. Shear forces increase the risk of keratosis and skin breakdown (see Section 10.4). Muscular weakness reduces dynamics during push-off. This prolongs the roll-off process, leading to prolonged duration of forefoot loading, with increased risk of overload injury in consequence. Whereas in physiological gait propulsion is mainly due to plantar flexion during the push-off phase (ankle strategy), in patients with diabetic neuropathy propulsion is produced mainly by the hip strategy using the gluteal muscles during the stance phase. This results in the typical gait pattern of these patients, characterized by slow, clumsy, and unsteady walking with small steps, placing the foot nearly flat on the ground. The uncertainty is apparent from the widened gait base and prolonged double stance time.

Skin lesions are the most important cause of ulcers, mainly due to excessive pressure and shear acting in a limited region. Laterally directed shear forces appear to be particularly dangerous. As pain sensation is lost, its protective function with the natural impulse to relieve pressure and spare the foot is also lost. In this way even small lesions may act as an entry portal for infection, which can readily spread due to the weakened immune system.[57] Other causes of skin lesions such as ischemia and mechanical destruction of internal and external structures and at the cellular level are discussed by Cavanagh et al.[60] Once an ulcer has developed, the consequences can be serious, including amputation. Although there is no clinical evidence yet to show that relief of pressure has a preventive effect,[61] there is a wealth of circumstantial evidence.[62] In this context pressure distribution measurement is an important tool and must accompany medical intervention. It has two main purposes[60]: (1) it supplements the clinical examination and provides evidence of functional deficits and incorrect loading; and (2) it can also be used to monitor treatment by documenting relief of pressure on the foot.

While a special role is attributed to mechanical causes in the development of ulcers, the situation is still unclear as regards development of the Charcot foot.[63] However, a biomechanical component in the chain of causation, at least in the initial phase, seems obvious. Assuming a bone structure, for instance in the tarsal bones, that is weakened by diabetes, even minor overloading can lead to microfractures. The consequence will be a shortening of these bones, leading to shortening of the longitudinal arch and thus to its flattening. This in turn results in increased loading of the arch (see Section 17.2.2) with an increased risk of further microfractures. It may in time lead to collapse of the arch.

Clinical management indicates mechanical unloading of the foot. If the patient's mobility is to be retained, this can be accomplished by a total contact cast. It is important that the cast should not only fit the foot, shank, and tibial condyles and provide a wide support area, but it should also immobilize the ankle. As the cast fully encloses the entire lower leg, it can take on up to 30% of the body weight.[64] An alternative is provided by therapeutic footwear, for example custom-made orthopedic shoes.[4] The orthopedic shoemaker can provide unloading in two ways: by means of insoles with a molded footbed to be worn in the shoe, and by modifying the shoe.

Molded insoles generally are formed from a plaster cast and thus provide an optimum fit to the shape of the foot to support it over its entire sole and not just over prominent regions. The insoles are made from materials of different hardness using the sandwich method. Soft materials are in contact with the sole, with the harder materials beneath. Because of the accurate fit, pressure is redistributed over the surface, with greater loading in the midfoot and reduced pressures in the heel, ball, and toe regions. This has little effect on gait (**Fig. 17.22**). Unloading effects of 25% or more may be achieved in both healthy persons and diabetic patients with insoles of this type.[51,65]

Shoe modifications consist mostly of a rocker under the heel and a rocker under the sole to facilitate roll-off during walking, especially when joint mobility is limited. The effect is more pronounced if the sole is stiffened. These modifications alter the gait pattern, in particular the time course of loading, as can be seen

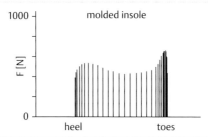

Fig. 17.22 Bar diagram representing the progression of the center of pressure from heel to toes for a person using a molded insole. Same person as in **Fig. 17.15**. The change in the time course of loading is negligible.

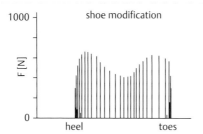

Fig. 17.23 Bar diagram representing the progression of the center of pressure (COP) from heel to toes for a person using shoe modifications. Same person as in **Figs. 17.15** and **17.22**. The modification produces a change in the time course of the COP, with much briefer loading in the forefoot and toes.

from the bar diagram in **Fig. 17.23**. Compared with **Figs. 17.15** and **17.22**, the bars in the toe and ball region appear more separated, indicating that the duration of loading is reduced in these regions; this may be interpreted as a temporal redistribution of pressure. In healthy persons the peak pressure in the ball of the foot is reduced by about 25%. In diabetic patients the reduction is smaller because their gait pattern is less dynamic.

These two orthopedic interventions, insoles and modifications of the shoe, are based on different mechanisms of unloading. They are additive in the region of the ball of the foot, so an unloading effect of 30% to 40% in this region can be achieved through pressure redistribution and gait alteration when the two measures are combined in patients. In the heel region, by contrast, the two mechanisms partly counteract each other, so that combining them achieves less unloading than when a molded insole is used on its own. In all cases, pressure distribution measurement provides important information for prevention and for treatment and treatment monitoring. However, the clinical question of the critical threshold above which ulceration occurs remains unanswered.[66] The large number of individually varying factors that influence the plantar pressure distribution makes it difficult to establish this critical threshold. This is particularly the case for peak pressure.

References

1. Procter P, Paul JPC. Ankle joint biomechanics. J Biomech 1982;15(9):627–634

2. Debrunner HU. Statische Anatomie und Gelenkmechanik des Fußes. Orthop Praxis 1980;16:422–426

3. Huson A. Functional anatomy of the foot. In: Jahss MH, ed. Disorders of the Foot and Ankle: Medical and Surgical Management. 2nd ed. Philadelphia: WB Saunders; 1991:409–431

4. Baumgartner R, Möller M, Stinus H. Orthopädieschuhtechnik. Geislingen: Maurer Verlag; 2011

5. Kummer B. Morphologie und Biomechanik der Sprunggelenke und des Fußes. In: Kummer B. Biomechanik: Form und Funktion des Bewegungsapparates. Cologne: Deutscher Ärzteverlag; 2005: 335–376

6. Debrunner HU, Jacob HAC. Biomechanik des Fußes. 2nd ed. Stuttgart: Enke; 1998

7. Mann RA. Overview of foot and ankle biomechanics. In: Jahss MH, ed. Disorders of the Foot and Ankle: Medical and Surgical Management. 2nd ed. Philadelphia: WB Saunders; 1991:385–408

8. Wu G, Siegler S, Allard P, et al; Standardization and Terminology Committee of the International Society of Biomechanics; International Society of Biomechanics. ISB recommendation on definitions of joint coordinate system of various joints for the reporting of human joint motion—part I: ankle, hip, and spine. J Biomech 2002;35(4):543–548

9. American Academy of Orthopaedic Surgeons. Joint Motion: Method of Measuring and Recording. Chicago: American Academy of Orthopaedic Surgeons; 1965

10. Kapandji IA. The Lower Limb. 5th ed. London: Churchill Livingstone; 1987. The Physiology of the Joints; vol 2

11. Isman RE, Inman VT. Anthropometric studies of the human foot and ankle. Bull Prosthet Res 1969;10:97–129

12. Inman VT. The Joints of the Ankle. Baltimore: Williams & Wilkins; 1976

13. Reinschmidt C, van den Bogert AJ, Lundberg A, et al. Tibiofemoral and tibiocalcaneal motion during walking: external vs. skeletal markers. Gait Posture 1997;6(2):98–109

14. Leitch J, Stebbins J, Zavatsky ABJ. Subject-specific axes of the ankle joint complex. J Biomech 2010;43(15):2923–2928

15. Lundberg A, Svensson OK, Németh G, Selvik G. The axis of rotation of the ankle joint. J Bone Joint Surg Br 1989;71(1):94–99

16. Hicks JH. The mechanics of the foot. I. The joints. J Anat 1953;87(4):345–357

17. McCullough MBA, Ringleb SI, Arai K, Kitaoka HB, Kaufman KR. Moment arms of the ankle throughout the range of motion in three planes. Foot Ankle Int 2011;32(3):300–306

18. Smith JW. The forces operating at the human ankle joint during standing. J Anat 1957;91(4):545–564

19. Scott SH, Winter DA. Internal forces of chronic running injury sites. Med Sci Sports Exerc 1990;22(3):357–369

20. Erdemir A, McLean S, Herzog W, van den Bogert AJ. Model-based estimation of muscle forces exerted during movements. Clin Biomech (Bristol, Avon) 2007;22(2):131–154

21. Komi PV, Fukashiro S, Järvinen M. Biomechanical loading of Achilles tendon during normal locomotion. Clin Sports Med 1992;11(3):521–531

22. Cheung JT, Zhang M, An KN. Effect of Achilles tendon loading on plantar fascia tension in the standing foot. Clin Biomech (Bristol, Avon) 2006;21(2):194–203

23. Hicks JH. The mechanics of the foot. II. The plantar aponeurosis and the arch. J Anat 1954;88(1):25–30

24. Gefen A. Stress analysis of the standing foot following surgical plantar fascia release. J Biomech 2002;35:629–637

25. Mittlmeier T, Klaue K, Haar P, Beck M. Charcot foot. Current situation and outlook [in German]. Unfallchirurg 2008;111(4):218–231

26. Jacob HAC. Forces acting in the forefoot during normal gait—an estimate. Clin Biomech (Bristol, Avon) 2001;16(9):783–792

27. Kaipel M, Krapf D, Wyss C. Metatarsal length does not correlate with maximal peak pressure and maximal force. Clin Orthop Relat Res 2011;469(4):1161–1166

28. Xiong SP, Goonetilleke RS, Jianhui Z, Wenyan L, Witana CP. Foot deformations under different load-bearing conditions and their relationships to stature and body weight. Anthropol Sci 2009;117:77–88

29. Carlsöö S, Wetzenstein H. Change of form of the foot and the foot skeleton upon momentary weight-bearing. Acta Orthop Scand 1968;39(3):413–423

30. Winter DA. A.B.C. (Anatomy, Biomechanics and Control) of Balance During Standing and Walking. Waterloo, Ontario: Waterloo Biomechanics; 1995

31. Hof AL, Gazendam MGJ, Sinke WE. The condition for dynamic stability. J Biomech 2005;38(1):1–8

32. Horak FB, Nashner LM. Central programming of postural movements: adaptation to altered support-surface configurations. J Neurophysiol 1986;55(6):1369–1381

33. Collins JJ, De Luca CJ. Open-loop and closed-loop control of posture: a random-walk analysis of center-of-pressure trajectories. Exp Brain Res 1993;95(2):308–318

34. Yavuz M, Botek G, Davis BL. Plantar shear stress distributions: comparing actual and predicted frictional forces at the foot-ground interface. J Biomech 2007;40(13):3045–3049

35. Chen WM, Vee-Sin Lee P, Park SB, Lee SJ, Phyau Wui Shim V, Lee T. A novel gait platform to measure isolated plantar metatarsal forces during walking. J Biomech 2010;43(10):2017–2021

36. Urry S. Plantar pressure-measurement sensors. Meas Sci Technol 1999;10:R16–R32

37. Putti AB, Arnold GP, Cochrane L, Abboud RJ. The Pedar in-shoe system: repeatability and normal pressure values. Gait Posture 2007;25(3):401–405

38. Gurney JK, Kersting UG, Rosenbaum D. Between-day reliability of repeated plantar pressure distribution measurements in a normal population. Gait Posture 2008;27(4):706–709

39. Melai T, IJzerman TH, Schaper NC, et al. Calculation of plantar pressure time integral, an alternative approach. Gait Posture 2011;34(3):379–383

40. Drerup B, Kraneburg S, Koller A. Visualisation of pressure dose, synopsis of peak pressure, mean pressure, loading time and pressure-time-integral. Clin Biomech (Bristol, Avon) 2001;16:833–834

41. Simoneau GG, Ulbrecht JS, Derr JA, Becker MB, Cavanagh PR. Postural instability in patients with diabetic sensory neuropathy. Diabetes Care 1994;17(12):1411–1421

42. Pedotti A. Simple equipment used in clinical practice for evaluation of locomotion. IEEE Trans Biomed Eng 1977;24(5):456–461

43. Mueller MJ, Zou D, Lott DJ. "Pressure gradient" as an indicator of plantar skin injury. Diabetes Care 2005;28(12):2908–2912

44. Zou D, Mueller MJ, Lott DJ. Effect of peak pressure and pressure gradient on subsurface shear stresses in the neuropathic foot. J Biomech 2007;40(4):883–890

45. Perry J. Gait Analysis: Normal and Pathological Function. Thorofare, New Jersey: Slack; 1992

46. Morag E, Cavanagh PR. Structural and functional predictors of regional peak pressures under the foot during walking. J Biomech 1999;32(4):359–370

47. Hillstrom HJ, Song J, Kraszewski AP, et al. Foot type biomechanics part 1: structure and function of the asymptomatic foot. Gait Posture 2013;37(3):445–451

48. Mootanah R, Song J, Lenhoff MW, et al. Foot type biomechanics part 2: are structure and anthropometrics related to function? Gait Posture 2013;37(3):452–456

49. Bosch K, Nagel A, Weigend L, Rosenbaum D. From "first" to "last" steps in life—pressure patterns of three generations. Clin Biomech (Bristol, Avon) 2009;24(8):676–681

50. Drerup B, Beckmann C, Wetz HH. Effect of body weight on plantar peak pressure in diabetic patients [in German]. Orthopade 2003;32(3):199–206

51. Drerup B. Normalisation of plantar pressure distribution with respect to gait velocity. In: Prendergast PJ, Lee TC, Carr AJ, eds. Proceedings of the 12th Conference of the European Society of Biomechanics. Dublin: Royal Academy of Medicine in Ireland; 2000:138

52. Segal A, Rohr E, Orendurff M, Shofer J, O'Brien M, Sangeorzan B. The effect of walking speed on peak plantar pressure. Foot Ankle Int 2004;25(12):926–933

53. Grieve DW, Gear RJ. The relationships between length of stride, step frequency, time of swing and speed of walking for children and adults. Ergonomics 1966;9(5):379–399

54. Drerup B, Szczepaniak A, Wetz HH. Plantar pressure reduction in step-to gait: a biomechanical investigation and clinical feasibility study. Clin Biomech (Bristol, Avon) 2008;23(8):1073–1079

55. Zhu HS, Wertsch JJ, Harris GF, Loftsgaarden JD, Price MB. Foot pressure distribution during walking and shuffling. Arch Phys Med Rehabil 1991;72(6):390–397

56. Brown HE, Mueller MJA. A "step-to" gait decreases pressures on the forefoot. J Orthop Sports Phys Ther 1998;28(3):139–145

57. Mittlmeier T, Haar P. The infected diabetic foot [in German]. Unfallchirurg 2011;114(3):227–235

58. Wrobel JS, Najafi B. Diabetic foot biomechanics and gait dysfunction. J Diabetes Sci Tech 2010; 4(4):833–845

59. Mueller MJ, Minor SD, Sahrmann SA, Schaaf JA, Strube MJ. Differences in the gait characteristics of patients with diabetes and peripheral neuropathy compared with age-matched controls. Phys Ther 1994;74(4):299–308, discussion 309–313

60. Cavanagh PR, Ulbrecht JS, Caputo GM. The biomechanics of the foot in diabetes mellitus. In: Bowker JH, Pfeiffer MA, eds. Levin and O'Neal's The Diabetic Foot. 6th ed. St. Louis: Mosby; 2001

61. Cavanagh PR, Bus SA. Off-loading the diabetic foot for ulcer prevention and healing. J Vasc Surg 2010; 52(3, Suppl)37S–43S

62. Owings TM, Apelqvist J, Stenström A, et al. Plantar pressures in diabetic patients with foot ulcers which have remained healed. Diabet Med 2009;26(11):1141–1146

63. Chantelau E, Onvlee GJ. Charcot foot in diabetes: farewell to the neurotrophic theory. Horm Metab Res 2006;38(6):361–367

64. Leibner ED, Brodsky JW, Pollo FE, Baum BS, Edmonds BW. Unloading mechanism in the total contact cast. Foot Ankle Int 2006;27(4):281–285

65. Bus SA, Haspels R, Busch-Westbroek TE. Evaluation and optimization of therapeutic footwear for neuropathic diabetic foot patients using in-shoe plantar pressure analysis. Diabetes Care 2011;34(7):1595–1600

66. Lavery LA, Armstrong DG, Wunderlich RP, Tredwell J, Boulton AJ. Predictive value of foot pressure assessment as part of a population-based diabetes disease management program. Diabetes Care 2003;26(4):1069–1073

18 Gait

The underlying causes of pathological gait vary widely. It may be that the muscles do not generate sufficient force, or they do not tolerate the strains required, or perhaps activation does not occur at the right time intervals. The left and right leg lengths may be different, or the geometry of the joints and the orientation of their axes of rotation may differ from normal. The main aims of gait analysis are (1) to classify a person's gait as normal or pathological, (2) to explore the causes of a pathological gait, (3) to check the effect of internal or external prostheses on gait, and (4) to assess the success of physiotherapy. To do these things, gait analysis documents the course of the motion in space and time. The muscle activation pattern is determined by the recording of electromyography (EMG) signals. Forces and moments acting on the segments of the lower extremity (foot, lower leg, and upper leg) can be calculated using the method of inverse dynamics. The pressure distribution under the sole of the foot and the energy consumption can also be measured. Walking is a complex movement, and one cannot expect that measurement of a single parameter will be enough to classify a person's gait as normal or pathological.

18.1 Gait Pattern

Inspection of the footprints (**Fig. 18.1**) conveys a first impression of an individual's gait pattern. The stride length is the sum of the left and right step lengths. Adults have a stride length in the order of 1.4 m.[1,2] During walking at a comfortable, self-selected speed, stride length is observed to be dependent on the leg length: on average, stride length increases with body height. For the purpose of comparisons, stride length is normalized for stature and the quotient of stride length/body height is used. After normalization, the stride lengths of men and women are almost identical.[3] In healthy persons the left and right step lengths are equal, each making up one half of the total stride length. In pathological gait, the left and right step lengths can be markedly different.

The line of progression runs through the center between the left and right footprints. In normal gait the prints of the right foot lie to the right of this line and the prints of the left foot to the left. If both feet are placed exactly on the line of progression, the gait pattern is conspicuously unusual. In pathological gait, it

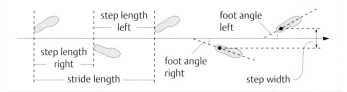

Fig. 18.1 Footstep pattern. Step length, step width, and foot angle are defined.

can even happen that both the right and the left foot cross the line of progression. The step width is defined as the distance between the centers of the heel prints of the right and the left foot, measured perpendicularly to the line of progression. In healthy persons the step width is around 10 cm.

The foot angle is the angle between the line of progression and the line connecting the center of the heel print and the second ray. In large cohorts, Dougan[4] and Patek[5] documented an average foot angle of 6°. In healthy persons, however, there was a wide variation in the range between +20° and –8°. Normally the angles of the left and right feet differed by 2° or more. Ducroquet et al[6] report normal foot angles of approximately 15°, but this value seems unrealistically high: Charlie Chaplin's unmistakable gait is characterized by foot angles of this magnitude. In a 9-month longitudinal study of 10 healthy adults, Brinckmann[7] observed that foot angles varied considerably, not just from step to step, but throughout the observation period. It follows that determining foot angle from one step alone at a single point in time will give an unreliable result.

Only limited information can be obtained from inspecting a footprint pattern. A marked difference between left and right step length or footprints that cross the line of progression point to a gait disorder, but the cause of the disorder cannot be discerned. Conspicuously short step lengths may be from a small person, or from a person of normal height walking slowly, or from a patient with Parkinson disease. The clinical significance of a deviation of the foot angle from the norm (and its potential influence on the orientation of the knee axis) is unknown. Recent technological advances have made it much easier to measure footprints optically and electronically, and we may expect this issue to be further explored in future cross-sectional and longitudinal studies.

18.2   Sequence of Steps in Time

Normal gait consists of a series of virtually identical steps succeeding each other in turn. In this cyclic motion, the basic unit is the so-called gait cycle, the time interval between successive heel strikes of the right or the left foot. **Fig. 18.2** shows a gait cycle starting at heel strike of the right foot. The stance phase (time interval of floor contact) commences at heel strike; it ends at toe-off. This is followed by the swing phase, which again is terminated by heel strike. In normal walking the stance phase makes up about 60% and the swing phase about 40% of the gait cycle. In pathological gait, values different from these are seen. Differences in leg length, for example, result in a shortening of the stance phase of the shorter leg.

At the beginning and in the middle of the gait cycle, on each occasion for about 10% of the gait cycle, both feet are in contact with the floor at the same time. The duration of this double support phase decreases as the velocity of walking increases. In running, the double support phase disappears and the stance and swing phase both assume the value of about 50% of the gait cycle. Unlike during walking, in running there are short time intervals in which both feet are off the ground. During these time intervals, both legs "fly"

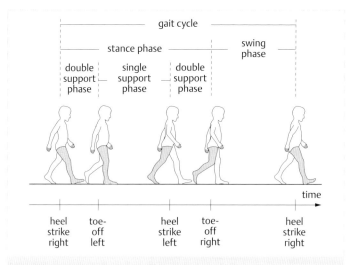

Fig. 18.2 Gait cycle, showing division into stance and swing phases (with reference to the right leg).

forward with the body. Because of this, the stride length when running can be increased beyond the maximum that is possible during walking, which is restricted for reasons of anatomy.

With S as stride length and T as duration of a stride, the velocity v in the direction of the line of progression is

(18.1) $$v = S/T \text{ [m/s]}$$

Normal walking speed is in the order of 1.3 m/s; slow and fast walking speeds are 0.8 m/s and 1.5 m/s, respectively.[1,2] Stride frequency v is given by

(18.2) $$v = 1/T \text{ [Hz]}$$

The stride frequency of slow walking is around 0.6 Hz; the stride frequencies of normal and fast walking are 0.9 and 1.0 Hz, respectively. For a given walking speed, persons of shorter stature have higher stride frequencies. This compensates their smaller step length, which is typical of shorter people.[1,2]

If, for a given walking speed, people are asked to choose their most comfortable stride frequency, these self-selected frequencies are observed to vary by only a small amount. Holt et al[8] provide a formula by which the duration of a stride may be approximately predicted:

(18.3) $$T \approx 2\pi \sqrt{\frac{I}{2 \cdot m \cdot g \cdot d}} \text{ [s]}$$

This empirical formula is derived from a pendulum model of the leg, modeling the whole leg as a rigid body and permitting no bending at the knee joint. In this formula g denotes the gravitational acceleration, I the

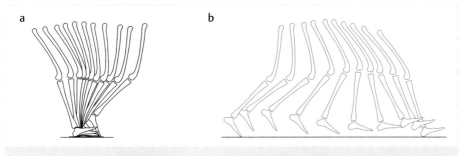

Fig. 18.3a, b Qualitative overview of the motion of the upper leg, lower leg, and foot during the stance phase (**a**) and the swing phase (**b**) of the gait cycle. (Adapted from Braune and Fischer.[9])

moment of inertia of the leg about an axis through its center of mass perpendicular to the sagittal plane, m the mass of the leg, and d the distance from the greater trochanter to the center of mass.

18.3 Kinematics

Fig. 18.3 shows an example from the pioneering experiments of Braune and Fischer[9] documenting the motion of the leg in the stance and swing phases. The locations and orientations of upper leg, lower leg, and foot were measured from a series of photographs by means of markers fixed on the skin; the contours of the bones shown in **Fig. 18.3** are merely shown for the purpose of illustration. At heel strike the hip joint is flexed. In the stance phase the hip joint is first extended and then flexed in preparation for the swing phase. At heel strike, the knee is flexed as well. In the stance phase it is extended and flexed again toward toe-off. The ankle joint changes the angle of its position from dorsiflexion at heel strike to plantar flexion at toe-off.

Today, the motion in walking is documented by optoelectronic methods. Light-emitting or light-reflecting markers are affixed to the segments of the body. The markers are observed by a set of video cameras, allowing reconstruction of their movement in three dimensions over time. At each instant in time, the location of the set of markers provides information on the relative position and orientation of the trunk, upper leg, lower leg, and foot segments. The change in position and orientation seen after a time lapse Δt (commonly ranging between 1/20 s and 1/50 s) allows the linear and angular velocities of the segments to be computed. The change in the velocities from one time interval to the next permits computation of the linear and angular accelerations of the segments.

Fig. 18.4 shows the temporal course of the angles in the sagittal plane of the hip, knee, and ankle during walking. The authors, Kerrigan et al, observed healthy adults of both sexes.[3] In the cohort investigated there were only minor differences between men and women. Strictly speaking, the motion of the segments of the lower extremity during walking is not confined to the sagittal plane; in reality it is three-dimensional, and in addition the leg may perform a rotation about its long axis. However, for many purposes the description of the motion of the leg as plane motion is an acceptable approximation.

Disease or injury can cause the angular motion to deviate from the healthy norm. For example, after reconstruction of an injured anterior cruciate ligament, some patients will avoid bending that knee in phases of high loading. In these patients, the reduced bending angle of the knee will be compensated by increased flexion of the hip. A bending deficit of the knee is also observed after partial excision of the

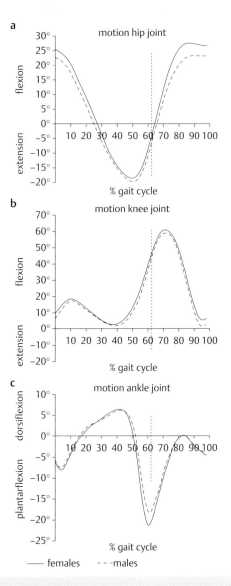

Fig. 18.4a–c Example of the angular motion of the hip (**a**), knee (**b**), and ankle (**c**) during a gait cycle, as measured in 99 healthy adults of both sexes aged between 20 and 40 years. The dotted lines mark the instant of toe-off at slightly over 60% of the gait cycle. (Adapted from Kerrigan et al.[3])

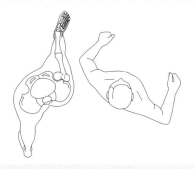

Fig. 18.5 Contrary rotations of hip and shoulder regions in walking. (Adapted from Ducroquet et al.[6])

meniscus. Weakness of the quadriceps, avoidance of its use, or inhibition of neuromuscular control have been suggested as possible causes.

During walking, a characteristic rotation of the trunk about a vertical axis can be observed. The anterior movement of the right leg in the swing phase is coupled with an anterior movement of the right hip. Seen from above, the pelvis is rotated anticlockwise (**Fig. 18.5**). To maintain the dynamic equilibrium, the shoulder must simultaneously be rotated in the opposite direction. The magnitude of the angular motion is in the order of ±5°.[10] If for some reason the compensatory movement of the shoulder cannot be performed, a striking alteration of the gait results.

18.4   Muscle Activity

EMG measurements show which muscles are activated in the course of the gait cycle. As an example **Fig. 18.6** shows the "on–off" pattern of the muscles at the hip.[11] The "on" time is defined as that time interval during which the EMG signal exceeds a particular threshold value. The threshold chosen could be, for example, 10% of the signal amplitude measured at peak activation of the muscle. In pathological gait the EMG pattern may differ markedly from normal: the activity of individual muscles may be increased, decreased, or vanishingly small. The time course of the activation may be modified, or unusual antagonistic activation may occur. Another important element in walking is the activation of the muscles of the trunk, especially of the back extensors and the oblique muscles. For example, the back extensors are always activated prior to heel strike. This prevents the trunk from tipping forwards upon heel strike.

18.5   Moment and Power of the Muscles

The moment and the power of the muscles that move a joint, and the force transmitted from one bone to another in that joint, cannot be measured directly. However, with knowledge of the kinematics and employing biomechanical models, it is possible to compute these parameters using the inverse dynamics

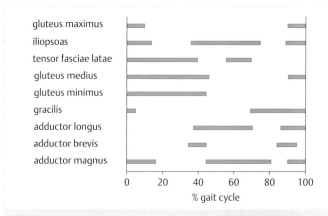

Fig. 18.6 Example of the "on–off" pattern of the electromyographic activity of the muscles of the hip joint during a gait cycle. (Adapted from Shiavi.[11])

approach (see Chapter 12). To explain the principle of this procedure in an accessible way, the following remarks are confined to the two-dimensional case. Modern, commercially available optoelectronic instrumentation measures and calculates in three dimensions.

For the purpose of calculation, the leg is modeled as consisting of three segments (upper leg, lower leg, and foot) connected by hinge joints (**Fig. 18.7**). The equations of motion state that the translational and rotational motion of each segment is effected by the sum of the forces and moments acting. Forces effecting an accelerated translation, and moments effecting an accelerated rotation, can be transmitted to any segment only from its adjoining segments. In addition, the gravitational force acts at the center of mass of each segment; this force is directed vertically downwards.

Let us assume the mass of the lower leg, the location of its center of mass, and the moment of inertia about its center of mass to be known. If the translational acceleration of the center of mass and the rotational acceleration are measured, it would be possible to calculate the sum of the forces and moments that effected the observed motion. It would, however, make little sense to perform such a measurement and calculation for the lower leg in isolation, for in that case then we would know only the sums of the forces and moments acting. What fraction of these sums were transmitted from the upper leg (across the knee) or from the foot (across the ankle) would remain unknown. For this reason, the calculation of the forces and moments always starts at one end of the kinematic chain of the segments, preferably at the foot segment. The force and moment transmitted to the foot from the floor can be measured using a force platform. If the sums of all forces and moments acting are determined from the motion data employing the method of inverse dynamics, the force and moment transmitted from the lower leg to the foot can be determined by subtraction. The procedure is now repeated for the lower leg segment. With knowledge of the motion data and of the force and moment transmitted from the foot, the force and moment transmitted from the upper leg via the knee can be specified. In the next step, the force and moment transmitted from the trunk to the upper leg via the hip joint are obtained.

In principle, the determination of forces and moments could equally well start at the other end of the kinematic chain of body segments. To do this, one would start at the head and arm segments, proceed to the trunk segment, and then to the leg segments. Apart from the gravitational force, no external forces act on the head, arms, and trunk, and thus no force measuring equipment would have to be employed. Because of the comparatively large mass of the trunk, however, and the fact that its description as a rigid body is only a rough approximation, the results of this measurement and calculation would be less precise.

In detail, the procedure is as follows:

Step 1. In the stance phase of the gait cycle, a force platform measures the vector $\mathbf{R}_1$ with components $\mathbf{R}_{1x}$ and $\mathbf{R}_{1y}$ of the force (ground reaction force) between floor and foot (**Fig. 18.7**). Since only

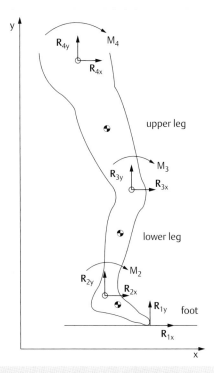

Fig. 18.7 Model of the leg employed for the calculation of the forces and moments transmitted between the foot, lower leg, upper leg, and trunk segments. Open circles: centers of rotation of the joints; segmented circles: centers of mass. The force $\mathbf{R}_1$ acts from the floor on the foot. $\mathbf{R}_2$–$\mathbf{R}_4$ and M_2–M_4 designate the forces and moments transmitted between the segments via the ankle, knee, and hip joints.

compressive forces (but no tensile forces) are transmitted between the floor and the foot, the moment M_1 transmitted from the floor on the foot is zero. With knowledge of the linear acceleration of the center of mass of the foot, the angular acceleration about the center of mass, the mass, and the moment of inertia, the net force and moment acting on the foot are calculated. If the vector $\mathbf{R}_1$ and the gravitational force are subtracted from the net force, the force $\mathbf{R}_2$ and the moment M_2 acting on the foot from the lower leg are obtained.

Step 2. The same algorithm is now applied to the lower leg segment. In mechanical equilibrium, the force and moment transmitted from the foot to the lower leg are opposite and equal to the force and moment transmitted from the lower leg to the foot; that is, they are $-\mathbf{R}_2$ and $-M_2$. With knowledge of the linear acceleration of the center of mass of the lower leg, the angular acceleration about the center of mass, the mass, and the moment of inertia, the net force and moment acting on the lower leg are calculated. If the vector $-\mathbf{R}_2$ and the gravitational force are subtracted from the net force, and the moment $-M_2$ is subtracted from the net moment, the force $\mathbf{R}_3$ and the moment M_3 acting on the lower leg from the upper leg via the knee joint are obtained.

Step 3. The same algorithm is now applied to the upper leg segment. The input data for the calculation are the force $-\mathbf{R}_3$ and the moment $-M_3$ transmitted from the lower leg to the upper leg as determined in step 2, the mass of the upper leg, its moment of inertia, and the linear and rotational acceleration measured. The result of this calculation gives the force $\mathbf{R}_4$ and the moment M_4 transmitted from the trunk via the hip joint to the upper leg.

The moments determined thus are the net moments generated by all the individual muscles and tendons spanning a joint. If more than a single muscle is active at the same time, the contribution of specific muscles to the net moment can only be determined if additional information is available (from EMG measurements, for example) or model assumptions are employed. For example, a small net moment may be a result of a low activity in the muscles involved, or, alternatively, it may mean that muscles have been activated antagonistically so that their moments partially compensate each other.

The power of muscles spanning a joint is equal to the product of moment and angular velocity:

(18.4) $$\text{power} = \text{moment} \cdot \text{angular velocity} \quad [\text{Nm/s} = \text{W}]$$

Power is measured in watts [W]. The power of a muscle is counted positive if the muscle shortens in the course of the motion; it is counted negative if the muscle elongates in the course of the motion.

To simplify comparisons between individuals, the moment and power of the muscles can be adjusted for body mass and stature and be quoted in Nm/(kg · m) and W/(kg · m), respectively. **Figs. 18.8** and **18.9** show the adjusted moment and power of the muscles of the hip, knee, and ankle during walking, measured in a cohort of adults of both sexes.[3] The course over time of moment and that of power look very different

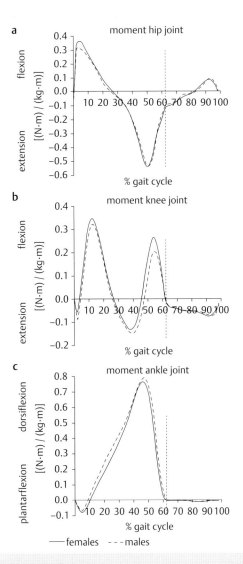

Fig. 18.8a–c Example of the calculated, adjusted moment of the muscles acting at the hip (**a**), knee (**b**), and ankle (**c**) in the course of a gait cycle. Observations from 99 healthy adults of both sexes aged between 20 and 40 years. To enable comparisons between individuals, the moment is divided by body height and body mass. The dotted lines indicate the instant of toe-off at approximately 60% of the gait cycle. (Adapted from Kerrigan et al.[3])

because the angular velocity changes in the course of the gait cycle. At those time points where either the moment or the velocity is zero, by definition the power is also zero. In the cohort investigated, the power of the muscles of the knee joint assumed a maximum value of approximately 0.4 W/(kg · m). For a person of

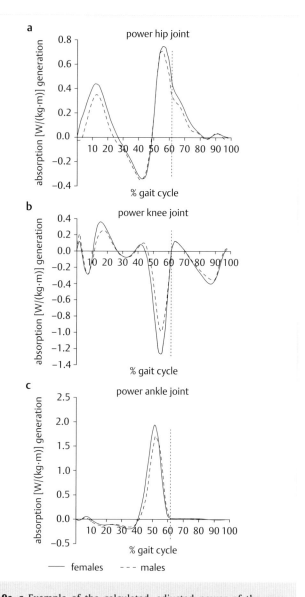

Fig. 18.9a–c Example of the calculated, adjusted power of the muscles acting at the hip (**a**), knee (**b**), and ankle (**c**) in the course of a gait cycle. Observations from 99 healthy adults of both sexes aged between 20 and 40 years. To enable comparisons between individuals, the power is divided by body height and body mass. The dotted lines indicate the instant of toe-off at approximately 60% of the gait cycle. (Adapted from Kerrigan et al.[3])

1.75 m body height and 65 kg mass, this corresponds to a power of 0.4 · 1.75 · 65 = 45.5 W. The power of muscles during particular phases or throughout the whole of the gait cycle is a sensitive indicator of the progress of healing after injury.

The joint force $\mathbf{R}$ between segments determined in gait analysis is the (net) sum of the compressive force between the articulating bones and the tensile force of the muscles, tendons, and ligaments that cross the joint. To calculate the compressive force acting on the articular surface, an anatomical model of the joint is needed. The model specifies the location of the center of rotation and the moment arms of the muscles. If more than one muscle is activated at a time, assumptions are required on how much of the total moment is generated by each of the different muscles (see Chapter 12). Examples of the compressive force on the articular surface of the hip and the femorotibial joint obtained from gait analysis are given in Chapters 13 and 14.

The concept of determining the forces and moments transmitted from one segment of the leg to the next using the inverse dynamics approach appears basically simple. In practice, however, intricate problems are encountered in both measurement and calculation. Sources of error and uncertainty include the following:

- The mass, location of the center of mass, and moment of inertia of the segments of the lower leg are known only imprecisely. The published reference data are derived from studies of small, unrepresentative groups.
- Against the assumptions made for the purposes of calculation, segments composed of bones and soft tissue are not rigid bodies but change their shape in the course of the gait cycle.
- Centers of mass and axes of rotation can be located only indirectly, by reference to external anatomical landmarks.
- The motion of segments is measured using markers fixed to the skin. Due to movement of the skin or the activation of muscles, these markers can move relative to the joints in an uncontrollable fashion.

Some studies simplify the determination of the moment exerted on the hip or the knee by including only the vector $\mathbf{R}_1$ of the ground reaction force in the calculation. The moments are then expressed as products of the magnitude of the ground reaction force and the perpendicular distance from the center of rotation of hip or knee to the line of action of this force (**Fig. 18.10**). However, this makes sense only for static or quasi-static applications where the inertial forces and moments of the segments can be neglected. In the dynamic case, moment and force depend not only on the vector of the ground reaction force, but also on the linear and angular accelerations of foot, lower leg, and upper leg.[12] Winter[12] illustrated this with an example: If the simplified concept were to be applied to the cervical spine, the moment on the cervical spine would amount to $L_c \cdot |\mathbf{R}_1|$. No sensible investigator would accept that a moment of this magnitude acts on the cervical spine during walking.

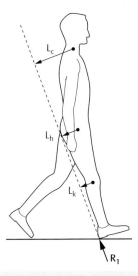

Fig. 18.10 Line of action of the ground reaction force **R**₁ and its moment arms L_k, L_h, and L_c in relation to the knee and hip joints and the cervical spine. (Adapted, with permission, from Winter.[12])

18.6 Application Point of the Ground Reaction Force

In the stance phase of walking, the point of application of the ground reaction force at any instant can be determined from the pressure distribution under the foot or from the data measured by a force platform (see Section 1.3.1). The migration of this point over the course of the gait cycle characterizes the temporal course of the loading of the different parts of the foot (see Section 17.4.2). Normally, the heel is the first to be loaded on contact between foot and floor, and in the course of the gait cycle the point of force application migrates distally up to the great toe. In pathological gait, it may be that the first contact occurs in the region of the ball of the foot (in talipes equinus [clubfoot], for example) or that in the stance phase the point of force application moves to and fro between the heel and the toe region.

18.7 Energy Consumption in Walking

In biomechanics, a distinction is made between internal and external work of the muscles. External work is performed, for example, when objects are lifted; this includes lifting one's own body when walking uphill. Internal work is the energy required to maintain a posture or to move the body. In a person walking on a level surface, the muscles perform internal work. The external work performed is almost zero, because on average the height of the body's center of mass above ground remains unchanged. When walking on a level surface, the only external work that can be performed is work to overcome friction between the body and the air (against a headwind) or between the feet and the floor (when walking through mud, for example).

One measure of the body's internal energy consumption would be its generation of heat, but measuring the generated heat would be technically complex. It is simpler to measure oxygen consumption and assume that the body's consumption of oxygen is proportional to the energy consumed. The energy consumption in walking can then be specified in various ways: as energy per unit time ("O_2 rate") or as energy per meter of walking distance ("O_2 cost"). The energy consumption per unit time is usually stated as volume of oxygen per minute per kilogram of body mass [mL O_2/(min · kg)]; the energy consumption per meter walking distance is stated as volume oxygen per meter per kilogram of body mass [mL O_2/(m · kg)]. The energy consumption is divided by the body mass to facilitate interindividual comparisons. Underlying this is the assumption of proportionality between energy consumption and body mass, which in reality need not be exactly the case.

Waters et al[2] published reference values for oxygen consumption per minute as a function of walking speed (**Fig. 18.11**). Consumption increased in proportion to speed; there was no difference between the sexes. Holt et al[13] showed that energy consumption was lowest during walking at the walker's own preferred stride frequency. If, while keeping a constant speed, stride frequency is reduced below or increased above the preferred frequency, oxygen consumption rises (**Fig. 18.12**). If stride length is kept constant, the oxygen consumption per unit of time rises continuously with stride frequency (**Fig. 18.13**). This result agrees with actual experience that any required deviation from what the individual perceives as comfortable walking requires additional physical effort.

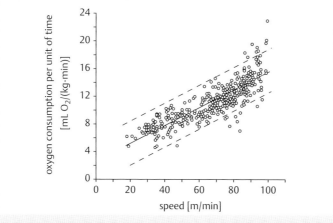

Fig. 18.11 Oxygen consumption per minute as a function of walking speed. (Adapted, with permission, from Waters et al.[2])

Waters et al[2] determined oxygen consumption per meter walking distance in children, teens, and adults as a function of walking speed (**Fig. 18.14**). At first sight the energy consumption seems to be greater at lower speeds. It must be remembered, however, that oxygen consumption is made up of the basal metabolic

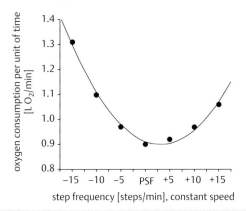

Fig. 18.12 Oxygen consumption per unit time at constant walking speed as a function of stride frequency. PSF, preferred stride frequency (as chosen by the individual walker). (Adapted from Holt et al.[13])

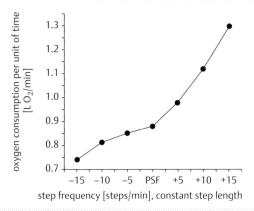

Fig. 18.13 Oxygen consumption per unit time at constant stride length as a function of stride frequency. PSF, preferred stride frequency. (Adapted from Holt et al.[13])

rate (energy consumption of the resting body per unit time) and the internal work required for walking. In walking slowly, more time is required to cover a given distance, and thus the contribution of the basal metabolic rate to the total oxygen consumption is higher.

According to Waters,[14] the energy efficiency of pathological gait can be defined as

$$(18.5) \qquad \text{efficiency } [\%] = \frac{\text{oxygen consumption per meter (normal gait)}}{\text{oxygen consumption per meter (pathologic gait)}} \cdot 100.0$$

If more oxygen is consumed in pathological gait than in normal gait, the efficiency falls below 100%. Experience shows that patients with gait disturbances, due for example to amputation, paralysis, or

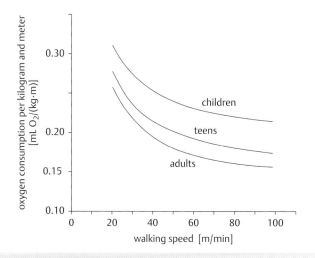

Fig. 18.14 Oxygen consumption per kilogram body mass and meter walking distance as a function of walking speed. (Adapted, with permission, from Waters et al.[2])

Parkinson disease, show energy efficiencies below 100%. Walking with different prostheses can likewise lead to different efficiencies. The reference values for healthy persons published by Waters[14] may serve in such cases as a benchmark for comparison.

18.8 Dominance of One Leg

It is well known that we do not use our left and right hands in the same fashion. The so-called dominant arm and dominant hand (in most cases the right ones) are used for writing, handshaking, pointing, and so on. As far as we know, the difference between sides (being right- or left-handed) is not acquired but congenital.

A difference between left and right is less striking in relation to the legs and feet than it is for the hands. Tests performed to determine a dominant side observe which foot is put forwards first in starting to walk,[15] which foot is used to kick a ball, or which foot takes the first step in walking up stairs. According to such tests, dominance of the right leg seems more prevalent than dominance of the left.[16] The dominance does not seem to lead to any discernable asymmetry of gait.

18.9 Falls

If the vertical projection of the center of mass of the body (the line of gravity) lies outside the base of support, the gravitational force exerts a moment in relation to the periphery of that base. The moment effects an accelerated rotation of the body about an axis lying inside the base. The body tips and the height of the center of mass above ground decreases. Potential energy is converted first to kinetic energy and then, on impact, to deformation and fracture energy and to heat. In erect stance, the base of support is given by the area under and between the feet. Postural control ensures that the line of gravity remains inside the base of support. Walking and stair climbing differ from standing still in that the line of gravity is located within the base of support only for very short time intervals. In walking, the line of gravity is for most of the time shifted to the side of the raised leg; in climbing stairs it is shifted forwards. In both cases there is a risk of falling. To prevent a fall, the raised foot must be put down quickly enough in the right place on the floor.

In erect stance, the height of the center of mass above the floor is equivalent to about two thirds of the body height. In any fall, an appreciable amount of energy will be released. For a person of 1.75 m body height and 65 kg body mass, whose center of mass after the fall is still 0.2 m above ground, the energy released equates to $(\frac{2}{3} \cdot 1.75 - 0.2) \cdot 65 \cdot 9.81 \approx 616$ Nm. This is enough energy to cause injury to bones and soft tissues. Falls from a sitting position are less frequent because the base of support is larger; they also usually have less serious consequences because the height of the fall is smaller.

18.9.1 Epidemiology of Falls

The risk of falling is not confined to the elderly: the young also fall. However, the probability of falling is higher in the elderly and accompanying injuries are more severe. For this reason, the majority of studies in the epidemiology of falls concentrate on persons over 65 years of age. Because of differences between the groups investigated, the numerical results of these studies vary somewhat. The discussion below is intended only to provide an overview.

The causes of falls are manifold. Reported risk factors include stumbling or slipping when walking; low force generation of the muscles of the leg; physical inactivity; impaired vision (visual acuity, spatial perception, image contrast); prolonged response time; impaired sense of balance; overweight; pain; medication; dementia, and distracted attention.[17] In a cohort of almost 3000 persons aged over 65 years, Prudham and Evans[18] found an incidence of 28 falls per 100 persons per year. The incidence increased with age. Initially women were affected more, but after the age of 85 years was passed, the probability of falling was equal among both sexes. No differences between fallers and non-fallers were found in terms of social class, type of housing, or living alone. Blake et al[19] obtained similar results in a survey of 1942 persons. In a cohort with a mean age of 75 years, Vellas et al[20] documented an incidence of 64 falls per month per 1000 persons; approximately 17% of the falls resulted in injury. Over 90% of the falls were "accidental." The persons had been standing or walking before they stumbled or tripped. Fewer than 3% reported "feeling faint" before they fell. In almost half of the cases, they had tripped over or against an object that led to an unexpected positioning of their legs or feet that could not be corrected quickly enough.

O'Neill et al[21] documented the direction of falls in a cohort of 1243 persons aged 50 years or over (**Fig. 18.15**). If the foot hits an obstacle while walking, a fall forwards may occur. If, by contrast, the leading foot slips forwards during heel strike, a backward fall may be expected.[22] During a forward fall, the arms are automatically stretched out to protect the face and head, and the impact then occurs in the region of hands and arms. In a backward fall, the impact preferentially occurs in the region of the pelvis. **Fig. 18.16** shows the body regions where the impact occurs.[20]

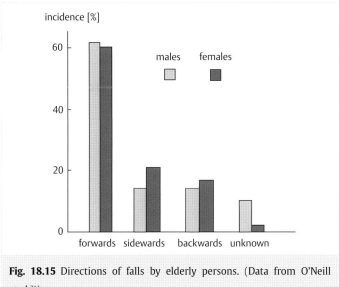

Fig. 18.15 Directions of falls by elderly persons. (Data from O'Neill et al.[21])

Not all falls result in injury requiring treatment. According to Sattin et al,[23] between 30% and 50% of falls (depending on the age of the person) result in injuries requiring hospitalization. In the study by Berg et al,[24] 5% of falls resulted in fractures and 9% in injury to the soft tissues requiring treatment. Slipping or falling sideways causes fractures mainly in the region of pelvis and hip. Forward falls are associated predominantly with fractures of the upper arm, lower arm, and wrist.[25]

18.9.2 Prevention of Injuries Due to Falling

Falls can result in serious, life-threatening injuries—and even after a fall that in fact did not cause damage, the fear of falling again can have a negative effect on quality of life. To mitigate the extent of these consequences, attempts can be made to reduce the incidence of falls by providing mechanical aids, or to reduce the severity of injuries by teaching appropriate fall techniques.

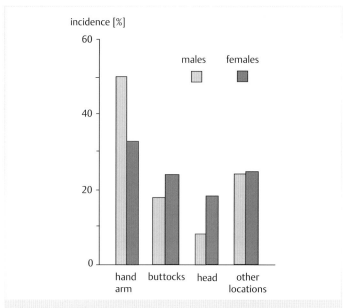

Fig. 18.16 Body regions where impact occurs after a fall. (Adapted, with permission, from Vellas et al.[20])

Reducing the Incidence of Falls

It has been shown experimentally that postural control may be compromised when attention is divided: that is, when cognitive tasks have to be performed simultaneously.[26,27] For example, in upright stance, elderly persons with a history of falling showed a marked increase in postural sway when they were given brain teasers to be solved. The authors conclude that the incidence of falls might be reduced by appropriate training. After a fall, people frequently report that they had "been in a hurry." If this is more than just an impression after the event, and hasty, haphazard motions did indeed contribute to the fall, it might be expected that targeted training of those at risk of falling would also lead to a reduced incidence of falls.

Weerdesteyn et al[28] conducted a 5-week physical exercise program for the prevention of falls. All the participants, who were aged 65 years, had a history of falls. The program involved balance and gait exercises and coordination training over an obstacle course (doorsteps, trip hazards, uneven pavement). In addition, walking in confined spaces with frequent alterations of speed and direction of walking was practiced. The incidence of falls in a 7-month period after the training program was compared with the incidence in the 6-month period preceding the program. The intervention led to a 46% reduction in falls.

Orthopedic Aids

In standing, the body's base of support is provided by the area beneath and between the feet. Using a cane can greatly enlarge this area in certain phases of the gait cycle (**Fig. 18.17**). The use of a walker can

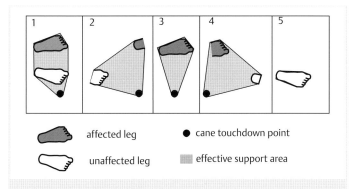

Fig. 18.17 Base of support over the course of a gait cycle when a cane is used. The cane is used contralaterally to the affected leg. (Adapted, with permission, from Bateni and Maki.[29])

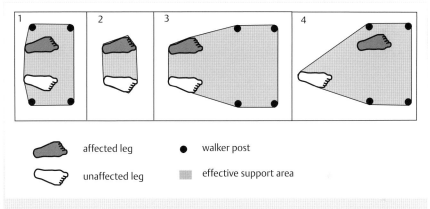

Fig. 18.18 Base of support over the course of a gait cycle when a walker is used. (Adapted, with permission, from Bateni and Maki.[29])

enlarge it still further (**Fig. 18.18**). Both the cane and the walker are effective aids in the prevention of falls. Problems that can arise in connection with these aids are overload injuries to the shoulders and arms, slipping of the cane if it is put down out of the vertical, disturbance of balance on lifting the walker, and unexpected contact of cane or walker with obstacles or unevenness of the floor.[29]

To prevent fractures in the region of the hip, so-called hip protectors have been developed. These hip protectors consist of a pair of undershorts with side pockets in the region of the greater trochanter; protective elements are inserted into these pockets.[30,31] Two different routes are followed. In one, a rigid element (or one that becomes rigid on impact) is designed to distribute the ground reaction force to a larger surface area of the body, thus relieving the major trochanter. In the other, an element manufactured from deformable foam is designed to damp the peak value of the impact force. Reports on the effectiveness of these hip protectors are conflicting. While some studies report a reduction of hip fractures by more than 50% (for example, Lauritzen et al[32] and Kannus et al[33]), others saw virtually no effect (for example, Kiel et al[34]). One obvious problem is that the protectors are not always put on correctly, or that they are not worn continuously because they are uncomfortable or are taken off at night.

Techniques for Falling to Reduce the Severity of Injury

A person falling forwards instinctively stretches out his or her arms. The risk of injury to the arms is accepted in order to avoid more serious injury to the face and head. DeGoede and Ashton-Miller[35] measured the force between hand and floor in healthy persons falling forwards from 1 m shoulder height and landing on both hands. Peak force values of more than 1000 N were seen when the test persons landed with an extended elbow joint. When they landed with the elbow flexed 10° the peak force was significantly lower. In theory, well-trained arm and shoulder muscles should be able to absorb the energy dissipated in a fall by contracting eccentrically. However, many elderly persons do not even have the force to perform a push-up. It is thus not realistic to expect them to achieve a soft landing from a fall using their arms: at most, activation of the muscles may help to reduce the force of the impact. The time interval between loss of balance and contact with the floor is in the order of 1 second. The time interval between the first floor contact and the occurrence of peak load on the hands or shoulders is less than 100 milliseconds. This interval is so short that neuromuscular reflexes during the impact can barely bring about any alteration. Everything that a person can do to prepare for impact has to happen within the first second after the loss of balance.[25]

Useful insights into how to reduce the severity of injuries due to falling may be anticipated from observing the course of falls of young, well-trained athletes. Especially in martial arts, falls are quite frequent, but they are only rarely associated with fractures. It must be assumed that the energy dissipated in a fall is absorbed essentially by eccentric contraction of the muscles. Documentations of the time course of falls show that the muscles of the upper and lower extremities carry out the crucial part of the damping of the impact force. As an example, **Fig. 18.19** shows the time course of a deliberately provoked slip resulting in a backward fall.[36] The step taken in an (unsuccessful) attempt to maintain balance and the rotational motion of arms and legs before finally the hip impacts the floor can all be seen. An example of a "controlled fall" in everyday life is sitting down on a chair.[37] The potential energy released by lowering the center of mass is absorbed by the extensors of the hip and the knee joint. A soft landing on the seat is the result.

Weerdesteyn et al[38] investigated whether martial arts fall techniques might be able to reduce the impact force of a fall. **Fig. 18.20** shows the example of a sideways fall from a kneeling posture. The first contact with the floor is with the pelvis; this is followed by a rolling motion and finally by arm contact with the floor. After brief training, young persons were able to reduce the pelvic impact force substantially when using this technique. However, it is still an open question whether the fall techniques illustrated in **Figs. 18.19** and **18.20** can be learned by elderly persons, and whether the learned techniques could be called upon quickly enough in unanticipated falls.

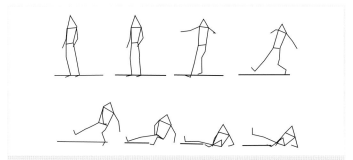

Fig. 18.19 Illustration of the temporal course of a deliberately provoked backward fall (seen obliquely from the side). (Adapted, with permission, from Hsiao et al.[36])

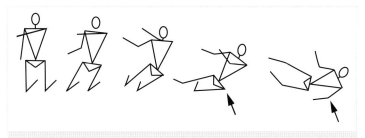

Fig. 18.20 Illustration of the temporal course of a sideways fall from a kneeling position as prescribed in Asian martial arts: floor contact is with the pelvis first, followed by rolling away via the arm and shoulder. (Adapted, with permission, from Weerdesteyn et al.[38])

References

1. Finley FR, Cody KA. Locomotive characteristics of urban pedestrians. Arch Phys Med Rehabil 1970;51(7):423–426

2. Waters RL, Lunsford BR, Perry J, Byrd R. Energy-speed relationship of walking: standard tables. J Orthop Res 1988;6(2):215–222

3. Kerrigan DC, Todd MK, Della Croce U. Gender differences in joint biomechanics during walking: normative study in young adults. Am J Phys Med Rehabil 1998;77(1):2–7

4. Dougan S. The angle of gait. Am J Phys Anthropol 1924;7:275–279

5. Patek SD. The angle of gait in women. Am J Phys Anthropol 1926;9:273–291

6. Ducroquet R, Ducroquet J, Ducroquet P. Walking and Limping. Philadelphia: Lippincott; 1968

7. Brinckmann P. The angle of gait [in German]. Z Orthop Ihre Grenzgeb 1981;119(5):445–448

8. Holt KG, Hamill J, Andres RO. The force-driven harmonic oscillator as a model for human locomotion. Hum Mov Sci 1990;9:55–68

9. Braune W, Fischer O. Der Gang des Menschen. Teil 1. Versuche am belasteten und unbelasteten Menschen. Abhandl Königl Sächs Gesellsch Wissensch XXXV, 1895

10. Murray MP. Gait as a total pattern of movement. Am J Phys Med 1967;46(1):290–333

11. Shiavi R. Electromyographic patterns in adult locomotion: a comprehensive review. J Rehabil Res Dev 1985;22(3):85–98

12. Winter DA. Biomechanics and Motor Control of Human Movement. 2nd ed. New York, NY: Wiley; 1990

13. Holt KG, Hamill J, Andres RO. Predicting the minimal energy costs of human walking. Med Sci Sports Exerc 1991;23(4):491–498

14. Waters RL. Energy expenditure. In: Perry J. Gait Analysis. Normal and Pathological Function. Thorofare, NJ: Slack; 1992:443–489

15. Nissan M, Whittle MW. Initiation of gait in normal subjects: a preliminary study. J Biomed Eng 1990;12(2):165–171

16. Sadeghi H, Allard P, Prince F, Labelle H. Symmetry and limb dominance in able-bodied gait: a review. Gait Posture 2000;12(1):34–45

17. Grabiner MD, Pavol MJ, Owings TM. Can fall-related hip fractures be prevented by characterizing the biomechanical mechanisms of failed recovery? Endocrine 2002;17(1):15–20

18. Prudham D, Evans JG. Factors associated with falls in the elderly: a community study. Age Ageing 1981;10(3):141–146

19. Blake AJ, Morgan K, Bendall MJ, et al. Falls by elderly people at home: prevalence and associated factors. Age Ageing 1988;17(6):365–372

20. Vellas BJ, Wayne SJ, Garry PJ, Baumgartner RN. A two-year longitudinal study of falls in 482 community-dwelling elderly adults. J Gerontol A Biol Sci Med Sci 1998;53(4):M264–M274

21. O'Neill TW, Varlow J, Silman AJ, et al. Age and sex influences on fall characteristics. Ann Rheum Dis 1994;53(11):773–775

22. Grabiner MD, Donovan S, Bareither ML, et al. Trunk kinematics and fall risk of older adults: translating biomechanical results to the clinic. J Electromyogr Kinesiol 2008;18(2):197–204

23. Sattin RW, Lambert Huber DA, DeVito CA, et al. The incidence of fall injury events among the elderly in a defined population. Am J Epidemiol 1990;131(6):1028–1037

24. Berg WP, Alessio HM, Mills EM, Tong C. Circumstances and consequences of falls in independent community-dwelling older adults. Age Ageing 1997;26(4):261–268

25. DeGoede KM, Ashton-Miller JA, Schultz AB. Fall-related upper body injuries in the older adult: a review of the biomechanical issues. J Biomech 2003;36(7):1043–1053

26. Woollacott M, Shumway-Cook A. Attention and the control of posture and gait: a review of an emerging area of research. Gait Posture 2002;16(1):1–14

27. Bloem BR, Grimbergen YA, van Dijk JG, Munneke M. The "posture second" strategy: a review of wrong priorities in Parkinson"s disease. J Neurol Sci 2006;248(1-2):196–204

28. Weerdesteyn V, Rijken H, Geurts AC, Smits-Engelsman BC, Mulder T, Duysens J. A five-week exercise program can reduce falls and improve obstacle avoidance in the elderly. Gerontology 2006;52(3):131–141

29. Bateni H, Maki BE. Assistive devices for balance and mobility: benefits, demands, and adverse consequences. Arch Phys Med Rehabil 2005;86(1):134–145

30. Holzer LA, Holzer G. The role of hip protectors in the prevention of hip fractures in older people [in German]. Wien Med Wochenschr 2007;157(15–16):381–387

31. Hönle W, Schuh A. Hip protectors. An overview [in German]. MMW Fortschr Med 2009; 151(Suppl 3):115–117

32. Lauritzen JB, Petersen MM, Lund B. Effect of external hip protectors on hip fractures. Lancet 1993;341(8836):11–13

33. Kannus P, Parkkari J, Niemi S, et al. Prevention of hip fracture in elderly people with use of a hip protector. N Engl J Med 2000;343(21):1506–1513

34. Kiel DP, Magaziner J, Zimmerman S, et al. Efficacy of a hip protector to prevent hip fracture in nursing home residents: the HIP PRO randomized controlled trial. JAMA 2007;298(4):413–422

35. DeGoede KM, Ashton-Miller JA. Fall arrest strategy affects peak hand impact force in a forward fall. J Biomech 2002;35(6):843–848

36. Hsiao ET, Robinovitch SN. Common protective movements govern unexpected falls from standing height. J Biomech 1998;31(1):1–9

37. Robinovitch SN, Hsiao ET, Sandler R, Cortez J, Liu Q, Paiement GD. Prevention of falls and fall-related fractures through biomechanics. Exerc Sport Sci Rev 2000;28(2):74–79

38. Weerdesteyn V, Groen BE, van Swigchem R, Duysens J. Martial arts fall techniques reduce hip impact forces in naive subjects after a brief period of training. J Electromyogr Kinesiol 2008;18(2):235–242

Further Reading

Perry J, Burnfield J. Gait Analysis: Normal and Pathological Function. 2nd ed. Thorofare, NJ: Slack; 2010

Part IV
Solved Problems

19 Solved Problems

19.1 Lifting Arm

19.1.1 Problem

A lever arm is employed to lift one side of a cement block of 500 kg mass (**Fig. 19.1**). What is the magnitude of the force exerted vertically by the hand?

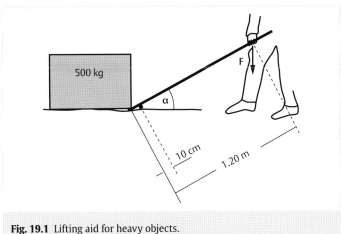

Fig. 19.1 Lifting aid for heavy objects.

19.1.2 Solution

In a symmetric, homogeneous block the gravitational forces under the right and left edges are equal, amounting to $250 \cdot g = 250 \cdot 9.81 = 2452.5$ N.

In equilibrium of moments it holds that

(19.1)
$$2452.5 \cdot 10 \cdot \cos\alpha = F \cdot 110 \cdot \cos\alpha \; [\text{N} \cdot \text{cm}]$$
$$F = 24525/110 = 222.95 \text{ N}$$

19.1.3 Remarks

The force exerted by the hand is directed vertically downwards. The effective lever arm of this force is not 110 cm but rather 110 cm · cos α.

19.2 Choosing the Point of Reference for Moments in the State of Mechanical Equilibrium

19.2.1 Problem

In the state of mechanical equilibrium the sums of all forces and moments are zero. When calculating the sum of the moments, the point of reference can be chosen freely; it does not necessarily have to be a "center of rotation." This statement is to be verified by calculating the force F_3 for a beam with center of rotation at point P (**Fig. 19.2**).

(a) Relate all moments to point P.

(b) Relate all moments to point X.

The force F_1 and the moment arms of F_1 and F_2 are given.

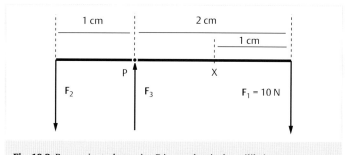

Fig. 19.2 Beam pivoted at point P in mechanical equilibrium.

19.2.2 Solution

(a) In relation to the fulcrum P, the equilibrium condition for the moments (inserting the magnitudes of the forces) reads

(19.2)
$$F_1 \cdot 2 - F_2 \cdot 1 = 0$$
$$F_2 = 2 \cdot F_1$$

In equilibrium of forces

(19.3)
$$\mathbf{F_1} + \mathbf{F_2} + \mathbf{F_3} = 0$$

For the coordinates of the forces it holds that

(19.4)
$$F_3 = -F_1 - F_2$$

If forces pointing downwards are counted as negative, one obtains for the force F_3

(19.5)
$$F_3 = -(-10)\,\text{N} - (-20)\,\text{N} = +30\,\text{N}$$

(b) In relation to point X, the equilibrium condition for the moments (inserting the magnitudes of the forces) reads

(19.6) $$F_1 \cdot 1 - F_2 \cdot 2 + F_3 \cdot 1 = 0$$

In equilibrium one obtains for the magnitude of the force F_3

(19.7) $$F_3 = F_1 + F_2$$

By insertion in Eq. 19.6 one obtains

(19.8)
$$F_1 \cdot 1 - F_2 \cdot 2 + (F_1 + F_2) \cdot 1 = 0$$
$$F_1 \cdot 2 - F_2 \cdot 1 = 0$$

This result is identical to the result of Eq. 19.2. The vector coordinate of F_3 is calculated as above from Eq. 19.4.

19.2.3 Remarks

Relating the moments to the center of rotation has the advantage that the sum of the moments contains fewer addends. The force acting at the center of rotation has no moment arm and thus the moment of this force does not contribute to the sum of moments. However, this only saves a step in the calculation; the result is unchanged. In other words, if an unknown force or an unknown moment is to be determined in mechanical equilibrium, it is not necessary to know the physical location of the center of rotation (the location of the axis of rotation).

In the above equations the signs sometimes cause confusion. This is because when a moment is defined as the product of moment arm and force, a sign convention has to be adhered to. In the above calculation the symbols for the forces in one case designate the magnitudes (in the sum of the moments) and in another case their vector coordinates (in the sum of the forces). For example, in the sum of the moments (Eq. 19.6) F_3 designates the magnitude of the force $\mathbf{F}_3$. It would be correct and unambiguous to use the notation $|\mathbf{F}_3|$, but this reads awkwardly. In equilibrium of forces (Eq. 19.4) F_3 designates the vector coordinate of $\mathbf{F}_3$. The numerical value of the vector coordinate can be positive or negative.

19.3   Calculating Inertial Force When Landing on the Floor after a Jump from a Low Wall

19.3.1 Problem

A person of 60 kg body mass jumps erect from a wall 0.5 m high onto the floor. Calculate the magnitude of the force between the floor and the feet under the following assumptions:

(a) Landing with straight legs within a time interval of 0.1 second to a complete stop.
(b) Landing with bent knees within a time interval of 1.0 second to a complete stop.

19.3.2 Instructions

In free fall from height h the velocity v is calculated from $v = \sqrt{2 \cdot h \cdot g}$ (the derivation of this formula will be found in any physics textbook). The gravitational acceleration g is 9.81 m/s². To calculate the acceleration during landing on the floor, the acceleration is assumed to be constant throughout the landing.

19.3.3 Solution

In the moment of touchdown on the floor the velocity is $v = \sqrt{2 \cdot 0.5 \cdot 9.81} = 3.13$ m/s. The acceleration is

(a) $a = v/t = 3.13/0.1 = 31.3$ m/s²

(b) $a = v/t = 3.13/1.0 = 3.13$ m/s²

Both gravitational and inertial forces act between the floor and the feet. This sum of forces is

(a) $F = 60 \cdot (9.81 + 31.3) = 2466.6$ N

(b) $F = 60 \cdot (9.81 + 3.13) = 776.4$ N

For comparison: when standing still the force between the floor and the feet is $F = m \cdot g = 60 \cdot 9.81 = 588.6$ N.

19.3.4 Remarks

In reality the velocity does not decrease linearly during the time interval of the landing. At the very beginning, the rate of the decrease will probably be small, it will then assume a maximum, and be small again towards the end. The value of the acceleration calculated from a = v/t is thus a lower limit of the actual maximum acceleration.

19.4 Calculating Energy Consumption in Walking

19.4.1 Problem

The energy consumption of an adult person of 60 kg body mass walking a distance of 1 km at a velocity of 50 m/min (comfortable walking speed) is to be determined. The energy consumption is quantified by means of the oxygen consumption. **Fig. 19.3** shows the data of Waters et al[1] on oxygen consumption as a function of walking speed. On a normal diet a consumption of 1 L of oxygen corresponds to an energy expenditure of approximately 5 kcal (kilocalories) or to approximately 20 kJ (kilojoules).

19.4.2 Solution

According to the diagram, an adult walking at 50 m/min consumes 0.18 mL of oxygen per kilogram of body mass and per meter of distance walked. For 60 kg body mass and a distance of 1000 m we obtain

$$\text{oxygen consumption} = 0.18 \cdot 0.001 \cdot 60 \cdot 1000 = 10.8 \text{ L } O_2$$

This corresponds to an energy consumption of $10.8 \cdot 5 = 54$ kcal. For comparison: The energy content of a chocolate is approximately 60 kcal; the energy content of 100 g peanuts is approximately 600 kcal.

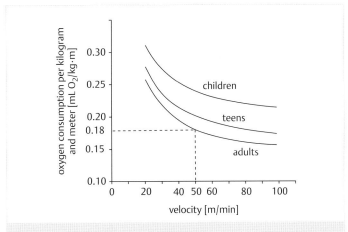

Fig. 19.3 Oxygen consumption per kilogram body weight and per meter distance walked. (Adapted, with permission, from Waters et al.[1])

19.4.3 Remarks

The conversion factor between oxygen and energy consumption cited above is valid for a normal diet. In people on special diets, deviation from this conversion factor can be expected as the chemical energy of the various components of the diet may differ.

For accurate measurement of the energy consumption of the body, its generation of heat would have to be measured. However, this is experimentally complicated. The study by Webb et al[2] is an example of a calorimetric measurement of this kind.

That the oxygen consumption increases at lower walking speeds (**Fig. 19.3**) is due to the fact that the curve shows the consumption of oxygen per meter walking distance. This consumption is made up of the resting metabolism and the energy specifically required for walking. At slower walking speeds, more time elapses for a given distance, and thus the relative contribution of the resting metabolism to the overall energy consumption increases. If, by contrast, the diagram showed the oxygen consumption per minute, the curve would look quite different, because at a slow walking speed less energy is consumed per unit time.

19.5 Calculating Mean Pressure

19.5.1 Problem

For a person of 60 kg mass (and thus a gravitational force of approx. 600 N) the following mean pressures are to be calculated (in pascals [Pa] and millimeters of mercury [mmHg]):

(a) On the soles of the feet when the person is standing still on both feet. The area of the sole is estimated as $8 \cdot 25 = 200$ cm².

(b) On the contact surface between the buttocks and thighs and the seat when the person is in a sitting position. Assumptions: The area of the contact surface is $25 \cdot 25 = 625$ cm². The mass of the head, trunk, and arms is 60% of the body mass.

(c) On the surface of the back when the person is lying supine. Assumptions: The mass of the trunk equals 50% of the body mass. The surface area of the back is approximately $30 \cdot 60 = 1800$ cm². The whole surface of the back is in contact with the mattress.

(d) On the surface of the back when lying supine. Assumptions: The mass of the trunk equals 50% of the body mass. The trunk is in contact with the mattress only in the region of the shoulder blades and the pelvis in four partial areas each of $8 \cdot 8 = 64$ cm².

19.5.2 Solution

The formula for mean pressure, which divides the force [N] by the base of support [m²], gives a result in pascals [Pa]. This must be converted into millimeters of mercury [mmHg]. The density of mercury is 13.546 g/cm³ ($= 13.546 \cdot 10^3$ kg/m³). A pressure of 1 mmHg equals the gravitational force of a mercury layer of 1 mm (10^{-3} m) thickness acting on an area of 1 m².

$$13.546 \cdot 10^3 \cdot 10^{-3} \cdot 9.81 = 132.886 \text{ N/m}^2 \approx 133 \text{ Pa}$$

Result: 1 mmHg corresponds to approximately 133 Pa.

(a) $p_m = 600/0.04$ N/m² $= 15000$ Pa. This corresponds to approximately 113 mmHg.

(b) $p_m = 360/0.0625$ N/m² $= 5760$ Pa. This corresponds to approximately 43 mmHg.

(c) $p_m = 300/0.18$ N/m² $= 1667$ Pa. This corresponds to approximately 13 mmHg.

(d) $p_m = 300/0.0256$ N/m² $= 11719$ Pa. This corresponds to approximately 88 mmHg.

19.5.3 Remarks

The arterial pressure in the skin of the sole of the foot ranges between 110 and 130 mmHg. It follows that when a person is standing still, the blood supply of the skin in some areas of the sole of the foot will be interrupted. The same is true of the blood supply of the skin of the buttocks and thighs where the arterial pressure ranges between 40 and 60 mmHg. In reality, however, the pressure distribution over this area is not uniform: the pressure under the ischial tuberosity is higher than the mean pressure. Persons who are too weak to change their sitting posture from time to time, or those sitting in a seat pan which does not allow for a change of the sitting posture, are at risk of injury to their skin. The arterial pressure in the skin of the back ranges between 20 and 40 mmHg. If the whole area of the back is supported by the mattress, there is no risk of interrupting the blood supply. However, this does not happen in practice. In reality, only small partial areas of the back are used for pressure transmission. To prevent injury to the skin, the pressure-transmitting area needs to be increased, for example by covering the mattress with very soft foam rubber or medical sheepskin.

19.6 Calculating Tibial Strength

19.6.1 Problem

The tibia is loaded by:

(a) A force acting longitudinally.

(b) A force acting perpendicularly at its middle, with the proximal and distal ends of the bone being fixed but not clamped (simulating a kick against the shinbone of a standing person).

(c) A torque about the long axis of the bone (such as generated for example by a lateral force **F** on the tip of a ski) (**Fig. 19.4**).

Calculate the forces resulting in fracture of the tibia.

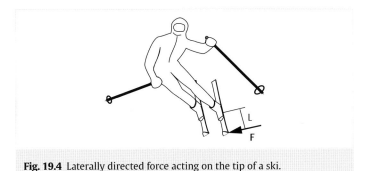

Fig. 19.4 Laterally directed force acting on the tip of a ski.

19.6.2 Instructions

Assumptions: The tibia has a tubular cross section with an outer diameter of 2.0 cm and an inner diameter of 0.9 cm. Its length is 35 cm. The distance L from the tip of the ski to the ankle joint is 1.0 m. The values for the ultimate compressive and tensile stresses of bone are 150 N/mm² and 120 N/mm² respectively (cf **Table 8.1**). The ultimate shear stress τ_{max} is 65 N/mm².

When loaded in compression, the stress is given by

(19.9)
$$\sigma = \frac{F}{A}$$

When loaded by a bending moment the tensile stress σ on the convex side of the tube is

(19.10)
$$\sigma = M/Z$$

where M designates the moment and Z the section modulus. For a tube with outer diameter D and inner diameter d, Z is calculated as

(19.11)
$$Z = \frac{\pi(D^4 - d^4)}{32 \cdot D}$$

When loaded in torsion the shear stress τ at the surface of the tube is calculated as

(19.12)
$$\tau = M/Z_p$$

where M designates the moment and Z_p the polar section modulus. For a tube with outer diameter D and inner diameter d, Z_p is given by

(19.13)
$$Z_p = \frac{\pi(D^4 - d^4)}{16 \cdot D}$$

19.6.3 Solution

Care must be taken to insert all variables in their correct dimensions. As σ and τ are given in newtons per square millimeter [N/mm²], it is advantageous to insert all lengths in millimeters.

(a) The stress is calculated from force / area

(19.14)
$$\sigma = \frac{F}{A} = \frac{4 \cdot F}{\pi(D^2 - d^2)} \, [N/mm^2]$$

Inserting for σ the ultimate value of 150 N/mm², one obtains F = 37581 N.

(b) For a tube supported (but not clamped) at both ends and loaded at its midpoint the bending moment M is

(19.15)
$$M = \frac{F}{2} \cdot \frac{L}{2} = F \cdot \frac{L}{4}$$

The stress is calculated from

(19.16)
$$\sigma = \frac{M}{Z} = \frac{F \cdot L \cdot 32 \cdot D}{4 \cdot \pi \cdot (D^4 - d^4)} \, [N/mm^2]$$

Inserting for σ the ultimate value of 120 N/mm², one obtains F = 1033 N.

(c) The moment amounts to

(19.17)
$$M = F \cdot L$$

With L = 1000 mm the stress is calculated from

(19.18)
$$\tau = \frac{M}{Z_p} = \frac{F \cdot 1000 \cdot 16 \cdot D}{\pi \cdot (D^4 - d^4)} \, [N/mm^2]$$

Inserting for τ the ultimate value of 65 N/mm², one obtains F = 98 N.

19.6.4 Remarks

In estimating the strength of a structure it is often assumed that the ultimate compressive and tensile stresses are equal. For bone, as generally for all brittle materials (glass, ceramics, cement), this assumption is not quite correct. In fact, the ultimate tensile stress of bone (approx. 120 N/mm²) is smaller than the ultimate compressive stress (approx. 150 N/mm²). Torsional strength on the other hand depends on the ultimate shear stress (approx. 65 N/mm²).

A comparison of the forces calculated above for the different loading modes demonstrates that, compared with loading in compression, loading in bending or torsion causes fracture at lower forces. For example, to break a matchstick into two, one does not press or pull on its ends (compressive or tensile load) but snaps it with a bending action (bending load). Under torsional load the shear stress is uniform along the length of the tube. At what place fracture eventually occurs depends on (small) irregularities in the material or the dimensions of the tube.

19.7 Calculating Stress Concentrations

19.7.1 Problem

A series of experiments is performed to determine the ultimate stress of cortical bone. For this purpose, rectangular prisms of width w = 2 mm and height h = 5 mm are cut from long bones. The prisms of length L = 30 mm are clamped at one end and loaded at the free end by a force **F** up to fracture (**Fig. 19.5**). The stress σ at the surface of the beam amount to $\sigma = L_1 \cdot F/Z$ with $Z = w \cdot h^2/6$. The ultimate tensile stress σ_{max} of cortical bone is approximately 150 N/mm².

(a) Calculate the force required to fracture the samples.

(b) Assume that someone inadvertently made a cut on the upper side of the beam with a sharp scalpel at L_1 = 15 mm. The stress at the location of the cut is $\sigma' = \sigma \cdot (1 + 2 \cdot \sqrt{d/r})$. In this formula σ denotes the initial stress (that is, without the cut), d denotes one-half of the depth of the cut, and r denotes the radius of the cut at its tip. With d = 0.25 mm and r = 0.025 mm, calculate the increase of the stress at the location of the cut of the damaged beam compared to the undamaged beam. Where will the beam fracture? What is the magnitude of the force that results in fracture?

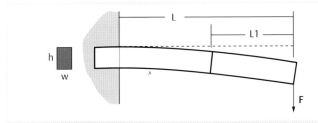

Fig. 19.5 Loading of a beam clamped at one end.

19.7.2 Solution

(a) The stress assumes its maximum value at the end where the beam is clamped. The force at the point of fracture is calculated from $F = \sigma_{max} \cdot Z/L = \sigma_{max} \cdot b \cdot h^2/L \cdot 6$. Inserting the data given above one obtains

(19.19) $$F = (150 \cdot 2 \cdot 25)/(30 \cdot 6) = 41.67 \text{ N}$$

(b) At the location of the cut the stress will be increased by a factor of $\sigma'/\sigma = (1 + 2 \cdot \sqrt{0.25/0.025}) = 7.32$. Without the cut the stress halfway along the beam would be equal to one-half of the stress at the clamped end (the stress rises in proportion to L_1). The cut increases the stress by a factor of more than 7. Thus the ultimate stress occurs first at the location of the cut. The bone sample fractures at the cut. The fracture force is equal to that of a bone sample whose ultimate stress has been reduced by a factor of 7.32.

(19.20) $$F = (150/7.32)(2 \cdot 25)/(15 \cdot 6) = 11.38 \text{ N}$$

19.8 Calculating Deformation Energy

19.8.1 Problem

(a) **Fig. 19.6** shows the force–deformation curve obtained from strength testing of a ligament.

(b) **Fig. 19.7** shows the moment–angle graph obtained from measuring passive rotation of the cervical spine.

In both cases the deformation energy is to be determined graphically in joules [J] and calories [cal].

19.8.2 Instructions

(a) The deformation energy is the energy required for the deformation achieved, that is, for the deformation from zero strain up to rupture. The deformation energy equals the area under the force–deformation curve. In **Fig. 19.6** this area is approximated by a triangle. To determine the area of the triangle, the base line and height have to be measured from the graph and converted into meters and newtons using the scales on the axes of the diagram. The area has the dimensions of energy (newton meters [Nm]). Conversion factor: 1 Nm is equivalent to 0.239 cal.

(b) The deformation energy equals the area enclosed by the hysteresis loop. In **Fig. 19.7** this area is (roughly) approximated by a rectangle. The sides of the rectangle have to be measured from the graph and converted into newton meters and radians. Conversion from degree to radian: 1° corresponds to 0.01745 rad. The area has the dimensions of energy, units newton meters [Nm].

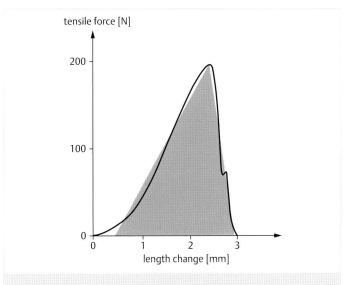

Fig. 19.6 Force–deformation curve of a ligament. (Adapted from Amiel et al.[3])

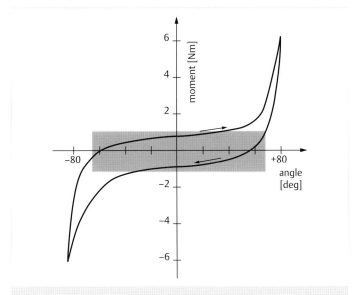

Fig. 19.7 Moment–angle graph obtained from measurement of passive rotation of the cervical spine. (Adapted from McClure et al.[4])

19.8.3 Solution

(a) Base line approximately 2.45 mm, height approximately 196.6 N, area approximately 0.24 Nm, equivalent to 0.06 cal.

(b) Range of motion approximately 134° corresponding to approximately 2.3 rad; moment approximately 2.22 Nm; area approximately 5.11 Nm, corresponding to 1.22 cal.

19.8.4 Remarks

The term "approximately" is used above, because the data can be extracted from the graphs only within certain error limits. Energy (work) is defined as force times distance or as moment times angle (the angle is dimensionless and must be inserted in units of radians). In both cases the dimension of the energy is newton meters. The description of the area under the curve as a triangle or a rectangle is a rough approximation. This suffices when determining the order of magnitude of the deformation energy. For a precise determination, the area has to be determined from the integral below the curve.

19.9 Vector Notation, with the Example of Relieving the Hip Joint by Using a Cane

19.9.1 Problem

In Chapter 13 it was deduced how the vertical component of the hip joint load changes when a cane is employed contralaterally. To keep the calculation simple, vector notation was not used. Instead, the reader had to keep a sign convention for moments in mind and cope with the confusion that F_y, W, H_y, and S sometimes designate the absolute values (magnitudes) and sometimes the positive or negative values of the forces. The advantage of using vector notation is that one does not have to keep additional conventions in mind. The effect on the hip joint load of using a cane is now to be deduced using vector notation.

19.9.2 Instructions

A right-handed xyz-coordinate system with its origin in the center of the femoral head (**Fig. 19.8**) is used: x-axis to the right, y-axis upwards, z-axis in forward direction. A three-dimensional coordinate system is required because with moment arm and force vector in the xy-plane, the vector of the moment points out of the xy-plane. Bold characters designate vectors, regular characters designate their coordinates.

19.9.3 Solution

The vectors of the moment arms and the forces are

$$(19.21) \quad \mathbf{L}_1 = \begin{bmatrix} L_1 \\ 0 \\ 0 \end{bmatrix} \quad \mathbf{F}_y = \begin{bmatrix} 0 \\ F_y \\ 0 \end{bmatrix} \quad \mathbf{D} = \begin{bmatrix} D \\ 0 \\ 0 \end{bmatrix} \quad \mathbf{W} = \begin{bmatrix} 0 \\ W \\ 0 \end{bmatrix} \quad \mathbf{E} = \begin{bmatrix} E \\ 0 \\ 0 \end{bmatrix} \quad \mathbf{S} = \begin{bmatrix} 0 \\ S \\ 0 \end{bmatrix} \quad \mathbf{H}_y = \begin{bmatrix} 0 \\ H_y \\ 0 \end{bmatrix}$$

Fy and **Hy** are the vertical components of the muscle force and joint load, respectively. The coordinates of the vectors in Eq. 19.21 may have positive or negative numerical values.

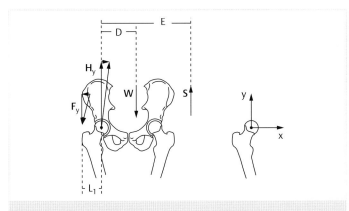

Fig. 19.8 Relieving hip joint load during slow gait by using a cane in the stance phase. D, moment arm of the gravitational force **W**; E, moment arm of the cane force **S**; F_y, muscle force; H_y, load on the hip joint; L_1, moment arm of the vertical component of the muscle force F_y.

The moment arms **D** and **E** (oriented oppositely to L_1) are given by

(19.22)
$$\mathbf{D} = -2\mathbf{L}_1 = \begin{bmatrix} -2L_1 \\ 0 \\ 0 \end{bmatrix} \quad \mathbf{E} = -4\mathbf{L}_1 = \begin{bmatrix} -4L_1 \\ 0 \\ 0 \end{bmatrix}$$

In equilibrium, the moments sum to zero:

(19.23)
$$\mathbf{L}_1 \times \mathbf{F} + \mathbf{D} \times \mathbf{W} + \mathbf{E} \times \mathbf{S} = 0$$

(19.24)
$$\begin{bmatrix} 0 \\ 0 \\ L_1 \cdot F_y \end{bmatrix} + \begin{bmatrix} 0 \\ 0 \\ -2L_1 \cdot W \end{bmatrix} + \begin{bmatrix} 0 \\ 0 \\ -4L_1 \cdot S \end{bmatrix} = 0$$

From this it follows that

(19.25)
$$L_1 \cdot F_y - 2L_1 \cdot W - 4L_1 \cdot S = 0$$
$$F_y = 2W + 4S$$

In equilibrium, the forces sum to zero:

(19.26)
$$\mathbf{H} + \mathbf{F} + \mathbf{W} + \mathbf{S} = 0$$

(19.27)
$$\begin{bmatrix} 0 \\ H_y \\ 0 \end{bmatrix} + \begin{bmatrix} 0 \\ F_y \\ 0 \end{bmatrix} + \begin{bmatrix} 0 \\ W \\ 0 \end{bmatrix} + \begin{bmatrix} 0 \\ S \\ 0 \end{bmatrix} = \begin{bmatrix} 0 \\ 0 \\ 0 \end{bmatrix}$$

From this it follows that

(19.28)

$$H_y + 2W + 4S + W + S = 0$$
$$H_y = -3W - 5S$$

with $W = -0.8 \cdot m \cdot g$

(19.29)

$$H_y = 2.4 \cdot m \cdot g - 5S$$

19.10 Vector Addition: Example of a Graphical Solution

19.10.1 Problem

In the stance phase of slow walking, a compressive force **H** acts on the femoral head; the greater trochanter is acted on by the tensile force **F** of the gluteus medius (**Fig. 19.9**). On the assumption that only these two forces are acting on the proximal part of the femur, what is the force acting on the femoral shaft at cross section A–A? (Graphical solution.)

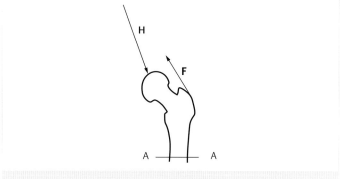

Fig. 19.9 Forces acting on the proximal part of the femur in the stance phase of slow gait.

19.10.2 Solution

The shaft is acted on by the vector sum of forces **H** and **F** (**Fig. 19.10**).

19.10.3 Remarks

Force **H** points approximately along the femoral neck. The sum of forces **H** + **F** acts on the femoral shaft; this force points approximately along the long axis of the femoral shaft. This example supports the hypothesis that bones are aligned such that they are loaded essentially in compression and only to a minor extent in bending. Bending is undesired because bending creates tensile stress in the material, and the tensile strength of bone is comparatively low.

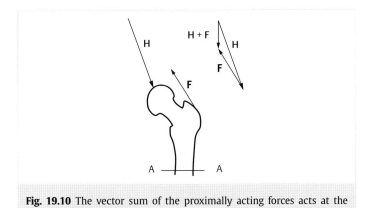

Fig. 19.10 The vector sum of the proximally acting forces acts at the cross section A–A.

19.11 Vector Addition: Another Example of a Graphical Solution

A bedridden patient is undergoing traction (**Fig. 19.11**). The set-up shown here is called "Russell's traction" after its inventor. The rope running over low-friction pulleys is tensioned by a weight. **W** denotes the vector of the gravitational force.

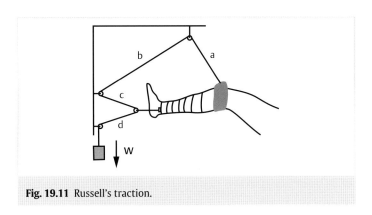

Fig. 19.11 Russell's traction.

19.11.1 Problem

What is the direction of the resultant force exerted on the upper leg? Does this direction change if the weight (and hence the magnitude of the gravitational force) is changed? Does the direction change if the patient slips towards the head end or towards the footboard of the bed? (The gravitational force of lower leg and foot is to be neglected.)

19.11.2 Solution

Due to the low-friction pulleys the tensile force (tension) has an identical magnitude W in each segment of the rope (**Fig. 19.12**). The resultant force on the upper leg is the sum of the forces acting in sections a, c, and d of the rope. The direction of the resultant force is left unchanged when the magnitude W of the gravitational force changes; the polygon of the vectors merely changes size. If the patient slips in the bed, the directions of the forces in sections a, c, and d change and so does the direction of their vector sum.

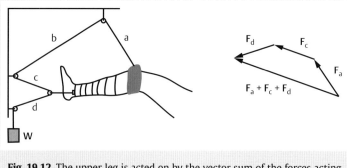

Fig. 19.12 The upper leg is acted on by the vector sum of the forces acting distal to the knee.

19.11.3 Remarks

The traction set-up discussed here is designed to generate a tensile force directed along the long axis of the femur, for example for the reduction of a fractured femur. Once the direction of the force has been properly adjusted, its magnitude can easily be changed according to treatment requirements. If the weight of the lower leg and the foot were to be taken into account, the downward-directed vector of this force would have to be added at the tip of vector $\mathbf{F}_d$.

19.12   Vector Addition: Graphical and Numerical Solutions

19.12.1 Problem

An example of traction treatment, such as is common in orthopedics or trauma surgery. Forces $\mathbf{F}_1$ and $\mathbf{F}_2$ act on the lower leg (**Fig. 19.13**). The weight of the lower leg is taken up by the support; the support is assumed to be friction-free. What additional force acts on the upper leg? Forces $\mathbf{F}_1$ and $\mathbf{F}_2$ are to be added graphically and numerically.

19.12.2 Graphical Solution

The length of the sum vector $\mathbf{F}_3$ has to be determined relative to the lengths of vectors $\mathbf{F}_1$ and $\mathbf{F}_2$. If, for example the lengths of $\mathbf{F}_1$ and $\mathbf{F}_2$ in the diagram are 5 cm and 2.5 cm, respectively (**Fig. 19.14**), the length

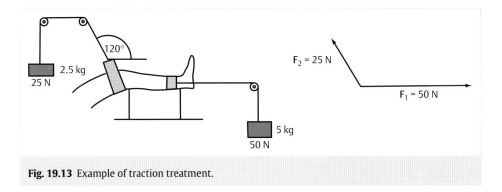

Fig. 19.13 Example of traction treatment.

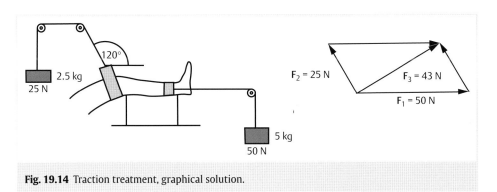

Fig. 19.14 Traction treatment, graphical solution.

of the vector $\mathbf{F}_3$ is read from the diagram to be approximately 4.3 cm. The magnitude of the force $\mathbf{F}_3$ is then approximately 43 N.

19.12.3 Numerical Solution

x-Axis horizontal, y-axis vertical; add the components of the vectors, then calculate the magnitude of the vector sum $\mathbf{F}_3$ and its angle from the x-axis.

(19.30)
$$F_{1x} = 50\,\text{N}$$
$$F_{1y} = 0\,\text{N}$$

(19.31)
$$F_{2x} = 25 \cdot \cos 120° = 25 \cdot (-0.5) = -12.5\,\text{N}$$
$$F_{2y} = 25 \cdot \sin 120° = 25 \cdot 0.866 = 21.65\,\text{N}$$

(19.32)
$$F_{3x} = 50 - 12.5 = 37.5\,\text{N}$$
$$F_{3y} = 0 + 21.65 = 21.65\,\text{N}$$
$$|\mathbf{F}_3| = \sqrt{37.5^2 + 21.65^2} = 43.3\,\text{N}$$

The angle of the vector sum $\mathbf{F}_3$ against the horizontal is

(19.33)
$$\alpha = \arctan(21.65 / 37.5) \approx 30°$$

19.12.4 Remarks

The magnitudes and directions of forces $\mathbf{F}_1$ and $\mathbf{F}_2$ are chosen in such a way that the line of action of the sum vector $\mathbf{F}_3$ points along the femur. The aim of the treatment is to exert a tensile force on the upper leg.

19.13 Decomposing a Vector into Components

In erect stance, the sacral base angle (angle of the midplane of the L5/S1 disk to the horizontal) is about 35°. In some persons, however, the angle is markedly larger or smaller (**Fig. 19.15**). In the following it is assumed that the L5 vertebra is loaded by two forces, the force of the extensors of the back and the weight of the body cranial to L5. The muscle force is directed approximately perpendicular to the plane of the disk, as the direction of the muscles follows the shape of the spine. The gravitational force points vertically downwards.

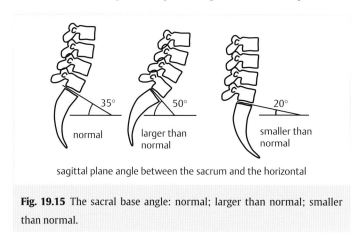

sagittal plane angle between the sacrum and the horizontal

Fig. 19.15 The sacral base angle: normal; larger than normal; smaller than normal.

19.13.1 Problem

The shear force in the plane of the L5/S1 disk is to be calculated for angles $\alpha = 35°, 50°$, and $20°$. Assumptions: The mass of the subject is 80 kg; 60% of the body mass is cranial to L5/S1; $g = 9.81$ m/s².

19.13.2 Solution

The weight $W = 0.6 \cdot m \cdot g$ acting on the L5/S1 disk is decomposed into two components $\mathbf{W} \cdot \cos\alpha$ and $\mathbf{W} \cdot \sin\alpha$ (**Fig. 19.16**). The magnitude of the ventrally directed shear force $W \cdot \sin\alpha$ for $\alpha = 35°$ is $0.6 \cdot 80 \cdot 9.81 \cdot 0.574 = 270.3$ N. For $\alpha = 50°$ and $\alpha = 20°$ one obtains 360.7 N and 161.1 N, respectively.

19.13.3 Remarks

In the intact lumbar spine the facet joints and the disks prevent anterior displacement of the vertebrae. If the sacral base angle is large, the pelvis can be tilted backwards and the lordosis reduced to lessen the shear load on the L5/S1 segment. The above calculation shows that if this angle is 35° the shear load is 25% smaller than if the angle is 50°. However, there are limits to how far the pelvis can be tilted. If the midplane

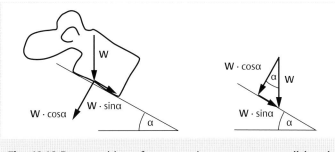

Fig. 19.16 Decomposition of a vector in components parallel and perpendicular to a given direction.

of L5/S1 were to be horizontal, the shear force would be zero, but the anterior coverage of the femoral head by the acetabulum would become unphysiologically small.

If a fracture of the vertebral arch in the pars interarticularis occurs (spondylolysis), it is usually followed by anterior gliding of the vertebra (spondylolisthesis). In such cases an attempt is made to reduce the lordosis—for example by means of a brace—to reduce the shear force. Individuals with back problems often assume a posture with reduced lordosis. Mechanically, such a posture (a) reduces the load on the facet joints, (b) enlarges the foramina, and (c) diminishes the radial bulge of the disks posteriorly and posterolaterally.

19.14 Composing a Moment from Partial Moments

19.14.1 Problem

Chapter 12 dealt with the estimation of the joint load in the dynamic case. For this purpose the force acting from the floor on the foot was decomposed into components $\mathbf{R}_{1x}$ and $\mathbf{R}_{1y}$ (**Fig. 12.14**). The total moment acting was taken as the sum of the moments generated by $\mathbf{R}_{1x}$ and $\mathbf{R}_{1y}$. The validity of the composition of a moment from partial moments is to be examined.

Together, the radius vector $\mathbf{r}$ and force vector $\mathbf{F}$ (**Fig. 19.17**) define the xy-plane. The moment is

(19.34) $$\mathbf{M} = \mathbf{r} \times \mathbf{F}$$

Can this moment be composed from partial moments?

(19.35)
$$\mathbf{M}_1 = \mathbf{r}_x \times \mathbf{F}_y$$
$$\mathbf{M}_2 = \mathbf{r}_y \times \mathbf{F}_x$$

19.14.2 Solution

Employing the three-dimensional unit vectors $\mathbf{e}_x$, $\mathbf{e}_y$, $\mathbf{e}_z$ one writes the partial moments as

(19.36)
$$\mathbf{M}_1 = x \cdot \mathbf{e}_x \times F_y \cdot \mathbf{e}_y = x \cdot F_y \cdot (\mathbf{e}_x \times \mathbf{e}_y) = x \cdot F_y \cdot \mathbf{e}_z$$
$$\mathbf{M}_2 = y \cdot \mathbf{e}_y \times F_x \cdot \mathbf{e}_x = y \cdot F_x \cdot (\mathbf{e}_y \times \mathbf{e}_x) = -y \cdot F_x \cdot \mathbf{e}_z$$

Vectors $\mathbf{r}$ and $\mathbf{F}$ are in the xy-plane. By definition, the z-component of the moment $\mathbf{M}$ (Eq. 19.34) reads

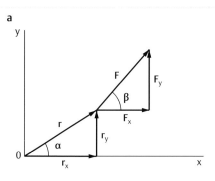

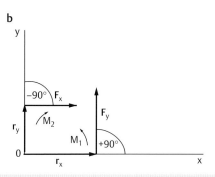

Fig. 19.17a, b Composition of a moment from partial moments.
a Moment of the force **F** acting at a point given by the radius vector **r**.
b Moments of the force components $\mathbf{F}_x$ and $\mathbf{F}_y$ acting at points given by the radius vectors $\mathbf{r}_y$ and $\mathbf{r}_x$, respectively.

(19.37) $$\mathbf{M} = \mathbf{M}_z = (x \cdot F_y - y \cdot F_x) \cdot \mathbf{e}_z$$

This is identical with the sum of the moments in Eq. 19.36.

Alternatively, the proof may be given by defining the moment using the magnitudes of the moment arm r and the force F, and the angle between moment arm and force

(19.38) $$M = r \cdot F \cdot \sin(\gamma) = r \cdot F \cdot \sin(\beta - \alpha)$$

(19.39) $$M_1 = r \cdot \cos(\alpha) \cdot F \cdot \sin(\beta) \cdot \sin(+90°) = x \cdot F_y$$
$$M_2 = r \cdot \sin(\alpha) \cdot F \cdot \cos(\beta) \cdot \sin(-90°) = -y \cdot F_x$$

The sum is equal to

(19.40) $$M_1 + M_2 = r \cdot F \cdot (\cos(\alpha) \cdot \sin(\beta) - \sin(\alpha) \cdot \cos(\beta))$$

With the subtraction theorem

(19.41) $$\sin(\beta - \alpha) = \sin(\beta) \cdot \cos(\alpha) - \cos(\beta) \cdot \sin(\alpha)$$

The sum of the moments (Eq. 19.40) equals the moment M (Eq. 19.38).

19.15 Locating a Center of Rotation: Graphical and Numerical Solutions

19.15.1 Problem

The angle of rotation φ and the location of the center of rotation x_F, y_F of a lumbar motion segment are to be determined from lateral radiographic views taken in flexion and extension. For this purpose the two views are superimposed in **Fig. 19.18** so that the outlines of the caudal vertebrae coincide. P and Q designate the "corners" of the cranial vertebra in the initial state; P′ and Q′ designate the corners in the final state.

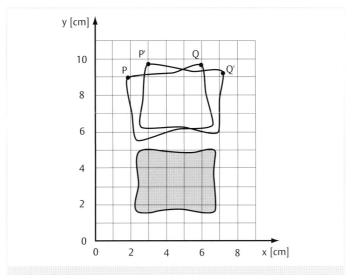

Fig. 19.18 Superimposed lateral radiographic views of a lumbar motion segment in flexion and extension.

19.15.2 Instructions

The graphical solution is performed according to the rule outlined in Chapter 6, **Fig. 6.3**. For the numerical solution Eqs. 6.16 to 6.20 and Eq. 6.14 are employed. The coordinates of the corner points are read from the diagram:

$$P(x_1 = 1.8\ y_1 = 9.0),\ P'(x'_1 = 3.0\ y'_1 = 9.7),\ Q(x_2 = 6.0\ y_2 = 9.6),\ Q'(x'_2 = 7.2\ y'_2 = 9.2)$$

19.15.3 Solution

Fig. 19.19 illustrates the graphical solution. The center of rotation is located approximately at the coordinates $x_F = 5.3$ and $y_F = 5.0$. To determine the angle of rotation, the angle φ between the lines PQ and P′Q′ is measured from the graph. It amounts to approximately $-15°$. By inserting the above coordinates in the equations of Chapter 6 (notation as there) one obtains

$$Z = -4.62,\ N = 17.34,\ \varphi = -14.92°,\ x_F = 5.07,\ y_F = 4.77$$

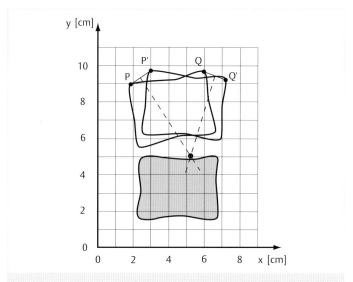

Fig. 19.19 Graphical solution for constructing the center of rotation.

19.15.4 Remarks

The small discrepancy between the graphical and the numerical solutions is not surprising. It is well possible that points P and P′ and points Q and Q′ are not marked at exactly the same locations on the vertebrae. Accuracy in drawing is limited, especially in the case of small movements. In the numerical solution, it is the reading of coordinates from the graph that is subject to error. Anyone who has written a computer program in Basic, Fortran, or Matlab in the (quite justifiable) attempt to avoid calculation errors, can test the sensitivity of the computed result to reading error by altering the input coordinates slightly. Other sources of error exist. In the graphs shown above the contours of the caudal vertebra coincide exactly, but in reality the projection and magnification may well be different in the flexion and extension views. Where this is the case, exact superposition of the images of the caudal vertebra is not possible, only a best fit.

19.16 Determining the Location of the Center of Mass, Experimentally and by Way of Calculation

19.16.1 Problem

The location of the center of mass of the body is to be determined from the lateral view of an athlete performing a high jump using the Fosbury flop technique (**Fig. 19.20**), experimentally and by way of calculation.

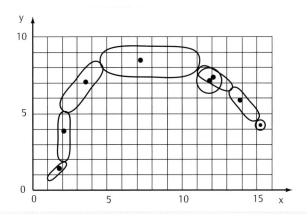

Fig. 19.20 Outline of a body executing a Fosbury flop. The full circles mark the location of the centers of mass of the body segments. (Adapted, with permission, from Kassat.[5])

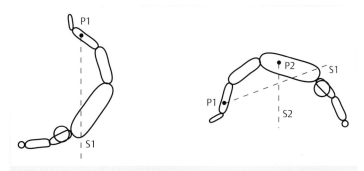

Fig. 19.21 Experimental solution, suspending the cutout from point P1 and then from point P2.

- *Experimental.* For this purpose the figure is cut out in rough outline. It is then suspended on a pin or a thread from any two points in succession, in such a way that it can rotate freely (**Fig. 19.21**). Each time, the perpendicular running through the point of suspension P is marked in by eye. The center of mass is located at the point where the two lines intersect.

- *By way of calculation.* The coordinates of all segmental centers of mass are read from **Fig. 19.20** (an estimate to one digit after the decimal point is sufficient). Use the data of Dempster[6] (**Table 11.3**) for the masses of the segments. (Note that the masses of the extremities listed in the table relate to one upper arm, one lower arm, etc.) The coordinates X_c, Y_c of the center of mass are calculated using the formula given in Chapter 11.

19.16.2 Experimental Solution

The center of mass is located at the intersection of the two lines S1 and S2.

19.16.3 Solution by Way of Calculation

Table 19.1 lists the masses of the body segments according to Dempster[6] and the coordinates X_c and Y_c of the segmental centers of mass read from the graph.

From this dataset the coordinates of the center of mass during the execution of a Fosbury flop are calculated as $X_c = 6.7$ and $Y_c = 7.1$. Marking these coordinates in **Fig. 19.20** shows that the center of mass is located below the trunk.

	Mass (as % of body mass)	X_c	Y_c
Head	7.9	11.8	7.2
Trunk	48.6	7.3	8.5
Upper arm	2.7	12.1	7.4
Lower arm	1.6	13.9	5.9
Hand	0.6	15.3	4.3
Upper leg	9.7	3.6	7.1
Lower leg	4.5	2.1	3.9
Foot	1.4	1.8	1.4

Table 19.1 Masses of body segments and coordinates (X_c,Y_c) of segmental centers of mass

Note: Masses of body segments from Dempster[6] (**Table 11.3**); coordinates of centers of mass read from **Fig. 19.20**.

19.16.4 Remarks

Experimental solution: The determination of the location of the center of mass with the help of the "paper doll" is only a rough approximation because not all segments of the body are of the same thickness.

Calculated solution: Accuracy in reading the coordinates of the segmental centers of mass from the graph is limited. In addition, it must be kept in mind that the segmental masses and the locations of their centers of mass as presented by Dempster[6] are only approximate reference values. Nevertheless, the main result remains: during the execution of a Fosbury flop, the body's center of mass may be located below the crossbar.

19.17 Determining the Moment Arm of a Tendon by Measuring the Rotational Motion of the Segment

Fig. 19.22 shows the model of a joint which can be moved in extension by tensing of the tendon. The tendon is in contact with the circular profile of the joint of radius L. If the end of the tendon moves through a distance x, the joint rotates through an angle α about point P. The distance x is equal to the length of the arc along which the tendon is unwound. It holds that

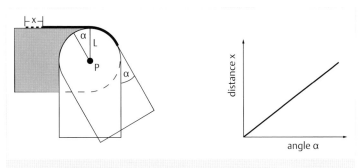

Fig. 19.22 Model of a joint moved by a tendon.

(19.42) $$x = 2\pi L \cdot (\alpha / 2\pi) = L \cdot \alpha$$

where α is inserted in radians.

A linear relation exists between x and α. If x is plotted against α, the slope of the line equals L, the moment arm of the tendon in relation to the center of rotation P. This method can be used to determine moment arms of tendons in joint specimens: the end of the tendon is moved and the angular motion of the joint is observed. If the moment arm changes in the course of movement (as is usually the case in human joints), the αx-diagram is not a straight line but a curve. At every point of the curve, the moment arm L is given by the slope of the curve.

An et al[7] used this method to determine the moment arms of the flexors and extensors of the metacarpophalangeal joints. **Fig. 19.23** shows the result of their observations for the tendons of the extensor indicis and lumbrical muscles.

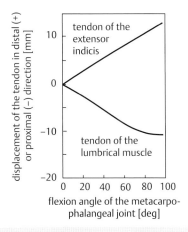

Fig. 19.23 Relationship between the rotational motion of the metacarpophalangeal joint and the linear displacement of the tendons of the extensor indicis and lumbrical muscles. (Adapted from An et al.[7])

19.17.1 Problem

The moment arms of the extensor indicis and lumbrical muscles at a flexion angle of 80° are to be determined.

19.17.2 Instructions

Tangents are drawn by eye on the curves of **Fig. 19.23**. The slopes $\Delta x / \Delta \alpha$ are read from the graph. The angular interval $\Delta \alpha$ has to be converted from degrees to radians. To this end the value in degrees is multiplied by the factor $2\pi/360$.

19.17.3 Solution

The slope of the curve of the extensor indicis is virtually constant throughout the range of angles investigated (**Fig. 19.24**). Read from the diagram, the slope $\Delta x / \Delta \alpha$ for the tendon of the extensor indicis is approximately 13 mm/100°. After conversion from degrees to radians one obtains for the moment arm a value of approximately

(19.43)
$$\frac{\Delta x}{\Delta \alpha} = \frac{13}{100 \cdot 2\pi / 360} \approx 7.5 \text{ mm}$$

The slope of the curve of the lumbrical muscle varies in the range of angles investigated (**Fig. 19.24**). At 80° of flexion the slope of the tangent $\Delta x / \Delta \alpha$ is approximately 5.3 mm/100°. After conversion from degrees to radians, one obtains for the moment arm a value of approximately

(19.44)
$$\frac{\Delta x}{\Delta \alpha} = \frac{5.3}{100 \cdot 2\pi / 360} \approx 3 \text{ mm}$$

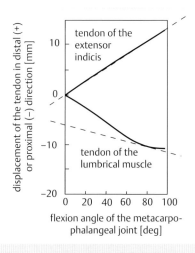

Fig. 19.24 Tangents drawn by eye to the curves of **Fig. 19.23**.

19.18 Calculating the Change in the Load on the Elbow Joint with the Bending Angle

19.18.1 Problem

In Chapter 12 the load on the elbow joint was calculated for the joint held at an angle of 90°. How does the load change when the arm is moved in extension (**Fig. 19.25**)?

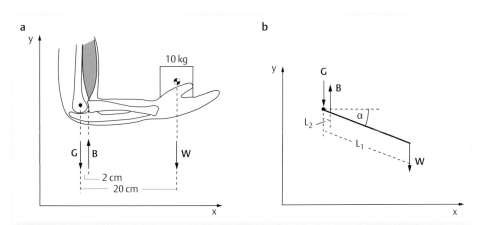

Fig. 19.25a, b The change in the load **G** on the elbow joint as the bending angle changes. **B**, muscle force; **W**, gravitational force.

a Lower arm held at 90°.

b Lower arm inclined at an angle α to the horizontal.

19.18.2 Solution

α denotes the angle between the lower arm and the horizontal. In equilibrium the moments sum to zero

(19.45)
$$-B \cdot L_2 \cdot \cos\alpha + W \cdot L_1 \cdot \cos\alpha = 0$$
$$B = W \cdot L_1 / L_2$$

In equilibrium the forces also sum to zero

(19.46)
$$\mathbf{G} + \mathbf{B} + \mathbf{W} = 0$$

or in terms of their coordinates

(19.47)
$$G + B + W = 0$$
$$G - W \cdot L_1 / L_2 + W = 0$$

Note that the magnitude of **B** is calculated as $B = W \cdot L_1 / L_2$. However, for the y-coordinate of **B** it holds that $B = -W \cdot L_1 / L_2$, because the vector **B** is oppositely directed to the vector **W**.

(19.48)
$$G = W \cdot (L_1 / L_2 - 1)$$

G does not depend on the angle α since Eq. 19.48 does not depend on α.

19.18.3 Remarks

For $\alpha = 90°$ the quotient of the effective moment arms $L_1 \cdot \cos\alpha \, / \, L_2 \cdot \cos\alpha = 0 \, / \, 0$ is undefined; that is, its value is indeterminate. This implies that in this case, in addition to the solution for **G** given above, other solutions exist, for example **B** = **0**, that is, **G** = −**W**.

19.19 Solving an Indeterminate System of Equations by Employing Additional Constraints (Demonstration)

If more than one muscle participates in satisfying mechanical equilibrium at a joint, the joint load cannot be derived from the equilibrium equations alone. This is because the number of unknowns is greater than the number of equations, so we are dealing with an indeterminate system. By employing additional constraints it is possible to select a single solution from the multitude of possible solutions of the indeterminate system. The following example has been outlined by Bean et al.[8]

19.19.1 Problem

At a joint two muscles maintain equilibrium against an external moment (**Fig. 19.26**). Muscle force F_1: moment arm $L_1 = 6$ cm, muscle cross section $A_1 = 10$ cm²; muscle force F_2: moment arm $L_2 = 2$ cm, muscle cross section $A_2 = 50$ cm²; external moment 5000 Ncm. The constraints are: (a) the muscle stress (force/cross-sectional area) must not exceed a limiting value of $\sigma_{max} = 40$ N/cm² and (b) muscles exert only tensile forces (muscle forces assume only positive values). Minimization of the joint load is chosen as the objective function. The paired values of muscle forces at which the joint load is as small as possible are to be calculated.

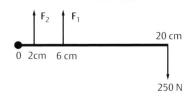

Fig. 19.26 Two muscle forces F_1 and F_2 maintain equilibrium against an external moment of 5000 Ncm.

19.19.2 Solution

In mechanical equilibrium (moments sum to zero) it holds that

(19.49)
$$F_1 \cdot 6.0 + F_2 \cdot 2.0 = 5000 \text{ [Ncm]}$$

or, rearranged,

(19.50) $F_2 = -F_1 \cdot 3.0 + 2500 \, [N]$

If F_2 is regarded as a dependent and F_1 as an independent variable, this is the equation of a straight line in an F_1F_2-coordinate system (**Fig. 19.27**). As muscle forces can assume only positive values, it suffices to consider the course of the straight line in the first quadrant. Every point on the line designates a potential pair of variables F_1, F_2 which fulfills the equilibrium condition for moments. However, due to the constraint of maximum muscle stress, not all pairs are permissible. At most, F_1 may assume a value of 400 N (10 cm² · 40 N/cm²) and F_2 a value of 2000 N (50 cm² · 40 N/cm²). All pairs F_1, F_2 of variables permissible under this constraint lie on the straight line between these two points (shown by the thick line in **Fig. 19.27**).

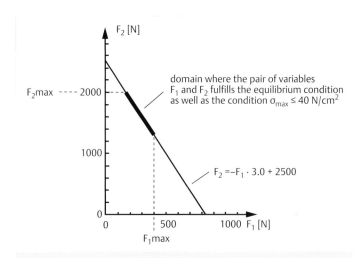

Fig. 19.27 F_2 in dependence on F_1: a straight line in the F_1F_2-coordinate system.

The joint load is lowest when the sum of the muscle forces is lowest. At one end of the permissible region, the sum of the muscle forces with $F_2 = 2000$ N and $F_1 = 167$ N (calculated from Eq. 19.50) is 2000 + 167 = 2167 N; at the other end, with $F_1 = 400$ N and $F_2 = 1300$ N (calculated from Eq. 19.50), it is 400 + 1300 = 1700 N. At this point the sum of the muscle forces $F_1 + F_2$ and hence the joint load assume the minimum value.

Instead of comparing different, permissible pairs of F_1 and F_2, the same result can be obtained directly. One calculates the sum of the forces and inserts into this expression the force F_2 obtained from Eq. 19.50

(19.51)
$$F_{Sum} = F_1 + F_2$$
$$F_{Sum} = F_1 - F_1 \cdot 3.0 + 2500 = -2F_1 + 2500$$

The sum of the forces depends linearly on F_1 and assumes its smallest possible value in the permissible region when F_1 assumes its maximum value.

(19.52)
$$\min(F_{Sum}) = -2 \cdot \max(F_1) + 2500 = -2 \cdot 400 + 2500 = 1700 \text{ N}$$

(It is pointed out that, when searching for a minimum value, the function being investigated is not differentiated in the usual way. A linear function can assume an extreme value, maximum or minimum, only if the region of the arguments is constrained.)

19.19.3 Remarks

The constraints enforce an unequivocal solution of the initially indeterminate system. The condition that F_1 and F_2 may assume only positive values is well founded as muscles can exert only tensile forces, not compressive forces. The condition that muscle stress may not exceed certain limits is also well founded, though there is no agreement what maximum value should be chosen. The condition that the joint load should be as low as possible makes sense, although its general validity has not been proven.

Alternatively, one could choose as constraint that the stress should be equal in both muscles. This constraint enforces an unequivocal solution. It is intuitively clear that at one end of the permissible region the stresses of the muscles are $\sigma_1 = 167/10 = 16.7$ N/cm² and $\sigma_2 = 200/50 = 40$ N/cm² and at the other end they are $\sigma_1 = 400/10 = 40$ N/cm² and $\sigma_2 = 1300/50 = 26$ N/cm². In between there will be a point where both stresses are equal. In principle this point could be found by trial and error along the line.

Instead of trial and error, the numerical value of the point where stresses are equal in both muscles can be calculated from Eq. 19.50, divided by the cross-sectional area of muscle 2.

(19.53)
$$\sigma_2 = -(3 \cdot 10/50) \cdot \sigma_1 + 2500/50 \text{ [N/cm}^2]$$
$$\sigma_2 = -(3/5) \cdot \sigma_1 + 50 \text{ [N/cm}^2]$$

With the requirement of equal stresses $\sigma_1 = \sigma_2$, one obtains

(19.54)
$$\sigma_2 = \sigma_1 = (50 \cdot 5)/8 = 31.25 \text{ N/cm}^2$$

19.20 Calculating the Load on the Femorotibial Joint

19.20.1 Problem

The load F_3 on the femorotibial joint in the posture shown in **Fig. 19.28** is to be estimated. Assumptions: Mass of the person 60 kg; one-legged stance with force $\mathbf{F}_1$ from the floor on the foot approximately equal to the body weight; only quadriceps activated exerting a force $\mathbf{F}_2$ on the patellar tendon; center of rotation of the joint (that is, the point of application of force $\mathbf{F}_3$) located at the center of the tibial plateau.

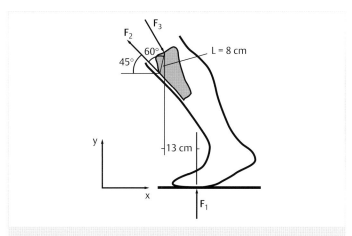

Fig. 19.28 Posture of the leg during walking up stairs. L is the distance between the points of application of the forces **F**$_2$ and **F**$_3$.

19.20.2 Solution

In equilibrium

(19.55)
$$F_2 \cdot 8 \cdot \sin(60°) = F_1 \cdot 13 \text{ Ncm}$$
$$F_2 = 60 \cdot 9.81 \cdot 13/8 \cdot 0.866 = 1104.5 \text{ N}$$

To determine the force **F**$_3$, the sums of the x- and y-coordinates of the forces are calculated.

x-Coordinates

(19.56)
$$F_{3x} = -F_{1x} - F_{2x}$$
$$F_{3x} = 0 - 1104.5 \cdot \cos(135°) = 781.0 \text{ N}$$

y-Coordinates

(19.57)
$$F_{3y} = -F_{1y} - F_{2y}$$
$$F_{3y} = -60 \cdot 9.81 - 1104.5 \cdot \sin(135°) = -1369.6 \text{ N}$$

The magnitude of **F**$_3$ is calculated from

(19.58)
$$|\mathbf{F}_3| = \sqrt{781.0^2 + 1369.6^2} = 1576.6 \text{ N}$$

19.20.3 Remarks

The model contains simplifications. The center of rotation is located at the center of the tibial plateau. This would be correct only if the femur actually rolled on the tibial plateau. In such a case the point of contact constitutes the instantaneous center of rotation. In reality, the motion of the knee joint is a combination of rolling and gliding. The center of rotation is positioned approximately 2 cm above the tibial plateau and in the dorsal third of the femoral condyle. It follows that the moment arm of the patellar tendon is in reality slightly larger than assumed here. Upon activation of the quadriceps, the anterior cruciate ligament will be loaded in dependence on the bending angle of the knee; this is neglected in the calculation. In one-legged stance it is not the entire body weight that must be supported: the weight of the lower leg and foot should really be subtracted. The error resulting from failure to do this is neglected in the calculation.

19.21 Calculating the Load on the Lumbar Spine

19.21.1 Problem

In a workplace, the work bench is too low, or the objects handled during work are positioned too far away, with the result that the worker adopts a forward-flexed posture (**Fig. 19.29**). What tension of the back extensors at the L5/S1 level is required to hold the trunk in this forward-flexed posture?

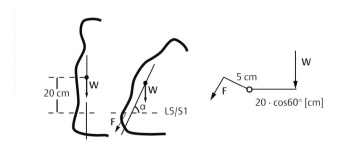

Fig. 19.29 Forward displacement of the center of mass of a human body in a forward-flexed posture. **F**, muscle force; **W**, gravitational force. (Adapted, with permission, from Chaffin et al.[9])

Assumptions: (a) The center of mass of the part of the body cranial to L5/S1 is located 20 cm above S1. (b) The total body mass is 80 kg; the body mass cranial to S1 is 60% of the total body mass. (c) The moment arm of the extensor muscles is 5 cm, independent of the flexion angle of the trunk. (d) The flexion angle α is 60°. The numerical value of the gravitational acceleration g is 9.81 m/s²

19.21.2 Solution

The weight of the body mass cranial to L5/S1 is 48 · 9.81 = 470.9 N. In equilibrium

(19.59)
$$F \cdot 5 = 20 \cdot \cos\alpha \cdot 470.9 \text{ Ncm}$$
$$F = 20 \cdot 0.5 \cdot 470.9/5 = 941.8 \text{ N}$$

The calculation shows that the additional load on the extensor muscles is larger than one times the body weight.

19.22 Calculating the Load on the Interphalangeal Joint of the Great Toe

Jacob[10] determined the insertion point and direction of the flexor hallucis longus tendon from measurements on specimens (**Fig. 19.30**).

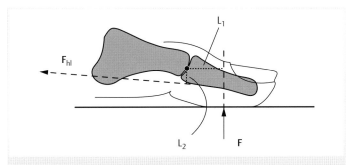

Fig. 19.30 Calculating the load on the interphalangeal joint. (Adapted, with permission, from Jacob.[10])

19.22.1 Problem

F designates the force on the great toe in the toe-off phase of gait. The center of rotation is assumed to be located at the center of the joint surface.

(a) The moment arm L_1 of the ground reaction force and the moment arm L_2 of the tendon are to be read from the graph (similar to the measurement of moment arms from a specimen). The force of the tendon is to be calculated as a multiple of force **F**.

(b) To obtain the load $\mathbf{F}_{ip}$ on the interphalangeal joint, the ground reaction **F** and the tendon force $\mathbf{F}_{hl}$ are to be added graphically.

19.22.2 Solution

(a) The quotient of the moment arms as read (with some reading error) from the graph (**Fig. 19.31**) is approximately 2.4/1. In equilibrium the force F_{hl} amounts to approximately 2.4 · F.

(b) The joint load is the sum of the forces **F** and $\mathbf{F}_{hl}$ acting distally to the joint. Measured from **Fig. 19.31** F_{ip} amounts to approximately 2.8 · F.

Jacob[10] obtained $F_{hl} = 2.2 \cdot F$ and $F_{ip} = 2.6 \cdot F$ in his study. There is adequate agreement between this result and the values read from the graph.

19.22.3 Remarks

Simplifications were required to solve this problem. The point of application of the force **F** shifts during toe-off. In the above problem the point of application is assumed to be under the central part of the toe.

Mean values were used for the direction of the tendon and its moment arms. The center of rotation was located in the center of the contact area of the joint. This is only approximately true as the joint motion is combined from rolling and gliding. It can be seen in **Fig. 19.31** that the force $\mathbf{F}_{ip}$ is oriented almost perpendicular to the joint surface. This is important for the function of the joint. As friction between cartilaginous surfaces is virtually zero, the joint surfaces cannot transmit shear forces (parallel to the joint surface). A shear force would place the joint capsule under load; this is tolerable only to a small extent.

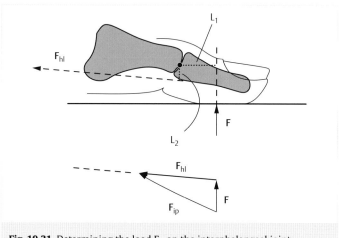

Fig. 19.31 Determining the load F_{ip} on the interphalangeal joint.

19.23   Locating the Center of Pressure under the Sole of the Foot

19.23.1 Problem

Pressure-sensitive insoles are employed to measure the pressure distribution under the sole of the foot. Commercially available insoles contain between 20 and 100 pressure transducers. To limit the computational cost, we consider an insole consisting of only four pressure transducers A to D (**Fig. 19.32**). From the measured pressures (**Table 19.2**), the areas of the transducers, and their locations, calculate

   (a) The magnitude of the force **F** from the floor onto the foot.
   (b) The point of application of that force, the so-called center of pressure.

19.23.2 Solution

   (a) The magnitude of force **F** equals the sum of the products of the areas and the pressures of transducers A to D

   (19.60) $$F = 18 \cdot 4 + 15 \cdot 2 + 25 \cdot 0.5 + 17 \cdot 6 = 216.50 \,\text{N}$$

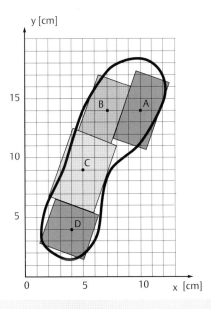

Fig. 19.32 Areas and locations of pressure transducers A to D beneath the sole of the foot.

Transducer	Area [cm²]	xy-coordinates of center [cm]	Pressure [N/cm²]
A	18	10/14	4
B	15	7/14	2
C	25	5/9	0.5
D	17	4/4	6

Table 19.2 Areas of the pressure sensors shown in **Fig. 19.32**, coordinates of their centers, and pressures measured

(b) The point of application of force **F** (the center of pressure) is calculated from the condition that the moments of force **F** in relation to the x- and y-coordinate axes must be equal to the sum of the moments of the four partial forces in relation to these axes

(19.61)
$$F \cdot x_c = 18 \cdot 4 \cdot 10 + 15 \cdot 2 \cdot 7 + 25 \cdot 0.5 \cdot 5 + 17 \cdot 6 \cdot 4 = 1400.50 \text{ Ncm}$$
$$F \cdot y_c = 18 \cdot 4 \cdot 14 + 15 \cdot 2 \cdot 14 + 25 \cdot 0.5 \cdot 9 + 17 \cdot 6 \cdot 4 = 1948.50 \text{ Ncm}$$

It follows that

(19.62)
$$x_c = 1400.50 / 216.50 = 6.47 \text{ cm}$$
$$y_c = 1948.50 / 216.50 = 9.00 \text{ cm}$$

19.23.3 Remarks

The equations for calculating the location of the center of pressure are identical to the equations used for calculating the location of the center of mass of four masses located at the geometric centers of the areas A to D. The result does not depend on the location and orientation of the xy-coordinate system: the identical physical point is always obtained.

19.24 Finding a Best Fit of Two Sets of Points by Translation and Rotation (Demonstration)

Reference points (landmarks) are fixed on a rigid body. If rotation matrix and translation vector are specified, the change of location of the reference points in the final state with respect to the initial state can be calculated exactly. In orthopedic biomechanics one is often confronted with the inverse problem: rotation matrix and translation vector are to be determined from the locations of reference points in the initial and the final state. This already complex task is further complicated by the fact that the locations of the points cannot be measured exactly, only with experimental errors. Consequently, there is no description of the motion (rotation matrix and translation vector) that will result in exact superimposition of the points in the initial and the final state. All one can do is search for a "best-fit" description that will superimpose them as closely as possible. In the following, the fitting procedure is described for both the two-dimensional and the three-dimensional case; the two-dimensional case is illustrated. Vector and matrix notation permit a largely uniform formulation of both the plane and the spatial problem.

19.24.1 Problem

Four reference points are fixed on the body (**Fig. 19.33**). (The minimum number of points in the plane case is two, and in the three-dimensional case it is three. In both cases it is an advantage to choose a larger number of reference points than the minimum.) A change of location is given, from which the rotation matrix and translation vector are to be determined.

Fig. 19.33a illustrates movement of the body in a plane from its initial location (open reference point symbols) to its final location (closed reference point symbols). The locations are described in an xy-coordinate system with the origin at O. The radius vectors of the reference points in the initial and final locations are $\mathbf{r}_i$ and $\mathbf{r}_f$; the radius vectors of the geometric centers of the reference points S_i and S_f are designated $\mathbf{R}_i$ and $\mathbf{R}_f$.

In a first step the body is translated from its initial location by the vector $\mathbf{t} = \mathbf{R}_i - \mathbf{R}_f$ (dashed outline, single-primed reference point numbers in **Fig. 19.33b**). The centers of mass are now superimposed. The relative vectors $\mathbf{p}'_i$ and $\mathbf{p}_f$ are still skewed.

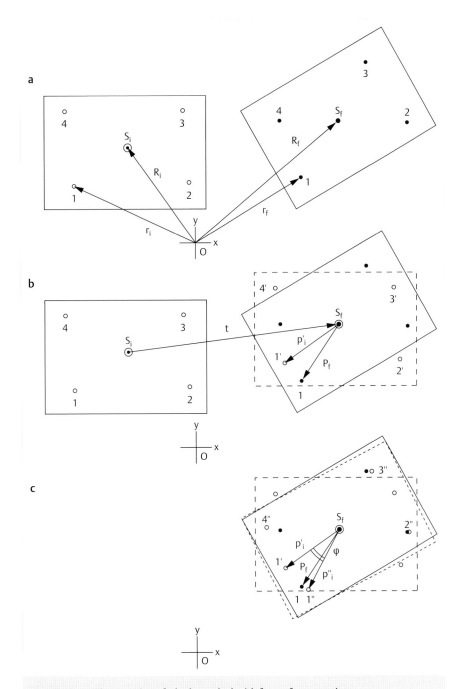

Fig. 19.33a–c Plane motion of a body marked with four reference points.

a Position of the body in the initial and the final state.

b Geometric centers of the reference points S_i and S_f are superimposed.

c The body is rotated to obtain a "best fit" of the reference points.

In a second step the body is rotated through an angle φ about the geometric center (pecked outline, double-primed reference point numbers in **Fig. 19.33c**). The rotated relative vectors $\mathbf{p}''_i$ are now fitted to the relative vectors $\mathbf{p}_f$ of the final location. Perfect superimposition cannot be achieved due to the measurement error in locating the reference points.

19.24.2 Procedure for Solution (Notation as in Chapter 7)

The radius vectors of the reference points are designated $\mathbf{r}_{ik}$ in the initial state, $\mathbf{r}_{fk}$ in the final state. The index k runs from 1 to n. The aim of the calculation is to superimpose the initial locations $\mathbf{r}_{ik}$ of the points as well as possible onto the final locations $\mathbf{r}_{fk}$. We imagine the fit as performed in two steps. In the first step the radius vectors $\mathbf{r}_{ik}$ are translated by a translation vector $\mathbf{t}$.

(19.63)
$$\mathbf{r}'_{ik} = \mathbf{r}_{ik} + \mathbf{t}$$

The geometric center of the reference points in the initial state is designated $\mathbf{R}_i$ and that after the translation is designated $\mathbf{R}'_i$. In the second step the translated points $\mathbf{r}'_i$ are rotated about their geometric center $\mathbf{R}'_i$ by the rotation matrix $\mathbf{D}$.

(19.64)
$$\mathbf{r}''_{ik} = \mathbf{D} \cdot (\mathbf{r}'_{ik} - \mathbf{R}'_i) + \mathbf{R}'_i$$

The quantity Q,

(19.65)
$$Q = \sum_k (\mathbf{r}''_{ik} - \mathbf{r}_{fk})^2 = \sum_k (\mathbf{D} \cdot (\mathbf{r}'_{ik} - \mathbf{R}'_i) + \mathbf{R}'_i - \mathbf{r}_{fk})^2$$

as a function of the translation vector $\mathbf{t}$ and the matrix $\mathbf{D}$, is to be minimized. First, it can be shown that the translation vector is given by $\mathbf{t} = \mathbf{R}_f - \mathbf{R}_i$. This means that the geometric center of the radius vectors in the initial state is to be shifted to the location of the geometric center of the radius vectors in the final state. If this value for $\mathbf{t}$ is inserted into Eq. 19.65 and the coordinates are expressed relative to the geometric center

(19.66)
$$\mathbf{p}'_{ik} = \mathbf{r}'_{ik} - \mathbf{R}'_i \quad \text{with} \quad \mathbf{R}'_i = \sum_k \mathbf{r}'_{ik}/n \quad \text{and} \quad \sum_k \mathbf{p}'_{ik} = 0$$

(19.67)
$$\mathbf{p}_{fk} = \mathbf{r}_{fk} - \mathbf{R}_f \quad \text{with} \quad \mathbf{R}_f = \sum_k \mathbf{r}_{fk}/n \quad \text{and} \quad \sum_k \mathbf{p}_{fk} = 0$$

then the minimum of Q is to be determined as a function of the rotation matrix $\mathbf{D}$:

(19.68)
$$Q = \sum_k (\mathbf{D} \cdot \mathbf{p}'_{ik} - \mathbf{p}_{fk})^2$$

In the two-dimensional case, only a single parameter, the angle of rotation φ, has to be fitted. In this case, there is an explicit solution:

(19.69)
$$\varphi = \arctan(S/C) \pm 180°$$

with

(19.70)
$$S = \sum_k (\xi'_i \cdot \eta_f - \eta'_i \cdot \xi_f)$$
$$C = \sum_k (\xi'_i \cdot \xi_f + \eta'_i \cdot \eta_f)$$

where ξ, η denote the relative coordinates of the vector $\mathbf{p}$ in the xy-plane.

In three dimensions, the rotation matrix $\mathbf{D}$ depends on three parameters (angles of rotation). For example, the matrix $\mathbf{D}$ can be represented according to Bryan–Cardan as a product of the three rotation matrices about three coordinate axes:

(19.71)
$$\mathbf{D} = \mathbf{D}_x(\phi_1) \cdot \mathbf{D}_{y'}(\phi_2) \cdot \mathbf{D}_{z''}(\phi_3)$$

The minimum condition for Q requires the solving of three nonlinear, coupled equations for the angles of rotation ϕ_1, ϕ_2, ϕ_3. An iterative procedure is best suited to this problem. Such a procedure starts with an approximation of the solution and delivers in its first step an improved solution; that is, a set of angles resulting in a smaller value of Q than the first approximation. This improved approximation is again used as input for a further improvement and so on, until Q becomes acceptably small. Due to measurement errors Q will never be exactly equal to zero. As iterative procedures are usually well suited to computer processing, they are in common use. The relevant formulae and algorithms (sequences of mathematical operations) are not listed here; for these, the reader is referred to textbooks on numerical methods. Once the parameters of three-dimensional motion, $\mathbf{t}$ and $\mathbf{D}$, are known, the motion can, according to Chasles' theorem, also be interpreted as helical motion. For this description the axis of rotation $\mathbf{n}$ and the angle of rotation φ (both determined from the rotation matrix $\mathbf{D}$) have to be specified. A point $\mathbf{r}_A$ on the axis and the translation vector $\mathbf{t}_p$ in the direction of the axis can then be calculated.

References

1. Waters RL, Lunsford BR, Perry J, Byrd R. Energy-speed relationship of walking: standard tables. J Orthop Res 1988;6(2):215–222

2. Webb P, Saris WH, Schoffelen PF, Van Ingen Schenau GJ, Ten Hoor F. The work of walking: a calorimetric study. Med Sci Sports Exerc 1988;20(4):331–337

3. Amiel D, Woo SL, Harwood FL, Akeson WH. The effect of immobilization on collagen turnover in connective tissue: a biochemical-biomechanical correlation. Acta Orthop Scand 1982;53(3):325–332

4. McClure P, Siegler S, Nobilini R. Three-dimensional flexibility characteristics of the human cervical spine in vivo. Spine 1998;23(2):216–223

5. Kassat G. Biomechanik für Nicht-Biomechaniker. Rödinghausen: Fitness-Contur; 1993

6. Dempster WT. Space Requirements of the Seated Operator. Geometrical, Kinematic and Mechanical Aspects of the Body with Special Reference to the Limbs. Wright-Patterson Air Force Base, Ohio: Wright Air Development Center; 1955. WADC Technical Report 55–159

7. An KN, Ueba Y, Chao EY, Cooney WP, Linscheid RL. Tendon excursion and moment arm of index finger muscles. J Biomech 1983;16(6):419–425

8. Bean JC, Chaffin DB, Schultz AB. Biomechanical model calculation of muscle contraction forces: a double linear programming method. J Biomech 1988;21(1):59–66

9. Chaffin DB, Andersson GBJ, Martin BJ. Occupational Biomechanics. 3rd ed. New York: Wiley; 1999

10. Jacob HA. Forces acting in the forefoot during normal gait—an estimate. Clin Biomech (Bristol, Avon) 2001;16(9):783–792

Notation

This section provides an overview of the notation conventions followed in this book.

Physical quantities and their units of measurement

Quantity	Symbol	Unit of measurement (dimension)
Length (distance, moment arm)	L, D, E, ...	m (meter)
Mass	m	kg (kilogram)
Time	t	s (second) or min (minute)
Area	A	m^2
Volume	V	m^3
Velocity (vector, magnitude)	**v**, v	m/s
Acceleration (vector, magnitude)	**a**, a	m/s^2
Angle	α, β, γ, ...	degree or radian
Angular velocity	ω	degree/s or radian/s
Angular acceleration	α	$degree/s^2$ or $radian/s^2$
Force (vector, magnitude)	**F, H, R**, ... F, H, R, ...	$kg \cdot m/s^2 = N$ (newton)
Moment (vector, magnitude)	**M**, M	$N \cdot m$
Mechanical work, energy	E	$N \cdot m = J$ (joule)
Momentum	**p**	$m \cdot \mathbf{v}$
Power	P	$N \cdot m/s = W$ (watt)
Gravitational acceleration	g	m/s^2
Gravitational force (weight)	$m \cdot g$	$kg \cdot m/s^2 = N$
Pressure	p	$N/m^2 = Pa$ (pascal)
Compressive or tensile stress	σ	$N/m^2 = Pa$
Shear stress	τ	$N/m^2 = Pa$
Strain	ε	Dimensionless
Moment of inertia	I	$kg \cdot m^2$
Radius of gyration	i	m
Section modulus	Z	m^3
Polar moment of inertia	I_p	m^4
Polar section modulus	Z_p	m^3
Modulus of elasticity, Young's modulus	E	N/m^2 or N/mm^2
Shear modulus	G	N/m^2 or N/mm^2
Poisson's ratio	μ	Dimensionless
Static friction coefficient	μ_s	Dimensionless
Kinetic friction coefficient	μ_k	Dimensionless

Prefixes for units of measurement

Symbol (name)	Multiplying factor
n (nano)	10^{-9}
μ (micro)	10^{-6}
m (milli)	10^{-3}
k (kilo)	10^{3}
M (mega)	10^{6}
G (giga)	10^{9}

Vectors and matrices

Item	Notation[a]
Vector	$\mathbf{F}$
Magnitude of a vector	$|\mathbf{F}|$ or F
Components of a vector in an xyz-coordinate system	$\mathbf{F_x}, \mathbf{F_y}, \mathbf{F_z}$
Coordinates of a vector in an xyz-coordinate system	F_x, F_y, F_z
Scalar product of two vectors	$\mathbf{F} \cdot \mathbf{G}$
Vector product (cross product) of two vectors	$\mathbf{F} \times \mathbf{G}$
Matrix	$\mathbf{D}$
Element of a matrix (i-th row, k-th column)	D_{ik}

[a] Illustrated by the example of vectors $\mathbf{F}$ and $\mathbf{G}$ and a matrix $\mathbf{D}$.

Index

Page numbers in *italics* refer to illustrations; those in **bold** refer to tables

A

abduction 134, *134*

abscissa 94

Achilles tendon 386, 387

acromioclavicular joint 362

actin filaments 182

– actin–myosin interaction 181–182

action potential 192

adduction 134, *134*

angular motion *see* rotation

anisotropic materials 36

– bone 147, *147*, 153–154

ankle joint 381–383

– extension movement *382*

– flexion movement *382*

– joint axes 383

– load calculation 259–266, *261*

– – foot held freely, no motion 261–264, *262*

– – foot with accelerated motion and floor contact 265–266, *266*

– – foot with accelerated motion and no floor contact 264–265, *265*

– loading of 384–386, *385*

– rotation 103, *104*

– – angular motion during gait cycle 417, *418*

ankle strategy 393, 405

anulus fibrosus *see* lumbar disks

aponeurosis, plantar 381, 386–387

architecture

– bone 142–144

– – adaptation 161–163, *162, 163*

– – in vicinity of joints 297–298, *298*

– muscles 197–202

artificial joints *see* prosthetic joints

aspect ratio 180

axis of rotation 135

– bone tissue 142–144

B

balance 390–394

– ankle strategy 393

– hip strategy 393

ball-and-socket joints 364, 368

– ankle 259

– hip 273, 287

– – pressure distribution 287–288, *287*

– range of motion 368–369, *368, 369*

– shoulder 364, 368

beams 57

– deformation and strength 57–63

– – bending, beam fixed at one end 59–61, *60*

– – compressive strength 58–59

– – tensile strength 58–59, *59*

– – torsion about long axis 61–63, *62*

bending moment 14, *14*

blood flow, viscosity relationship 28

body segments

– center of mass 247–248, **247**

– length 245–246, **246**

– mass 244–245, **245**

– mean density 244, **245**

– moment of inertia 248, **248**

– volume 245, **246**

body-fixed coordinate system 115

bone

– adaptation to mechanical demands 161–169

– – bone density 163–167, *164*, *165*, **165**, *166*, *167*

– – control signals for remodeling 168–169

– architecture 142–144

– – adaptation 161–163, *162*, *163*

– – in vicinity of joints 297–298, *298*

– – macroscopic findings 143–144

– – microscopic findings 142–143

– – ultramicroscopic findings 142

– cortical 143–144

– – material properties 148–151, **149**, *150*

– – microfissures 151, *151*

– deformation and strength testing 54–57

– – compressive strength 55–56, *56*

– – three-point loading experiment 54, *55*

– – torsional strength 54–55, *55*

– density determination 155–159, *156*, *157*, *158*

– – clinical applications 159–161, *160*

– growth 144–145

– imaging 156–157

– – computed tomography (CT) 157–159, *158*

– – dual energy X-ray absorptiometry (DXA) 157, *157*

– – dual photon absorptiometry (DPA) 157

– – radiography 156, *156*

– mechanical demands on *141*

– primary spongy 143

– shape adaptation 144, *145*

– stress and strain 146–148

– trabecular 143–144

– – material properties 151–155, *152*, *153*, *154*

– – porosity 152–153, *153*

– – trabeculae orientation 162–163, *163*

– woven 143, 146

– *see also* fractures

bone mineral content 157

bone mineral density 157

– age dependence 339, *339*, *340*, *341*

– gender differences 339, *339*, *340*, *341*

– lumbar vertebrae 160, 338–343

– physical activity relationships 163–166, *164*, *165*, **165**, *166*, *167*

– strength relationship 159–160, *160*, 338–339

– vibration effects 166–167, *168*

boundary friction 172

breaking strain 47

breaking stress 47

Brinell hardness 44

brittle materials 47, *47*

Bryan–Cardan angles 117–118, *117*

– calculation 129–130

C

cardiorespiratory endurance training 213–215

Cartesian coordinates 93–94, *94*

cartilage 141–142

– adaptation 172–173

– age-related changes 173

– – hip joint 292–293

– frictional properties 172

– mechanical properties 170–172, *170*, *171*

– partial loading effect 173, *173*

– structure 169–170, *170*

center of gravity 236

center of mass (COM) 8, 236, *308*, 392–394, *392*

– body segments 247–248, **247**

– determination 236–239, *237, 238, 239, 240,*
    462–464, *463,* **464**

center of pressure (COP) 22–24, *23,* 392–394, *394*

– location of 474–476, *475,* **475**

center of rotation 14–15, *15,* 89–91, 95–98

– lumbar spine segments 345, *345*

cervical spine, passive rotation *56,* 57

Charcot arthropathy 388, 407

Chasles' theorem 124

chemical energy 29

Chopart joint 381, 388

collagen

– bone 142, 143

– cartilage 169–170, *170*

– muscle 186

– scar tissue 228

– skin 225

collateral ligaments, knee joint 302–303, *302*

COM *see* center of mass

compression test 39–40, 48

compressive force 5, *6*

– beam 58–59

compressive stress 25

– cartilage 170–171, *170*

– ultimate compressive stress 48

– – bone *153*

– *see also* pressure

compromise axis 306–307, *306, 307*

computed tomography (CT) 157–159, *158*

– quantitative (QCT) 158–159

connectin *see* titin

coordinate system

– body-fixed 103

– joint 135–137, *137*

– space-fixed 103

COP *see* center of pressure

coronal plane 133, *133*

cortical bone 143–144

– material properties 148–151, **149,** *150*

– microfissures 151, *151*

cosine 70–72, **72**

creep 41, *42*

– skin 229

cruciate ligaments 301–303, *301, 302,* 316

– loading of 316–322, *318, 320,* **321**

cuneiform bones 381

D

deformation 4, *5,* 24, *25*

– cartilage 170–172, *171*

– compressive test 39–40

– elastic 41

– plastic 41, *42,* 56–57

– structures 51

– – beams 57–63

– – experimental determination 52–63

– tensile test 36–39, *37*

– torsional 54–55, *55,* 61–63, *62*

– viscoelastic 41, *41,* 54, 56–57

deformation energy 57, *58*

– calculation 450–452, *451*

dermis 225, *225*

diabetic foot 406–409, *406, 409*

dual energy X-ray absorptiometry (DXA) 157, *157*

dual photon absorptiometry (DPA) 157

Duchenne limp 276, *277*

dystrophin 183, *184*

E

eigenvalue 119

eigenvector 119

elastic cartilage 169

elasticity 41
– implant materials **38**
– modulus of *37*, 38–40
– superelasticity 43–44, *44*
– tendons 191
elastin mesh, skin 225, 227
elbow joint 363
– load calculation 255–259, *255, 256, 257, 258*
– – change in load with bending angle 467–468, *467*
electromyography (EMG) 196–197, 267–268
– gait cycle analysis 419, *420*
– lumbar spine load calculation 330
EMG *see* electromyography
endurance training 213–215
energy 29–30
– chemical energy 29
– consumption in walking 426–429, *427, 428, 429*
– – calculation 444–445, *445*
– deformation 57, *58*
– – calculation 450–452, *451*
– kinetic energy 29
– potential energy 29
epidermis 224–225, *225*
epimysium 179
Euler angles 116–117, *116*, 128
– calculation 129
extension 134, *134*
external friction 27, *27*
external rotation 134, *134*
external work 30
extracellular matrix 169

F

failure of materials 47–50
falls 429–435
– avoidance 34, *34*
– controlled falling 34
– epidemiology 430–431
– – causes 430
– – direction of falls 431, *431*
– injury prevention 431–435
– – falling techniques 434–435, *435*
– – orthopedic aids 432–434, *433*
– reducing incidence of 432
fatigue fractures 50, 150–151, *150*
– lumbar vertebrae 337
fatigue strength 49, *49*
– lumbar vertebrae 337
femoropatellar joint load 313–316, *313, 314, 315*
– contact area 298–299
femorotibial joint *298*
– contact regions *303*
– load on 307–313, *308, 309, 311*
– – calculation 470–472, *471*
– – deep kneel 309, *310*
– – gait analysis 311–312, *312*
– – menisci 312–313, *313*
– – one-legged stance 309–311, *310*
femur
– compressive loading 161, *162*
– force on shaft during walking 454, *454, 455*
– strength related to bone density 159–160, *160*
fibrocartilage 145, *146*, 169
fixed point 98
flexion 134, *134*
floating axis 136
fluid film lubrication 172
fluids
– friction in 28
– pressure in 21
– viscosity 28
foot 380–381, *380, 384*

– center of pressure location 474–476, *475*, **475**

– deformation 390

– diabetic foot 406–409, *406, 409*

– friction between foot and floor 47

– kinematic chain 381–383, *382*

– shear stress 21

– statics 383–390

– – internal forces in the arch 386–388, *387, 388*

– – internal forces in the forefoot 389–390, *389*

– *see also* plantar pressure distribution

force 3–9, 69

– compressive 5, *6*

– friction 27–28

– gravitational 8

– inertial 7, *7*

– – calculation when landing from jump 443–444

– muscular force generation 181–183, *181, 182, 183*, 193

– shear 5, *6*

– tensile 5, *6*

– – beam 58–59, *59*

force couple 13

force–deformation diagram 52–54

– ligament *53*

– lumbar vertebrae 336, *337*

– muscle *54*

– skin *53*

force sensors 395

forefoot 381

– internal forces in 389–390, *389*

forward dynamics 269

fractures

– compressive 55–56, *56*

– fatigue 50, 150–151, *150*, 337

– healing 145–146, *146*

– – primary healing 146

– – secondary healing 146

– lumbar vertebrae 337, 342–343, *343*

– – vertebral arch 343–344, *344*

free body diagram 257, *257*

free moment 13

friction 27, 45–47

– between foot and floor 47

– boundary 192

– external 27, *27*

– hydrodynamic 192

– internal 28

– joints 45, *46*, 172, 299

– kinetic 27–28, 45

– skin 229, **229**

– solid state 192

– static 27–28, 45

friction force 27–28

G

gait 414

– dominance of one leg 429

– energy consumption in walking 426–429, *427, 428, 429*

– – calculation 444–445, *445*

– gait pattern 414–415, *414*

– – shuffling gait 404–405

– – step-to gait *404*, 405–406, *406*

– ground reaction force application point 426

– kinematics 417–419, *417, 418, 419*

– muscle activity during 419, *420*

– – moment and power of muscles 419–425, *421, 423, 424, 426*

– plantar pressure distribution relationship 404–406, *404, 405, 406*

– sequence of steps in time 415–417, *416*

gait analysis

– hip joint load 280–283, *280, 282, 283*

– knee joint load 310–312, *312*

gait line 400

gastrocnemius muscle *306*, 307, *317, 318*

gimbal lock 137, *138*

girdle

– pelvic 362, 365

– shoulder 362, *363*, 364

glenohumeral joint 363

glenoid cavity 364

gravitational acceleration 8

gravitational force 8

great toe, interphalangeal joint load
    calculation 473–474, *473, 474*

ground reaction force

– application point 426

– plantar pressure distribution and 400–401, *402*

H

Hagen–Poiseuille law 28

hamstring muscles *306*, 307, *317*, 318–319, *318, 320*

hard materials 47, *47*

hardness 44–45

– muscle 45

heel strike 5, *6*

– momentum change 31, *31*

helical axis theorem 124

– finite helical axis 304, *305*

– instantaneous helical axis 304–305

helical motion 121, 124

high cycle fatigue 49

hindfoot 381

hip joint 272

– angular motion during gait cycle 417, *418, 419*

– load on 272–285

– – cane use influence 277–279, *278*, 452–454, *453*

– – determination by instrumented joint prosthesis 283–285, **284**

– – determination of by gait analysis 280–283, *280, 282, 283*

– – gait technique influence 276, *277*

– – stance phase of slow gait 272–276, *273, 274*

– – surgical intervention influence 279–280, *279*

– model 289–290, *289, 290*

– osteoarthritis cause 292–294

– pressure distribution calculation 285–292, *286, 287, 291*

hip strategy 393, 405

homogenous materials 36, 146

Hooke's law 4, *5*, 38

– generalized 147–148

Hounsfield units 158

hyaline cartilage 169–170, *170*

– adaptation 172–173

hydrodynamic friction 172

hyperkeratosis 230, *230*

hypermobility 33, 367

hypotenuse 70

hypoxia 230

hysteresis loop 41, *41*

– complete 42, *43*

I

identity matrix 111

imaging parameters 99–101, *100, 101*

indeterminate mechanical systems 266

– solving by employing additional constraints 468–470, *468, 469*

inertial force 7, *7*

– calculation when landing from jump 443–444

inhomogenous materials 36, 146

instability 33–34, 365–367

– segmental 367

internal friction 28

internal rotation 134, *134*

internal work 30, *30*

interphalangeal joint of the great toe, load
      calculation 473–474, *473, 474*

intra-abdominal pressure related to lumbar spine
      load 331–332, *331*

inverse dynamics 265

ischemia 230

– skin tolerance 231, *231*

isotropic materials 36, 146–147

J

joint coordinate system 135–137, *137*

joint load 250

– calculation 253

– – ankle joint, dynamic case 259–266, *261, 262,*
      265, 266

– – beam balance in static equilibrium 253–254,
      253, 254

– – elbow joint, static case 255–259, *255, 256,*
      257, 258

– – more than one active muscle 266–269

– mechanical equilibrium 250–252, *251*

joints

– bone architecture around 297–298, *298*

– friction 45, *46*, 172, 299

– hypermobility 33

– incongruency 141, 297

– motion in space, description 135–137, *137*

– muscle power 32–33, *32*

– stability 33

– *see also* joint load; prosthetic joints; *specific*
      joints

K

kinetic energy 29

kinetic friction coefficient 27–28, 45, **46**

knee joint 297, *317*

– center of rotation determination 300–301, *300*

– cruciate ligament load 316–322, *318, 320,* **321**

– femoropatellar joint load 313–316, *313, 316, 317*

– femorotibial joint load 307–313, *308, 309, 311*

– – deep kneel 309, *310*

– – gait analysis 311–312, *312*

– – menisci 312–313, *313*

– – one-legged stance 309–311, *310*

– force-transmitting area 298, *299*

– motion 135–137, *137*, 300–307

– – angular motion during gait cycle 417, *418*

– – as a pure hinge joint 300–301

– – as guided by the cruciate ligaments 301–303,
      301, 302

– – based on condylar shape 303–304, *303, 304*

– – compromise axis 306–307, *306, 307*

– – in terms of a helical axis 304–305, *305*

– muscles 307, *307*

L

landmarks 88

lifting and carrying recommendations 332–336,
      333, 334, 335

ligaments

– force–deformation diagram 52–53, *53*

– knee joint motion guidance 301–303, *301, 302*

– long plantar *380*, 381

– role in joint stability 300

– rupture 53

line of action 9, *10*

line of gravity 34, 384

linear motion *see* translation

Lisfranc joint 381, 388

load, mechanical 3

load–deformation graph 57, *58*

low cycle fatigue 49

lumbar disks 347–352

– intradiskal pressure related to radial bulge 350–352, *350, 352*

– mechanical function *347, 348*

– pressure distribution 348–350, *348, 349*

– prolapse 352–356

– – epidemiological studies 354–356

– – heavy spinal loading relationship 354–356, **355, 356**

– – mechanical cause hypotheses 353–354

lumbar spine

– bone and bone mineral density 337–343

– – age dependence 339, *339, 340, 341*

– – gender differences 339, *339, 340, 341*

– – measurement 340–341, *341*

– load on 326–336

– – calculation example 472, *472*

– – EMG-based model calculations 330

– – intra-abdominal pressure relationship 331–332, *331*

– – lifting and carrying recommendations 332–336, *333, 334, 335*

– – plane model calculation 326–329, *327, 328*

– – ten-muscle model 329, *330*

– – three-dimensional model calculations 329–330

– segmental motion 344–347

– – description as combination of rotation and translation 346, *346*

– – description as pure rotation 344–345

– vertebral fractures 337, 342–343, *343*

– – vertebral arch 343–344, *344*

– vertebral strength 336–344

– – age-related changes 341–342, *342*

– – bone density relationship 337–338, *338*

– – bone mineral density relationship 160, *160,* 338–339

– – compressive strength 160, *160,* 336–339, *337, 339,* 341–343, *342*

– *see also* lumbar disks

M

material fatigue 49, *49*

matrix

– definition of 86

– identity matrix 111

– multiplication 86–87

– notation 86–87, 101–102

– orthogonal 111

mean density 244, **255**

– body segments **245**

mean pressure *18,* 19–20

– calculation 445–447

– hip joint 20, *20,* 285, *286*

– plantar surface of the foot *18,* 19, 445–447

mechanical equilibrium 250–252, *251*

mechanical load 3

mechanical stress 24–27, *26*

– bone 147–148

– compressive 25

– – *see also* pressure

– dimension 38

– stress–strain diagram 37, 47–48, *48*

– ultimate stress 47–48, **48,** 148

– – bone 149, *150,* 153, *153*

– *see also* shear stress

mechanical work 28–30

microfissures, cortical bone 151, *151*

midfoot 381

modulus of elasticity *37*, 38–40

– bone 149, *150*, 153

– implant materials **38**

– skin 226–229

Mohs qualitative hardness scale 44

moment 9–17, *10*, *13*, 83–85, *84*

– composition from partial moments 459–460, *460*

– effect of 11, *11*, *12*

– muscle 204–206

– – determination 420–422, *421*, *423*, *425*, *426*

– reference point 442–443, *442*

moment arm 9, 205, *205*

– knee 308–309, *308*

– tendon, determination of 464–466, *465*, *466*

moment of inertia 60, 240

– body segments 248, **248**

– determination of 240–244, *241*, *242*

– polar 62, 63

momentum 30–31, *31*

motion

– in a plane 133–135, *133*, *134*

– relative motion of two bodies 130–133, *131*

– *see also* rotation; translation

motoneurons 193

motor unit 193–195, *194*

muscle fibers 179–180, *180*, 193, 197

– types 193, **193**

muscles

– activation during gait cycle 419, *420*

– – motion and power of muscles 419–425, *421*, *423*, *424*, *426*

– architecture 197–202, *198*, *199*

– – functional significance 200–202, **200**, *201*, *202*

– co-activation of several muscles 268–269

– electromyography (EMG) 196–197

– endurance training 213–215

– force generation 181–183, *181*, *182*, *183*, 193

– force regulation 192–196

– – recruitment 195–196, *195*

– – temporal summation 195

– force–deformation diagram 54, *54*

– force–frequency curve *192*

– force–length relationship 183–187, *185*, *201*, 206

– – passive force–length curve 186–187

– force–velocity relationship 187–188, *187*, *201*

– hardness testing 45

– insertion related to center of rotation 202, *202*

– mechanics 203–207

– – concentric contraction 203

– – eccentric contraction 203–204

– – isometric contraction 203

– – mechanical efficiency 204

– – moment 204–205, 420–422, *421*, *423*, 425

– – moment arm 205, *205*, *426*

– – stretch–shortening cycle 204

– morphology 179–183, *180*

– parallel muscles 197, *198*

– pennate muscles 197, 198–199, *198*

– physiological cross-sectional area (PCSA) 199–200

– power 32–33, *32*, 207–208, *208*

– – during gait cycle 419–425, *424*

– strength 207

– strength training 207–212

– – muscular hypertrophy *208*, 209–210, *209*

– – neural adaptation *208*, 210–212

– theoretical modeling of muscle behavior 188–190, *189*

myofibrils 180–184

myofilaments 180–181

myosin filaments 181

– actin–myosin interaction 181–182

N

neural adaptations to strength training *208*, 210–212

– evidence for 210–212

neutral fiber 59

neutral zone 57

Newton's second law 3, *4*

Newton's third law 5, *6*

nucleus pulposus *see* lumbar disks

O

ordinate 94

orthogonal matrix 111

orthonormal base 107

osteoarthritis

– hip joint 292–294

– mechanical factors 292–294

osteoblasts 142–143

osteoclasts 142, 143

osteocytes 142, 143

oxygen consumption in walking 427–429, *427, 428, 429*

– calculation 444–445, *445*

P

parallel muscles 197, 198

parallelogram law of vector addition 76, *77, 78*

parallelogram of forces 77, *78*

patellar tendon 313–314, *313, 317*

PCSA *see* physiological cross-sectional area

pelvic girdle 362

pennate muscles 197, 198–199, *198*

physical activity

– bone mineral density relationship 163–167, *164, 165,* **165**, *166, 167*

– cartilage thickness relationship 172–173

physiological cross-sectional area (PCSA) 199–200

pedography 395

plantar aponeurosis 381, 386–387

– tensile force in 387–388, *387*

plantar pressure distribution 21, 394–406

– during push-off 389–390

– ground reaction force and 400–401, *402*

– influencing factors 401–406

– – gait 404–406, *404, 405, 406*

– – walking speed *402*, 403–404, *403*

– – weight 402–403

– measurement 395–400

– – data interpretation 398–400, *398, 400*

– – force–time integral 399

– – peak pressure *398*, 399

– – point of force application 400, *400*

– – pressure gradient analysis 400

– – pressure–time integral 399

– – requirements 395–398, *396, 397*

– – temporal mean value 399

plastic deformation 41, *42,* 56–57

Poisson's ratio 39

polar moment of inertia 62, 63

polar section modulus 62, 63

posturography 390–394, *391, 392, 394*

potential energy 29

power 31–33

– muscle power 207–208, *208*

– – during gait cycle 419–425, *424*

– – in joint 32–33, *32*

pressure 17–24

– center of 22–24, *23*

– – location 474–476, *475*, **475**

– definition 17, *18*

– in a fluid 21

– in a gas 21

– joint surface 20

– mean pressure *18*, 19–20

– – calculation 445–447

– – hip joint 20, *20*, 285, *286*

– – plantar surface of the foot *18*, 19,
    445–447

– prosthetic limb 21

pressure distribution 18–21, *18*, *20*

– plantar 21, 394–406

pressure ulcers 231

primary spongy bone 143

projected area 19

pronation 134, *134*

prosthetic joints

– hardness of materials 44

– hip, load measurement 283–284

– knee

– – load measurement 312, **312**

– – stability 15-16, *16*

– shoulder, load measurement 376–378, *378*

– wear debris 45

prosthetic limbs

– hardness of materials 44–45

– shaft pressure distribution 21

– stability 15–16, *16*

Pythagoras' theorem 75

Q

quadriceps muscle *306*, 307, *317*, 318–319, *318*,
    319, *320*

quantitative computed tomography
    (QCT) 158–159

R

radiography 156, *156*

radius rotation 363–364, *364*

radius vectors 108, *109*

relative motion of two bodies 130–133, *131*

right hand rule 82, *83*

rotation 89–90, *89*

– axis of 135

– combined translation and rotation 90–92, *91*,
    97–99, *98*, 120–124, *120*, *121*, *123*

– – Chasles' theorem 124

– error influences in description 92–93, *93*

– external 134, *134*

– finding a best fit of two sets of points
    476–479, *477*

– in a plane 95–96, *96*

– – imaging parameters 99–101, *100*, *101*

– – matrix notation 101–102

– in three-dimensional space 103–106,
    112–124

– – Bryan–Cardan rotations 117–118, *117*

– – coordinate transformations 108–111, *110*

– – coordinates and vectors 106–108, *107*, *108*

– – Euler rotations 116–117, *116*

– – parameter calculation from reference point
    coordinates and images 125–133, *125*, *128*

– – rotation about an arbitrary axis 118–119, *119*

– – sequence of rotations 113–115, *114*

– – single rotations about coordinate axes
    112–113, *113*

– internal 134, *134*

rotator cuff 365, *367*, 369

Russell's traction 455–456, *455*

S

sacral base angle 458–459, *458*, *459*

sagittal plane 133, *133*

sarcomeres 180–182, *180*, *183*, 193

– force–length relationship 185–187, *185*

– *see also* muscles

scalar quantities 69

scapula movement 362, 364–365, *364*

scapulohumeral rhythm *364*, 365

scapulothoracic joint 362

scar tissue 228, *228*

screw home motion 304

section modulus 60

– polar 62, 63

segmental instability 367

shear force 5, *6*

shear modulus 40

shear stress *26*, 40

– plantar surface of the foot 21

– skin injury 231–234, *233*

shoe modifications 408

Shore hardness 44–45

shoulder 362

– dislocation 367

– gimbal lock 137, *138*

– link chain 362–365, *363*, *364*

– loading 370–378

– – dynamic three-dimensional calculations 374–376, *376*

– – measurement by instrumented joint prosthesis 376–378, *378*

– – static plane model calculations 370–372, *371*

– – static three-dimensional model calculations 372–374, *373*, *374*

– muscles 365, **365**, *366*

– shoulder girdle 362, *363*, 364

– stability 365–369

shuffling gait 404–405

sine 70–72, **72**

skeletal age 145

skeletal muscle *see* muscles

skin 224

– anatomy 224–225, *225*

– injury caused by mechanical loading 230–234

– – pressure injury 230–231, *231*, *232*

– – shear injury 231–234, *233*

– mechanical properties 226–229

– – compression test 229

– – force–deformation diagram 53–54, *53*

– – friction properties 229, **229**

– – modulus of elasticity 226–229

– reaction to mechanical loading 229–230, *230*

– scar tissue 228, *228*

soft materials 47, *47*

solid-state friction 172

space-fixed coordinate system 115

spine *see* cervical spine; lumbar spine; vertebrae

stability 33–34

static friction coefficient 27–28, 45, **46**

static mechanical equilibrium *see* mechanical equilibrium

step-to gait pattern *404*, 405–406, *406*

sternoclavicular joint 362

stiffness 52

– torsional 52

stiffness matrix 147

strain 38

– bone 147–148

– ultimate strain 47, **48**

stress *see* mechanical stress

stress concentrations 63–65, *63*, *64*, *65*

– calculation 449–450, *449*

stress fractures *see* fatigue fractures

stress relaxation 42, *43*

– skin 229

stress–strain diagram *39*, 47–48, *48*

– skin 226, *226*, *227*, *228*

structures 51

– deformation and strength 51–63

– – beams 57–63

– stiffness 52

– – torsional 52

– strength decrease due to stress
        concentrations 63–65

– – calculation 449–450, *449*

subtalar joint 381, *382*

– inversion movement *382*

– joint axis 383

superelastic materials 43–44, *44*

supination 134, *134*

T

talocalcaneal joint 381

talocrural joint 381, *382*

– joint axis 383

talonavicular joint 381

tangent 70–72, **72**

tendons 190–192

– energy storage 191–192

– force–length characteristic 190, *190*

– moment arm determination 464–466, *465*, *466*

tensile force 5, *6*

– beam 58–59, *59*

tensile test 36–39

– ultimate tensile stress 47–48, **48**

tibia

– motion relative to femur 130–133, *131*

– strength calculation 447–449

titin 183, 186–187

torque 14, *14*

torsional deformation

– beam 61–63, *62*

– bone 54–55, *55*

torsional stiffness 52

tough materials 47, *47*

trabecular bone 143–144

– age-related changes 151–152, *152*

– material properties 151–155, *152*, *153*, *154*

– – intercept length 154, *154*

– – star length and star volume 154, *154*

– – volume orientation 154, *154*

– porosity 152–153, *153*

– trabeculae orientation 162–163, *163*

traction treatment 455–458, *455*, *456*, *457*

translation 88–89, *89*

– combined translation and rotation 90–92, *91*,
        97–99, *98*, 120–124, *120*, *121*, *123*

– – Chasles' theorem 124

– error influences in description 92–93, *93*

– finding a best fit of two sets of points
        476–479, *477*

– in a plane 94–95, *95*

– – imaging parameters 99–101, *100*, *101*

– – matrix notation 101–102

– in three-dimensional space 103–106,
        111–112, *112*

– – coordinate transformations 108–111, *110*

– – coordinates and vectors 106–108, *107*, *108*

– – parameter calculation from reference point
        coordinates and images 125–133, *125*, *128*

transverse plane 133, *133*

trigonometric functions 70–73

trunk rotation during walking 419

U

ulna rotation 363–364, *364*

ultimate strain 47, **48**

ultimate stress 47, **48**, 148

– bone 149, *150*, 153, *153*

– compressive 48, *153*

unit circle 72, *72*

V

vectors 69, 454–458

– addition of 76–80

– – graphical procedure 67, *68*, *69*, 76–79, 454–457, *454*, *455*, *456*, *457*

– – numerical procedure 79–80, *80*, 457–458

– – parallel vectors 77–78, *77*

– – parallelogram law 76, *77*, *78*

– components 69, 74

– coordinates 74

– decomposition into addends 80–81, *81*, 458–459, *459*

– designation 69–70

– multiplication of 81–85

– – scalar product 81

– – vector product 82–85, *82*

– null vector 79

– origin of 76

– radius vectors 108, *109*

– representation of 73–76, *73*, *75*

– – coordinates 74–75, *75*

vertebrae

– bone and bone mineral density 160, 339–343

– – age dependence 339, *339*, *340*, *341*

– – gender differences 339, *339*, *340*, *341*

– – measurement 340–341, *341*

– compressive strength 55–56, *56*

– – age-related changes 341–342, *342*

– – bone density relationship 337–338, *338*

– – bone mineral density relationship 160, *160*, 338–339

– – lumbar vertebrae 160, *160*, 336–339, *337*, 341–343, *342*

– fracture 336–337

– – lumbar vertebrae 337, 342–344, *343*, *344*

– rotation 104–106, *105*

– *see also* lumbar spine

vibration effect on bone mineral density 166–167, *168*

viscoelastic deformation 41, *41*, 54, 56–57

viscoelastic materials 48, 54

– bone 149

viscosity 28

W

walking *see* gait

wear debris 45

wheelchair propulsion 375–376, *376*

windlass mechanism 388, *388*

Wolff's law 161

work *see* mechanical work

woven bone 143, 146

Y

Young's modulus 38